Schizophrenia

Part One
Descriptive Aspects

REPRINTED FROM
Schizophrenia

SECOND EDITION

EDITED BY

STEVEN R. HIRSCH
DANIEL R. WEINBERGER

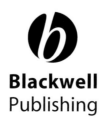

Blackwell
Publishing

ISBN 1-4051-1412-6

Printed and bound in Denmark by
Narayana Press, Odder

The views expressed in this publication are those of
the authors and not necessarily those of Astra Zeneca

Contents

1 Concepts and classification of schizophrenia

J.K. Wing and N. Agrawal

Each account of the concept of 'schizophrenia' reaches into the past from a viewpoint in a contemporary present. Berrios and Hauser (1988) commented that such accounts were unhistorical because we still lived in a Kraepelinian world. That was fair comment at the time and could be applied to many emerging disciplines whose concepts became temporarily stuck. It is also true that most people who have been concerned with such concepts over a professional lifetime find that the accumulation of new knowledge requires them to take a critical look back along several progressively different sightlines. This chapter is limited to the past two centuries, but a comment by John Locke over 300 years ago illustrates the confusion arising from terms used to describe severe deviations from mental health.

> Locke was 'astonished at the Obstinacy of a worthy man, who yields not to the Evidence of reason, though laid before him as clear as Day-light . . . I shall be pardoned for calling it by so harsh a name as *Madness*, when it is considered that opposition to Reason deserves that Name and is really Madness; and there is scarce a man so free from it, but that if he should always on all occasions argue or do as in some cases he constantly does, would not be thought fitter for *Bedlam*, than for Civil Conversation. I do not here mean when he is under the power of an unruly Passion, but in the calm steady course of his Life.' (Locke 1959)

Locke carefully distinguished 'madness' in the sense of unreasonableness, which was as common in his time as in ours, and the effects of being overpowered by 'an unruly passion', which was rare. His terminology is upside down to current readers but his distinction is clear and surprisingly modern.

Nevertheless, Michel Foucault would have none of it. To him, madness was always a form of opposition to 'established' reason. He thought that the way people react to it was a function of the historical epoch in which they lived (Foucault 1967). Such issues have not gone away, but one of the strongest tendencies in modern psychiatry is towards accepting Locke's basic differentiation between 'unreasonableness', which is common, and illness, which is rare. The international acceptance of specified definitions for mental disorders, with 'schizophrenia' as perhaps the outstanding example, may, however, have created an undue confidence in the durability of the global concepts. It is less likely that definitions of the constituent 'symptoms', about which people understandably complain and which are the most obvious and accessible phenomena, will change much in the foreseeable future. However, there is a gradual acceptance that standardized definitions of symptoms, plus new means of investigating brain functions, might eventually lead to the combination, break-up or abandonment of some current disease concepts, schizophrenia conceivably among them.

Even to the sceptical eye of the present authors, there has been sufficient advance in knowledge during the past decade to make another retrospective worthwhile, both for its own sake and because of the possible implications for future development.

Early concepts

Griesinger

There has been no time since attempts at classification began when controversy about the nature of 'schizophrenia' was absent. However, there have been periods when a sort of orthodoxy was accepted. One of these was based on Griesinger's teaching that only what we would now call affective and schizoaffective disorders constituted a 'primary' disease process (Griesinger 1861). What we now call chronic schizophrenic impairments could develop secondarily, but only after earlier affective episodes. Griesinger eventually came to agree that there could be a primary psychosis, even in the absence of these preliminaries, and thus 'abandoned the classification system of mental disorders hitherto traditional for him and his time' (Janzarik 1987). Thirty years of confusion about the relationships between a multiplicity of syndromes followed.

Kraepelin

It was not until the publication of the fifth edition of Kraepelin's textbook (1896/1987) that a firm line of demarcation was drawn between dementia praecox and affective psychosis and a sort of consensus again achieved. Both Griesinger's and Kraepelin's concepts were couched in terms of 'disease entities', following the lines of successful developments in medicine at that time. The discovery of the anatomical and physiological concomitants of clinically identified syndromes, often with a 'natural' history and a pathology, and sometimes with what appeared to be a single causal agent such as the tubercle bacillus or the cholera vibrio, proved irresistible to the neuropsychiatrists who were also carving more specific syndromes out of the global concepts of dementia, delirium and insanity that preceded them. Because cause was unknown, although variously postulated, classification depended largely on the course and outcome of groups of symptoms.

Kraepelin introduced a simple distinction between conditions characterized by mental deterioration such as the catatonia and hebephrenia of his contemporary Kahlbaum (1874/1973), which with paranoid deterioration became subdivisions of the disease, and more periodic forms of mania and melancholia, such as the *folie circulaire* of Falret (1854). His follow-up data suggested a mental state profile recognizable at the time of presentation and a 'generally regular and progressive' course. The chief symptoms were auditory and tactile hallucinations, delusions, thought disorder, incoherence, blunted affect, negativism, stereotypies and lack of insight. The phenomena were expressed as psychological rather than physical abnormalities, with catatonic symptoms, for example, being described in terms of disorders of the will. Paranoia was regarded as a separate disorder, characterized by incorrigible delusions often circumscribed in topic, a general absence of hallucinations, and a chronic but non-deteriorating course. Kraepelin also adopted Kahlbaum's model – general paralysis of the insane – as his prototype for a disease based on unity of cause, course and outcome. The nature of the disease was obscure although probably related to 'a tangible morbid process in the brain'.

A sympathetic and illuminating account of the development of Kraepelin's ideas up to 1913 has been provided by Berrios and Hauser (1988). They point out that his concept was neither as simple nor as rigid as is generally assumed and that it continued to develop. Indeed, Kraepelin (1920) eventually came to agree that dementia praecox and manic-depressive psychosis could coexist and, thus, that a unitary psychosis could not be ruled out.

Bleuler

The term 'schizophrenia' stems from Eugen Bleuler (1911/1950), who acknowledged in his preface his indebtedness to Kraepelin for 'grouping and description of the separate symptoms' and to Freud, whose ideas Bleuler used to 'advance and enlarge the concepts of psychopathology'. He retained the separation from manic-depressive psychosis while pointing out that affective symptoms could coexist. His concept was based on an assumption that the manifold external clinical manifestations masked an inner clinical unity that 'clearly marked [them] off from other types of disease'. Moreover, he argued that 'each case nevertheless reveals some significant residual symptoms common to all'. The end results were identical, 'not quantitatively but qualitatively'.

Bleuler's primary symptom was cognitive: a form of 'thought disorder', loosening of the associations. It provided links to Kraepelin's 'dementia' and to the biological origins of the disease, but also, through 'psychic complexes', to disorders of affectivity, ambivalence, autism, attention and will. These essential symptoms could be observed in every case. Catatonia, delusions, hallucinations and behavioural problems he regarded as accessory psychological reactions, not caused by the biological process or processes.

A substantial subgroup was designated 'simple schizophrenia', in which no accessory symptoms (the most easy to recognize) need be present. Diem (1903/1987), who worked with Bleuler, gave a description of two cases that he thought were caused by simple dementing forms of dementia praecox. Both were apparently normal as children, but as young men they began inexplicably to lose volition and purpose, ending as vagrants. Delusions and hallucinations were absent. Although no early developmental history was provided, these two people certainly became severely impaired in psychological and personal functioning and fitted Bleuler's severe version of simple schizophrenia. Bleuler's own examples are less easy to recognize. Among the lower classes, they 'vegetate as day labourers, peddlars, even as servants'. At higher levels, 'the most common type is the wife . . . , who is unbearable, constantly scolding, nagging, always making demands but never recognizing duties'. Beyond this 'simple' form of the disease, the largest subgroup was labelled 'latent schizophrenia': 'irritable, odd, moody, withdrawn or exaggeratedly punctual people'. Bleuler thought it 'not necessary to give a detailed description' of the manifestations in this group but there is a clear merger with subsequent concepts of schizoid and schizotypal personality (e.g. Kendler 1985).

This is in contrast to Kraepelin, whose account even of the 'mild' form of the course sounds severe. Thus, although Bleuler separated those with the disease from those without, the concept was in effect dimensional. Although accepting much of Kraepelin's formulation, Bleuler substantially widened the concept, while continuing to describe his concept as a disease entity. The simple and latent forms, whose vaguely defined primary symptoms could be elaborated through 'psychic complexes', were thus able to carry the weight, power and putative severity of a widely recognized diagnosis. Under the influence of contrasting types of theory – one psychoanalytical, the other biological – Bleuler's least differentiated subgroups came to exert an undue influence on the way that the diagnosis of schizophrenia was made and used in the USA and USSR during the 1970s (Wing 1978, chapter 6).

The phenomena of schizophrenia

Many attempts have been made to carry forward, refine or break up the syndromes described by the two conceptual giants. One motive was to improve earlier formulations of the fundamental characteristics that might underlie all the others. Berze (1914/1987), for example, drew on Griesinger's 'lowered mental energy' to postulate a basic factor, described in terms of a primary insufficiency of mental activity. This negative factor was responsible for the secondary positive phenomena as in Bleuler's theory, but without the psychic complexes. The mechanism was similar to that in Jackson's (1869/1932) theory of a hierarchy of levels of functional organization in the nervous system. A (negative) loss of function higher up can result in a (positive) disturbance of functions lower down. Gruhle (1929) pointed to the difficulty of applying such explanations to the phenomena of schizophrenia. He also made the unexceptionable, but rarely heeded, comment that some experiences and behaviours in schizophrenia cannot easily be fitted into either category. Gruhle distinguished between sets of primary negative and primary positive features, each specifiable descriptively.

Thus, issues connected with theories of 'negative' and 'positive' abnormalities have been hotly debated since at least the time of Griesinger. A more recent attempt to examine the relationships between symptoms in long-term schizophrenia used a profile of four measures:

1 flatness of affect;
2 poverty of quantity and/or content of speech;
3 incoherence of speech; and
4 specific types of coherently expressed delusions and hallucinations.

Affective flattening was particularly associated with poverty of speech, less so with incoherence and least with coherently expressed delusions. There was no evidence that the three types of speech abnormality were mutually exclusive categories (Wing 1961).

In a study comparing three hospitals with different social environments, poverty of content and quantity of speech were classified together with social withdrawal, flat affect, slowness, underactivity and low motivation as a 'negative' syndrome. Incoherence of speech was included with delusions, hallucinations, overactivity and socially embarrassing behaviour as a 'positive' syndrome (Wing & Brown 1961).

Crow (1985) gave added point to the descriptive separation by suggesting that different neural mechanisms might underlie the two syndromes, which he designated types I and II. Whether there are two, three or more syndromes has continued to be strongly debated, but now with fresh impetus to validate such clinical constructions by demonstrating biological differences. Crow has subsequently suggested that the 'first-rank symptoms' provide clues to the process of separation of the two hemispheres of the brain 'that is the species-defining characteristic of the brain of *Homo Sapiens*' (Crow 1998).

Positive symptoms

In the preface to the second edition, published in 1919, of his book on general psychopathology, Karl Jaspers wrote:

We trail around with us a great number of vague generalities. I have tried to clarify them as far as possible. But the deep intentions, which sometimes find expression through them, should not simply be set aside and let fall because full clarification has not been attained . . . .

Jaspers did indeed provide illumination at both levels (1946/1963). In order to clarify the key problem of delusion formation he discriminated between phenomena that can be understood in terms of some antecedent factor such as social beliefs or abnormal affects (overvalued and delusion-like ideas), and those that are based on irreducible experiences, not comprehensible in such terms. 'There is an immediate intrusive knowledge of the meaning and it is this which is itself the delusional experience.' In the examples he quotes, Jaspers makes it clear that such experiences are direct and sudden in onset, and not congruent with affect.

He and Kurt Schneider kept up a regular correspondence during the years 1921–55 (Janzarik 1984). Schneider (1959, 1976) composed a list of experiences that could, in practice, be used to differentiate schizophrenia from manic-depressive psychosis with reasonable reliability. His 'first-rank' symptoms included:

• thoughts experienced as spoken aloud, or echoed, or removed, or broadcast or alien;
• voices heard commenting on the patient's thoughts or making references in the third person;
• experiencing bodily functions, movements, emotions or will as under the control of some external force or agency;
• delusional atmosphere; and
• delusional perception.

Any of these experiences could be elaborated according to the personal preoccupations of the individual concerned, including those that were socially shared. Schneider did not suggest that the first-rank symptoms carried any special theoretical or prognostic significance but did think (correctly: World Health Organization 1973) that most clinicians would make a diagnosis of schizophrenia if they were present in the absence of evident brain disease.

This still left a small group of seemingly inexplicable delusions that did not fit Schneider's primary criteria. For example, Kraepelin had regarded paranoia as a separate category. In 1918, Kretschmer (1966/1974) published a monograph on a group of disorders characterized by delusions that developed following a specific stress occurring to someone with a sensitive personality. These conditions could become chronic but were not accompanied by deterioration. Other, usually monothematic delusional disorders have been separated from schizophrenia. For example, a single delusion that other people think the individual smells, or that some part of the anatomy is distorted or missing, in the absence of any apparent basis in affective, or any other, disorder. One such symptom can ruin the sufferer's whole life. Acute delusional or hallucinatory states of brief duration, with no subsequent development of schizophrenic symptoms, were classified by French psychiatrists as *bouffées délirantes*, following Magnan (1893). This rich vein of clinical description facilitated subsequent attempts to operationalize the concepts.

Negative symptoms

Another line of development followed the ideas of Kahlbaum (1874/1973), who had been the first to describe both hebephrenia and catatonia, and of Kraepelin, who included catatonia as a form of dementia praecox. Bleuler gave a detailed description of catatonic signs but regarded them as 'accessory' phenomena and tended to interpret them in psychoanalytical terms.

Fisher (1983) noted that, 'prior to 1900, when neurological and psychiatric syndromes were being delineated, the symptoms of psychomotor retardation, slowness, apathy and lack of spontaneity were universally regarded as manifestations of abulia'. Much of the literature was concerned with the most severe state, akinetic mutism. Kleist (1960) and Leonhard (1957; Fish 1958) delineated narrow clinical syndromes intended to serve as indicators of equally specific brain abnormalities, but were unable to convince sceptics who pointed to the lack of evidence of specific pathology.

More recently, there has been a recrudescence of interest in motor disorders associated with psychological abnormalities. Rogers (1992) has reviewed the history of the concept of catatonia and its long-standing separation from extrapyramidal neurological disorders (dyskinesias and parkinsonism). He pointed to the occurrence of both kinds of symptom in schizophrenia, affective disorders, obsessive–compulsive disorder and mental handicap.

The motor phenomena observed in schizophrenia before the advent of psychotropic medication included reduced and increased speech and behaviours, abnormalities of non-verbal means of communication, symptoms such as negativism, ambitendence, forced grasping, echopraxia and echolalia, opposition, automatic obedience, mannerisms, posturing and stereotypies. This list is taken from the tenth edition of the Present State Examination (PSE) (WHO 1999). Some of these phenomena, such as automatic obedience, forced grasping and negativism, can be interpreted as disturbances of volition. Extrapyramidal and catatonic signs were highly correlated in a sample of patients with schizophrenia examined by McKenna *et al.* (1991). More specifically, there were 'independent associations between tardive dyskinesia and "positive" catatonic phenomena (i.e. those distinguished by the presence of an abnormality), and between parkinsonism and "negative" catatonic phenomena (i.e. those featuring the absence or diminution of a normal function)'.

The concept of autism

Bleuler (1919) regarded autism as one of the fundamental features of schizophrenia. He described it as an *active* withdrawal from contact with reality in order to live in an inner world of fantasy. Gruhle (1929) pointed out that it was just as likely to be forced on the patient by the cognitive disorder. Kanner (1943) recognized, in a flash of genius, a syndrome worth separating from the then amorphous mass of 'subnormality' and 'psychosis' in children. His observations were precise and brilliant, but at the same time he adopted the much less exact term 'autism' to describe it, thus linking it to Bleuler's concept. Within a year, Asperger (1944/1991) independently described a behaviour pattern he called 'autistic psychopathy', now referred to as Asperger's syndrome. Both Kanner's and Asperger's syndromes had in common a range of disorders of development present from birth or early childhood (Wing 1981, 2000; Tantam 1988; Frith & Frith 1991; Gillberg 2002). The results of an epidemiological study in south-east London (Wing & Gould 1979) showed typical examples of each syndrome, but identified many more children who shared features of both, or who met some but not all the diagnostic criteria for either. The authors developed the hypothesis of an autistic spectrum, characterized by a triad of impairments affecting the development of social interaction, communication and imagination, associated with a narrow repetitive pattern of activities.

The chief feature of the triad was social impairment, which could be manifested in several ways. Three groups were particularly evident.

1 Aloofness and indifference to others, e.g. avoiding social contact except for simple needs or to obtain pleasure from physical stimulation such as tickling. Those in this group tended to be the most disabled because of intellectual, behavioural and language impairments.

2 Passive acceptance of approaches from others but little or no spontaneous social interaction.

3 Initiating contacts in an odd one-sided way, unaffected by the reaction of the person approached. Those in this group tended to have less global impairment but behaviour was markedly abnormal.

The borders between groups are not neatly differentiated and can change over time; for example, some children change from aloofness to passivity, or to active but odd participation, as they grow up. Psychological examination has suggested that affected children and adults have an inborn difficulty that limits their understanding of other people's thoughts and feelings (Frith 1989). This lack is one part of a more general and fundamental problem shared by all those with the spectrum, which limits the attribution of meaning to experiences (Wing 1982; Frith 1989; Frith & Happé 1994). This hypothesis comes closer to Gruhle's view that autism is a consequence of cognitive disorder rather than of an 'active withdrawal' as suggested by Bleuler, and is in striking contrast to Jasper's description of the intrusion of abnormal meaning in the primary delusions of schizophrenia.

The diagnosis of autistic spectrum disorders in adults depends on characteristics of early development that are rarely considered by psychiatrists when taking histories from adult patients. For some diagnostic categories used in adult psychiatry, the ICD-10 criteria overlap with those in the autistic spectrum. For example, the criteria for schizoid and schizotypal personality disorders are closely similar to those for Asperger's syndrome as defined in ICD-10 and DSM-IV. Sula Wolff (1995) followed up children with 'schizoid personality disorder' and came to consider that they were better placed in the autistic spectrum, representing the most able individuals who fit Asperger's descriptions.

Many of the features of catatonia, as recently described by Joseph (1992), Bush *et al.* (1996) and by Rogers (1992), are identical to those found in autistic spectrum disorders, especially in younger and more severely disabled children. Follow-up into adult life has shown that a small proportion of those with autistic disorders, at any level of ability, have marked exacerbation of catatonic features in adolescence or early adult life. Some become severely incapacitated as a result (Wing & Shah 2000).

The narrow repetitive range of activities characteristic of autistic spectrum disorders can be mistaken for obsessive–compulsive disorder but the more common misdiagnosis is that of schizophrenia, although the diagnostic criteria for the latter are substantially different from those of autism. Such mistakes tend to be based on a misinterpretation of the social aloofness and passivity, or the odd speech and ideas that are found in people with active but odd social interaction. There is no evidence that medications, whether 'typical' or 'atypical', have a useful effect on the core symptoms of autism, although their tranquillizing effects are sometimes useful. The 'management' of autistic spectrum disorders depends on the provision of an appropriately structured environment, with well-programmed activities that encourage the use of any potential skills.

The concept of disease

Disease as entity or as deviation from normal functioning

Kendell (1987) has pointed out that none of the four types of psychosis – schizophrenic, affective, good prognosis acute and chronic paranoid – discussed above has been clearly demonstrated to be a disease entity. Does it matter? Kraepelin and Bleuler thought it did. But even so well 'validated' a disease as tuberculosis cannot be said to be an 'entity' in the sense that everyone with the bacillus in the bloodstream has the same (or any) symptoms, let alone the same course or outcome.

Cohen (1961) argued that the concept of disease that 'still dominates our textbook descriptions, as illustrated by the so-called classical pictures of typhoid fever, influenza, disseminated sclerosis and the rest, is little more helpful in diagnosis than would be a composite portrait of a football team in revealing whether any one individual is a member'.

Throughout medicine, but particularly during the past 50 years, rigid disease categories have been replaced by more useful concepts that are constantly evolving in the light of the experimental evidence. As disease concepts evolve in the light of the successes and failures of hypothesis testing, it becomes obvious that some diseases previously thought to be 'entities' are actually linked and that the fundamental processes involve deviations or blockages in the functioning of normal homeostatic cycles. Hypertension, diabetes and coronary heart disease are obvious examples, but so, increasingly, are most well-known diseases. Different defining formulae that use the same name have to fight against each other for survival. Which is more successful at any one time depends on the weight of evidence its protagonists can provide.

The evidence must also include the epidemiology of schizophrenia: the genetics, age and sex distribution, excess of births in the winter months and the possibility that the course and even the incidence varies both geographically and over time.

Hierarchy in psychiatric disorders

Some sense can be made of the relationships between psychiatric disorders if dimensional as well as categorical concepts are borne in mind. Both are useful so long as it is recognized that it is essential to move easily between them. The ancient hierarchies divided mental faculties into conative, cognitive and affective. If brain function is profoundly impaired, there can be no or only negligible function of will. Movement, thought and emotion will then be absent or distorted.

It is possible that each of the three faculties can be impaired independently of the others and that the conventional hierarchical system of diagnosis would have more than just practical use if based on three or four dimensions (the extra one representing motor functions). Positive and negative aspects would then be represented at every level.

At the moment, in practice, diagnoses tend to be made as follows:
• At the top are disorders such as dementia, which, at least in the early stages, can be associated with any other type of problem. For example, 'schizophrenic symptoms' occurring in the course of Huntington's disease or temporal lobe epilepsy or severe learning disability tend to be discounted for the purpose of diagnosis.
• Similarly, disorders in the autistic spectrum, if diagnosed on the developmental history and the spectrum, should not be given a primary diagnosis of schizophrenia.

- In general, schizophrenic symptoms, in the absence of 'organic' disorder, take precedence in diagnosis and for treatment over bipolar psychoses if both are present.
- Affective psychoses in turn take precedence over unipolar depression and the anxiety that is so commonly associated with all the above disorders.
- Symptoms such as fatigue, worry and muscular tension are regarded as non-specific.

The hierarchy is generally non-reflexive, i.e. each disorder tends to manifest the symptoms of those lower down (Foulds 1965; Sturt 1981) but not those of disorders higher up. By the same token, *all* disorders can be seen in cross-section as well as longitudinally, manifesting a complex of symptoms, some negative and some positive, and many 'non-specific' for the 'diagnosis'. Both perspectives are legitimate for different purposes (Wing 1978, chapter 3; 1991).

Other types of theory

A review of the history of concepts of schizophrenia would not be complete without a reference to theories of 'not-schizophrenia', although these tend to be logically self-destructive. Most are variants of those by Goffman (1961), Laing and Esterson (1964), Scheff (1966) and Szasz (1971), which have been dealt with elsewhere (Wing 1978, chapter 5).

This is far from saying that there are no other components to the aetiology of schizophrenia than those that involve purely biological elements. In fact, from the time of Kraepelin, concepts of disordered attention or arousal have suggested that environmental events may influence symptoms for better or worse. Certainly, some sufferers have learned for themselves how to cope with symptoms without losing control, and many carers have found, without help from professionals, how to provide an optimal environment (Creer & Wing 1974; Wing 1975). Interactive biosocial theories that suggest how environmental over- and understimulation may act to improve or exacerbate the positive and negative impairments (Wing 1978) cannot be taken seriously by those who reject any deviation from a purely biological approach. Thus, an absolute biologism is as limiting and ultimately sterile as an absolute rejection of biology.

The value of cognitive–behaviour therapy for the enhancement, in some cases, of the effects of the new medications during recovery from an attack of schizophrenia, and the acquisition of a degree of control over symptoms during convalescence and between attacks, is not only a success of the past decade but a pointer to the future. Tools for assessing claims of efficacy for such treatment methods are available, and must be applied according to strict rules by disinterested investigators.

Excluding clinical concepts that cannot be expressed clearly and numerically does not mean they are clinically valueless. Some may in time prove to be significant, but they have to wait until someone with the clinical intuition of Alzheimer, Asperger, Kanner or Kurt Schneider clarifies them.

Some critics of formulations such as schizophrenia (e.g. Bentall *et al.* 1988) have suggested that there is no need to do

more than study symptoms, pointing to evidence that symptom-based therapies can provide relief and greater autonomy to sufferers and their families. It has yet to be demonstrated how far control of one symptom will generalize to others, how long relief lasts and what proportion of sufferers can benefit. A more specific disadvantage is that concentrating on single symptoms, instead of – rather than as well as – syndromes, may divert attention from the *clinical context* of the symptoms, with a resulting detriment to problems that are multifaceted and interconnected.

Empirical approaches to the classification of schizophrenia

Many of the clinical concepts of schizophrenia summarized so far, selected from a range that could be broadened to include dozens more authors, have been unsatisfactory in several ways:
- their symptomatic and syndromic components overlap but are not identical;
- they cannot be stated in precisely reproducible terms;
- the weights given to individual symptoms when formulating a diagnosis are not specified but left to clinical interpretation;
- other criteria, such as course, are of uncertain value for classification; and
- until recently there has been little convincing evidence for specific pathologies or physical causes in the large majority of cases.

Testing clinical concepts

New syndromes can be derived from symptom lists by the application of statistical techniques. There is a long line of such studies, many of them initiated in the 1950s and 1960s in order to overcome the unreliability then being demonstrated in day-to-day clinical diagnosis (e.g. Lorr 1966). They were successful in achieving reasonable reliability, but the usefulness of the statistical syndromes was not demonstrated, except in the sense that the factors often looked very similar to the diagnoses they tried to leave behind.

Kendell (1989) addressed the problem in a more practical way. He suggested utilizing statistical methods to refine syndromes, which could then be tested against outcome and used to generate or test biological hypotheses. His own studies (Kendell & Brockington 1980) did not demonstrate a point of statistical discontinuity between schizophrenic and affective psychoses. This could be due in part to fluctuation over time; cross-sections cannot display the clinical picture that eventually emerges. In addition, the hierarchies that run through psychiatric classification ensuring that disorders higher up, such as dementia, schizophrenia and bipolar disorder, which tend to be co-morbid with symptoms of disorders lower down, must also be considered. A high proportion of people with schizophrenia in the International Pilot Study of Schizophrenia (WHO 1973) would have been classified by the PSE computer program known as CATEGO as having affective disorders if symptoms discriminating for schizophrenia had been left out (Wing *et al.* 1974). Moreover, some at least of the affective symptoms so common in acute schizophrenia must be reactive to the stress of the primary experiences.

From concepts to classification

The clinical concepts, especially those of Kraepelin and Bleuler, can be recognized as early attempts to classify schizophrenia, but there were differences in their approach to defining schizophrenia as an entity. While Kraepelin emphasized the value of onset and course as well as descriptions in diagnosis and classification of schizophrenia, Bleuler and Schneider preferred a cross-sectional approach based on patients' current mental state, emphasizing fundamental and characteristic distinguishing symptoms. Recent recognizable international classification systems such as DSM and ICD have attempted syntheses of these concepts to foster international consensus.

Early DSM and ICD classifications (such as DSM-II and ICD-8) included a very broad definition of psychosis based on severity of social and personal dysfunction, thereby allowing for considerable overlap with personality disorders. This, in addition to the prevalent influence of the psychoanalytic movement in the USA, led to significant differences in the interpretation of diagnostic guidelines and definitions of concepts of psychosis and schizophrenia. These differences were clearly reflected in studies such as the US–UK study (Kendell *et al.* 1971), which displayed the range of concepts of schizophrenia from a broad one in the USA to a very narrow one in Europe.

One obvious line of development, therefore, has been to try to provide comprehensive, accurate and technically specifiable means of describing and classifying the component concepts (phenomena) in order to allow more meaningful comparisons between clinicians, academic schools, research laboratories and public health statistics.

Standards for symptom definition and combination

In the case of schizophrenia, the first essential is to provide differential definitions of the symptoms and signs, based as far as possible on deviations from normal psychological functioning. The descriptions of Jaspers and Kurt Schneider are well suited to such an exercise. These descriptions influenced attempts of clinical standardization in the form of development of definitions and structured interviews and diagnostic criteria such as the PSE (Wing & Brown 1970), Schedule for Affective Disorders and Schizophrenia (SADS) (Endicott & Spitzer 1978) and Research Diagnostic Criteria (RDC) (Spitzer *et al.* 1975). The 10th edition of PSE (now with other materials called Schedule for Clinical Assessment in Neuropsychiatry (SCAN); Wing *et al.* 1998, WHO 1999) is a more recent attempt of clinical standardization, as is the Diagnostic Interview for Social and Communication Disorders (DISCO) for social and communication

disorders (Leekam *et al.* 2002; Wing *et al.* 2002). The definitions of symptoms and the algorithms for standardized diagnosis they provide make it possible to undertake more reliable and comparable clinical studies and more specific tests of biological functioning. These developments influenced further revisions of ICD and DSM concepts and classifications of schizophrenia. The American diagnostic classification (DSM) in the next revision of DSM-III and -IIIR made the concept of schizophrenia one of the narrowest, whereas the concept in ICD-9 remained very broad. However, in their most recent revisions, DSM-IV and ICD-10 have tried to bridge these differences by bringing the criteria closer.

Modern classifications of schizophrenia and their limitations

ICD-10 and DSM-IV provide the criteria for diagnosing schizophrenia and other psychotic disorders. At best, they can only be considered an 'arbitrary but well informed consensus on the definition of schizophrenia aimed at reliable communication' (Andreasen & Carpenter 1993). These reflect our current understanding of the concept of schizophrenia.

These diagnostic concepts must be considered provisional constructs intended to fulfil the need for international communication and research. Therefore, a need for constant revision based on epidemiological, pathophysiological, aetiological validation and evaluation of emerging neurosciences and genetic data cannot be denied. This must be an ongoing process. These classification systems currently use descriptive diagnostic criteria based on the intensity and duration of systems. They are operationalized to a variable extent (more in DSM-IV than in ICD-10) with explicit exclusion and inclusion criteria.

The conditions recognized by applying the criteria laid down in DSM-III, and its successors DSM-IIIR and DSM-IV (American Psychiatric Association 1993), and also in ICD-10 (WHO 1993), are not described as diseases but as disorders. The rules for schizophrenia laid down in the Diagnostic Criteria for Research in subchapter F20 of ICD-10 are far from describing a disease concept. They list most of the symptoms described by Kraepelin but do not include a long-term course or a particular outcome, or refer to a pathology or a cause. The distinction from bipolar disorder if both are present is limited to a clinical judgement as to which type of symptom occurs first. Schizophrenia in ICD-10 is not a disease but a disorder. The introduction explains that this terminology is adopted:

> so as to avoid even greater problems inherent in the use of terms such as 'disease' and 'illness'. 'Disorder' is not an exact term, but it is used here to imply the existence of a clinically recognizable set of symptoms or behaviour that in most cases is associated with distress and with interference with functions.

An article in the *Schizophrenia Bulletin* illustrated the position clearly (Flaum & Andreason 1991). The authors listed DSM-IIIR and ICD-10 criteria, and three further versions then under consideration for DSM-IV. It is unlikely that a disease concept will change its nature by choosing two of one kind of item and three of another, rather than three of the first kind and two of the second. In fact, in the version eventually adopted (DSM-IV), the chief distinctions from ICD-10 (the requirement for a 6-month course and deterioration in social functioning) remain. Nevertheless, the coding system for DSM-IV is still mapped to that of ICD-9. However, both sets of criteria should be applied, using standardized instruments such as SCAN/PSE10 and the Composite International Diagnostic Interview (CIDI) (Robins *et al.* 1988) in research and public health projects, in order to foster international comparisons and comparisons with locally favoured alternatives.

ICD-10 and DSM-IV concepts of schizophrenia and related disorders

Although attempts have been made to bridge the gap between ICD-10 and DSM-IV and move them closer, significant differences still persist concerning the definition, duration and subtypes of schizophrenia and the nomenclature of various other psychotic disorders classified with schizophrenia. ICD-10 classifies schizotypal disorder, persistent delusional disorder, acute and transient psychotic disorders, induced delusional disorder and schizoaffective disorders together with schizophrenia (Table 1.1). DSM-IV does not include the category of schizotypal disorders with psychotic disorders but classifies it along with cluster A personality disorders (see Chapter 7).

Induced delusional disorder in ICD-10 is called shared psychotic disorder in DSM-IV; persistent delusional disorder in ICD-10 is called delusional disorder in DSM-IV (Table 1.2). The major difference is in the category of acute and transient psychotic disorder of ICD-10, which overlaps with brief psychotic disorder and schizophreniform disorder of DSM-IV.

The other major difference is in the classification of psychotic illness secondary to substance misuse and to general medical conditions, which are classified together with schizophrenia in DSM-IV but are classified with disorder due to psychoactive substance misuse (F10–F19) and organic mental disorder (F00–F09), respectively, in ICD-10.

ICD-10 avoids criteria based on social and occupational dysfunction for the diagnosis of schizophrenia on the basis that it is difficult to equate these criteria between different cultures. This is a major inclusion criterion in DSM-IV that is essential for the diagnosis of schizophrenia.

Diagnostic criteria for schizophrenia

ICD-10 requires either one of the Schneiderian first-rank symptoms, or bizarre delusions, or two or more symptoms including persistent hallucinations, thought disorder, catatonic behaviour, negative symptoms or significant and persistent behavioural change. These features are required to be present for a 1-month duration or longer. ICD-10 recognizes that there may be a prodromal phase associated with schizophrenia, but as a prodrome typical of and specific to schizophrenia could not be described reliably it is not included in the diagnostic criteria. The 1-month duration of schizophrenia according to ICD-10 does not include the prodromal phase (Table 1.3).

ICD-10 requires exclusion of substance use or organic brain disease if they may be causing features of schizophrenia. As described earlier, the presence of the schizophrenia-like symptoms caused by either organic brain disease or substance use are classified along with organic mental disorder and substance misuse disorders, respectively, in ICD-10, not with schizophrenia.

DSM-IV requires, for the diagnosis of schizophrenia, 1 month's duration of characteristic symptoms with at least two of the symptoms of delusions, hallucinations, disorganized speech, grossly disorganized catatonic behaviour or negative symptoms (Table 1.4). However, only one of these is required if delusions are bizarre or third-person auditory hallucination or running commentary are present. This criterion brings the DSM-IV diagnosis of schizophrenia closer to that of ICD-10. In

Table 1.1 Brief outline of ICD-10 classification of schizophrenia and other psychotic disorders.

F20	Schizophrenia
F21	Schizotypal disorder
F22	Persistent delusional disorder
F23	Acute and transient psychotic disorders
F24	Induced delusional disorders
F25	Schizoaffective disorder
F28	Other non-organic psychotic disorders
F29	Unspecified non-organic psychosis

Table 1.2 Brief outline of DSM-IV classification of schizophrenia and other psychotic disorders.

295.x	Schizophrenia
295.4	Schizophreniform disorder
295.7	Schizoaffective disorder
297.1	Delusional disorder
298.8	Brief psychotic disorder
297.3	Shared psychotic disorder
293.x	Psychotic disorder due to (specify medical condition):
.81	with delusions
.82	with hallucinations
293.x	Substance-induced psychotic disorders:
.xx	onset during intoxication
.xx	onset during withdrawal
297.1	Delusional disorder
298.8	Brief psychotic disorder
297.3	Shared psychotic disorder
298.9	Psychotic disorder NOS

NOS, not otherwise specified.

Table 1.3 ICD-10 diagnostic criteria for schizophrenia.

Characteristic symptoms
At least one of:
    Thought echo, thought insertion/withdrawal/broadcast
    Passivity, delusional perception
    Third person auditory hallucination, running commentary
    Persistent bizarre delusions
or two or more of:
    Persistent hallucinations
    Thought disorder
    Catatonic behaviour
    Negative symptoms
    Significant behaviour change

Duration
More than 1 month

Exclusion criteria
Mood disorders, schizoaffective disorder
Overt brain disease
Drug intoxication or withdrawal

Table 1.4 DSM-IV diagnostic criteria for schizophrenia.

Characteristic symptoms
At least one of:
    Bizarre delusions
    Third person auditory hallucinations
    Running commentary
or two or more of:
    Delusions
    Hallucinations
    Disorganized speech
    Grossly disorganized behaviour
    Negative symptoms

Duration
1 month of characteristic symptoms
With 6 months of social/occupational dysfunction

Exclusion criteria
Schizoaffective or mood disorders
Direct consequence of substance use or general medical condition
Pervasive developmental disorders

addition to this criterion, DSM-IV requires a total duration of at least 6 months, including 1 month of active symptoms and social and occupational disfunction during this time. This criterion is significantly different from ICD-10 as the duration required is only 1 month in ICD-10 and social and occupational dysfunction is not required at all. DSM-IV recognizes the prodrome of schizophrenia and the duration of prodrome is included in the total 6-month duration required for its diagnosis. Specific exclusion criteria are similar to those of ICD-10, including those of schizoaffective and mood disorders and exclusion of disorders secondary to general medical condition and substance misuse. In the DSM-IV, schizophrenia-like illness secondary to a general medical condition or substance misuse is classified in the chapter on schizophrenia and related psychotic disorders. This is in contrast with ICD-10, as described above, and avoids hierarchical assumptions.

Course and subtypes of schizophrenia

Both ICD-10 and DSM-IV provide broadly similar classifications of longitudinal course. The subtypes of schizophrenia included in both ICD-10 and DSM-IV are paranoid, catatonic, undifferentiated and residual schizophrenia. Hebephrenic schizophrenia is called disorganized type in DSM-IV. The requirement for the subtypes is similar in both classification systems, although they are more clearly operationalized in DSM-IV.

Common subtypes in ICD-10 and DSM-IV

- Paranoid
- Catatonic
- Hebephrenic (disorganized in DSM-IV)

- Residual
- Undifferentiated

Additional subtypes in ICD-10

- Simple
- Postschizophrenic depression

ICD-10 also includes subcategories of simple schizophrenia and postschizophrenic depression as subtypes of schizophrenia. ICD-10 clarifies retention of simple schizophrenia as a subtype of schizophrenia, with the requirement of certain described features for at least 2 years because of its continued use in some countries and because of the uncertainty about its nature, which will require additional information for resolution. Diagnosis of postpsychotic depression requires a clear diagnosis of schizophrenia within the past 12 months with the presence of some features of schizophrenia and predominant depressive symptoms, which meet a threshold of depressive episode, for 2 weeks.

In addition to a categorical description of schizophrenia subtypes, DSM-IV offers a dimensional alternative in its Appendix B:
- psychotic dimension;
- disorganized dimension; and
- negative dimension.
ICD-10 does not give a description of any dimensions yet as these are difficult to define.

Diagnostic criteria for related psychotic disorders

Schizotypal disorder in ICD-10 is classified in the 'Schizophrenia and other psychotic disorders' section as this disorder is described as possessing many of the characteristic features of schizophrenia without its obvious delusions and hallucinations. The diagnosis requires the presence of more than three of the characteristic features without meeting the criteria for schizophrenia itself. In contrast, DSM-IV classifies the condition with the cluster A personality disorders, such as schizoid and paranoid.

Persistent delusional disorder of ICD-10 and delusional disorder of DSM-IV have similar diagnostic criteria except for differences in the duration of illness required, which is 3 months in ICD-10 and only 1 month in DSM-IV. Both classifications define this condition by the presence of a non-bizarre persistent delusion or set of related delusions. DSM-IV, in addition, specifies seven subtypes of this condition.

Any disorder of acute onset with typical schizophrenic features or other psychotic features lasting for more than 1 day to less than 1 month is classified in DSM-IV as brief psychotic disorder. This disorder is associated with a return to the premorbid level of functioning with good prognosis and may or may not be associated with marked stressors. This condition in ICD-10 is classed as acute and transient psychotic disorder. If the disorder persists for more than 1 month with schizophrenia-like symptoms, it is classified as schizophrenia in ICD-10, whereas in DSM-IV it will be classed as schizophreniform disorder. It will only be reclassified as schizophrenia if it lasts for more than 6 months. If the acute and transient psychosis has features of schizophrenia and has non-bizarre delusions, DSM-IV will class it as delusional disorder after 1 month whereas ICD-10 will class it as persistent delusional disorder only after a 3-month duration.

Schizoaffective disorder is diagnosed according to ICD-10 when both definite affective symptoms and schizophrenic symptoms are prominent simultaneously or within a few days of each other within the same episode of illness. In addition, DSM-IV requires the presence of typical schizophrenic features for at least 2 weeks along with the presence of prominent mood features. A substantial proportion of the illness should be characterized by the presence of mood features. Both classifications subdivide the disorder into manic or bipolar type and depressive type.

Induced delusional disorder is a rare disorder defined in ICD-10 as a condition in which two or more people share the same delusion or delusional system, support each other in this belief and have an unusually close relationship. The dominant person usually develops the illness first and induces the delusion later in the passive person. The DSM-IV diagnostic criteria for this illness are the same, although the disorder is called shared psychotic disorder.

Both ICD-10 and DSM-IV, while providing the basis for an effective communication between the professionals and a basis for research, also confer the disadvantages of creating an impression of discrete entities by imposing a framework on what are in fact complex and overlapping phenomena. These classification systems are complex, difficult to follow in day-to-day practice and the criteria are constantly revised; consequently, the research based on these systems becomes rapidly obsolete and difficult to apply in a clinical setting. Nevertheless, it is very hard to imagine working in a complex field such as schizophrenia and related psychotic disorders and not having a reasonable level of shared understanding of modern widely used concepts and definitions.

Conclusions

This review began with 'unitary psychosis'. Has this ceased to exist because there is no code for it in ICD-10 or DSM-IV? Should those who regard basic schizophrenic phenomena as symptoms of dysfunctions in the central nervous system classify them under F06.2 (organic schizophrenia-like disorder) or F20 (schizophrenia)? Another problem of the same order concerns the significance of the difference between G93.3 (postviral fatigue syndrome) and F48, which includes fatigue syndrome.

Being able to pose these questions does not demonstrate the futility of providing standardized definitions for international use. The examples do not inspire confidence but the effort to provide reference criteria is essential. It does demonstrate that, whether called 'diseases' or 'disorders', we are dealing with constantly changing concepts. That is not all. The same is true of 'syndromes' and of 'symptoms'. They, too, are concepts that must compete with each other. The more precisely they, and the predictions that follow from them, are stated, the more easily they can be refuted if they are wrong. It may pay, in the short term, to be vague; however, a greater distraction from the search for knowledge is that some protagonists, even when using an impeccably sceptical approach in their scientific work, tend to use the terminology of 'disease entities' and seem to want to believe that the Snark or the Boojum really exist. Others react against each such provocation and waste their time and wit in polemic.

Such arguments are inevitable and will continue. However, looking back from this new vantage point, it is still possible to discern a pattern amid the noise.

References

American Psychiatric Association (1993) *Diagnostic and Statistical Manual of Mental Disorders*, 4th edn. APA, Washington, DC.

Andreasen, N.C. & Carpenter, W.T. (1993) Diagnosis and classification of schizophrenia. *Schizophrenia Bulletin* **19**, 199–211.

Asperger, H. (1944/1991) Autistic psychopathy in childhood. In: *Autism and Asperger Syndrome*. Cambridge University Press, Cambridge. Translated and annotated by U. Frith, from: Die 'Autistischen Psychopathen' im Kindesalter. *Archiv für Psychiatrie und Nervenkrankheiten* **117**, 76–136.

Bentall, R.P., Jackson, H.F. & Pilgrim, D. (1988) Abandoning the concept of schizophrenia. *British Journal of Psychology* **27**, 303–324.

Berrios, G.E. & Hauser, R. (1988) The early development of Kraepelin's ideas on classification: a conceptual history. *Psychological Medicine* **18**, 813–821.

Berze, J. (1914/1987) Primary insufficiency of mental activity. In: *The Clinical Roots of the Schizophrenia Concept* (eds J. Cutting &

M. Shepherd), pp. 51–58. Translated from Chapter 4 of *Die primäre Insuffizienz der psychischen Aktivität*. Deuticke, Leipzig.

Bleuler, E. (1911/1950) Dementia praecox or the group of schizophrenias. New York: International Universities Press. Translated by J. Zinkin from Dementia Praecox oder der Gruppe der Schizophrenien. In: *Handbuch der Geisteskrankheiten* (ed. G. Aschaffenburg). Deuticke, Leipzig.

Bleuler, E. (1919) *Das Autistisch-Indisziplinierte Denken in der Medizin und Seine Überwindung*. Springer, Berlin.

Bush, G., Fink, M., Petrides, G. *et al.* (1996) Catatonia. I. Rating scale and standardised examination. *Acta Psychiatrica Scandinavica* **93**, 129–136.

Cohen, H. (1961) The evolution of the concept of disease. In: *Concepts of Medicine* (ed. B. Lush), pp. 159–169. Pergamon, Oxford.

Creer, C. & Wing, J.K. (1974) *Schizophrenia at Home*. National Schizophrenia Fellowship, London. [Reprinted with a new preface, 1988.]

Crow, T.J. (1985) The two syndrome concept: origns and current status. *Schizophrenia Bulletin* **11**, 471–486.

Crow, T.J. (1998) Nuclear schizophrenic symptoms as a window on the relationship between thought and speech. *Schizophrenia Research* **28**, 127–141.

Diem, O. (1903/1987) The simple dementing form of dementia praecox. In: *The Clinical Roots of the Schizophrenia Concept* (eds J. Cutting & M. Shepherd), pp. 25–34. Translated from Die einfach demente Form der Dementia Praecox. *Archiv für Psychiatrie und Nervenkrankheiten* **37**, 81–87.

Endicott, J. & Spitzer, R.L. (1978) A diagnostic interview: the Schedule for Affective Disorders and Schizophrenia. *Archives of General Psychiatry* **35**, 837–844.

Falret, J. (1854) *Leçons Cliniques de Médicine Mentale*. Baillière, Paris.

Fish, F.J. (1958) Leonhard's classification of schizophrenia. *Journal of Mental Science* **104**, 103.

Fisher, C.M. (1983) Abulia minor versus agitated behavior. *Clinical Neurosurgery* **31**, 9–31.

Flaum, M. & Andreason, N.C. (1991) Diagnostic criteria for schizophrenia and related disorders: options for DSM-IV. *Schizophrenia Bulletin* **17**, 143–156.

Foucault, M. (1967) *Madness and Civilisation*. Tavistock, London.

Foulds, G.A. (1965) *Personality and Personal Illness*. Tavistock, London.

Frith, C.D. & Frith, U. (1991) Elective affinities in schizophrenia and childhood autism. In: *Social Psychiatry. Theory, Methodology and Practice* (ed. P.E. Bebbington), pp. 65–88. Transaction, New Brunswick.

Frith, U. (1989) *Autism: Explaining the Enigma*. Blackwell, Oxford.

Frith, U. & Happé, F. (1994) Autism: beyond theory of mind. *Cognition* **50**, 115–132.

Gillberg, C. (2002) *A Guide to Asperger Syndrome*. Cambridge University Press, Cambridge.

Goffman, E. (1961) Asylums. *Essays on the Social Situation of Mental Patients and Other Inmates*. Penguin, Harmonsworth.

Griesinger, W. (1861) *Die Pathologie und Therapie der Psychischen Krankheiten*. Krabbe, Stuttgart.

Gruhle, H.W. (1929) Psychologie der Schizophrenie. In: *Psychologie der Schizophrenie* (eds J. Berze & H.W. Gruhle). Springer, Berlin.

Jackson, J.H. (1869/1932) Certain points in the study and classification of diseases of the nervous system. Reprinted in: *Selected Writings of John Hughlings Jackson*, Vol. 2. (ed. J. Taylor). Hodder and Stoughton, London.

Janzarik, W. (1984) Jaspers, Kurt Schneider und die Heidelberger Psychopathologie. *Nervenarzt* **55**, 18–24.

Janzarik, W. (1987) The concept of schizophrenia: history and problems. In: *Search for the Causes of Schizophrenia* (eds H. Häfner, W.F. Gattaz & W. Janzarik). Springer-Verlag, Heidelberg.

Jaspers, K. (1946/1963) *General Psychopathology*. Manchester University Press, Manchester. Translated by J. Hoenig & M. Hamilton from *Allgemeine Psychopathologie*. Springer Verlag, Heidelberg.

Joseph, A.B. (1992) Catatonia. In: *Movement Disorders in Neurology and Neuropsychiatry* (eds A.B. Joseph & R.R. Young), pp. 335–342. Blackwell Scientific, Boston.

Kahlbaum, K. (1874/1973) *Catatonia*. Johns Hopkins University Press, Baltimore. Translated by Y. Levij & T. Priden from *Die Katatonie oder das Spannungs-Irresein*. Hirschwald, Berlin.

Kanner, L. (1943) Autistic disturbances of affective contact. *Nervous Child* **2**, 217–250.

Kendell, R.E. (1987) Diagnosis and classification of functional psychoses. *British Medical Bulletin* **43**, 499–513.

Kendell, R.E. (1989) Clinical validity. *Psychological Medicine* **19**, 45–55.

Kendell, R.E. & Brockington, I.F. (1980) The identification of disease entities and the relationship between schizophrenic and affective psychoses. *British Journal of Psychiatry* **137**, 324–331.

Kendell, R.E., Cooper, J.E., Gourlay, A.J. *et al.* (1971) Diagnostic criteria of American and British psychiatrists. *Archives of General Psychiatry* **25** (2), 123–130.

Kendler, K.S. (1985) Diagnostic approaches to schizotypal personality disorder: a historical perspective. *Schizophrenia Bulletin* **11**, 538–553.

Kleist, K. (1960) Schizophrenic symptoms and cerebral pathology. *Journal of Mental Science* **106**, 246–255.

Kraepelin, E. (1896/1987) Dementia praecox. In: *The Clinical Roots of the Schizophrenia Syndrome* (eds J. Cutting & M. Shepherd), pp. 15–24. Cambridge University Press, Cambridge. Translated from *Lehrbuch der Psychiatrie*, 5th edn, pp. 426–441. Barth, Leipzig.

Kraepelin, E. (1920) Die Erscheinungsformen des Irreseins. *Zeitschrift für Neurologie und Psychiatrie* **62**, 1–29.

Kretschmer, E. (1966/1974) The sensitive delusion of reference. In: *Themes and Variations in European Psychiatry* (eds S.R. Hirsch & M. Shepherd). Wright, Bristol. Translated from *Der sensitiver Beziehungswahn*. Springer, Heidelberg.

Laing, R.D. & Esterson, A. (1964) *Sanity: Madness and the Family*. Tavistock, London.

Leekam, S.R., Libby, S.J., Wing, L. *et al.* (2002) The diagnostic interview for social and communication disorders. Algorithms for ICD 10 childhood autism and autistic spectrum disorders. *Journal of Child Psychology and Psychiatry* **43**, 325–327.

Leonhard, K. (1957) *Aufteilung der Endogenen Psychosen*. Akademie Verlag, Berlin.

Locke, J. (1959) *Essay Concerning Human Understanding*, Vol. 1, 2nd edn (ed. A.C. Fraser). Dover, New York.

Lorr, M. (1966) *Explorations in Typing Psychotics*. Pergamon, London.

McKenna, P.J., Lund, C.E., Mortimer, A.M. & Biggins, C.A. (1991) Motor, volitional and behavioural disorders in schizophrenia. II. The 'conflict of paradigms' hypothesis. *British Journal of Psychiatry* **158**, 328–336.

Magnan, V. (1893) *Leçons Cliniques Sur les Maladies Mentales*. Battaille, Paris.

Robins, L.N., Wing, J., Wittchen, H.U. *et al.* (1988) The Composite International Diagnostic Interview: an epidemiological instrument suitable for use in conjunction with different diagnostic systems and in different cultures. *Archives of General Psychiatry* **45**, 1069–1077.

Rogers, D. (1992) *Motor Disorder in Psychiatry: Towards a Neurological Psychiatry*. Wiley, New York.

Scheff, T.J. (1966) *Being Mentally Ill*. Aldine, Chicago.

Schneider, K. (1959) *Clinical Psychopathology*. Translated by M.W. Hamilton. Grune & Stratton, New York.

Schneider, K. (1976) *Klinische Psychopathologie*, 11th edn. Thieme, Stuttgart.

Spitzer, R.L., Endicott, J. & Robins, E. (1975) *Research Diagnostic Criteria: Rationale and Reliability*. Hodder and Stoughton, London.

Sturt, E. (1981) Hierarchical patterns in the distribution of psychiatric symptoms. *Psychological Medicine* **11**, 783–794.

Szasz, T. (1971) *The Manufacture of Madness*. Routledge, London.

Tantam, D. (1988) Asperger's syndrome. *Journal of Child Psychology and Psychiatry* **29**, 245–255.

Wing, J.K. (1961) A simple and reliable subclassification of chronic schizophrenia. *Journal of Mental Science* **107**, 862–875.

Wing, J.K., ed. (1975) *Schizophrenia from Within*. National Schizophrenia Fellowship, London.

Wing, J.K. (1978) *Reasoning About Madness*. Oxford University Press, London.

Wing, J.K. (1991) Social psychiatry. In: *Social Psychiatry: Theory, Methodology and Practice* (ed. P.E. Bebbington), pp. 3–22. Transaction, New Brunswick.

Wing, J.K. & Brown, G.W. (1961) Social treatment of chronic schizophrenia: a comparative survey of three mental hospitals. *Journal of Mental Science* **107**, 847–861.

Wing, J.K. & Brown, G.W. (1970). *Institutionalism and Schizophrenia*. Cambridge University Press, London.

Wing, J.K., Cooper, J.E. & Sartorius, N. (1974) *The Description and Classification of Psychiatric Symptoms: an Instruction Manual for the PSE and CATEGO System*. Cambridge University Press, London.

Wing, J.K., Sartorius, N. & Üstün, T.B. (1998) *Diagnosis and Clinical Measurement in Psychiatry: the SCAN System*. Cambridge University Press, Cambridge.

Wing, L. (1981) Asperger's syndrome. *Psychological Medicine* **11**, 115–129.

Wing, L. (1982) Development of concepts, classification and relationship to mental retardation. In: *Psychoses of Uncertain Aetiology* (eds J.K. Wing & L.G. Wing), pp. 185–190. Cambridge University Press, Cambridge.

Wing, L. (2000) Past and future research on Asperger Syndrome. In: *Asperger Syndrome* (eds A. Klin, F. Volkmar & S. Sparrow). Guildford Press, New York.

Wing, L. & Gould, J. (1979) Severe impairments of social interaction and associated abnormalities in children: epidemiology and classification. *Journal of Autism and Developmental Disorder* **9**, 11–29.

Wing, L. & Shah, A. (2000) Catatonia in autistic spectrum disorders. *British Journal of Psychiatry* **176**, 357–362.

Wing, L., Leekam, S.R., Libby, S.J. *et al.* (2002) The diagnostic interview for social and communication disorders. *Journal of Child Psychology and Psychiatry* **43**, 307–325.

Wolff, S. (1995) *Loners: The Life Path of Unusual Children*. Routledge, London.

World Health Organization (1973) *The International Pilot Study of Schizophrenia*. WHO, Geneva.

World Health Organization (1993) *The ICD-10 Classification of Mental and Behavioural Disorders: Diagnostic Criteria for Research*. WHO, Geneva.

World Health Organization (1999) *Schedules for Clinical Assessment in Neuropsychiatry*. World Health Organization, Geneva.

Descriptive psychopathology

J. Cutting

Introduction

In schizophrenia the apparatus of the mind disintegrates, severely and pervasively. It does so, moreover, in such a fashion that an experienced clinician can distinguish the condition from all other psychiatric disorders by the pattern of what is left after the mayhem. What we encounter in an individual suffering from schizophrenia are two sets of features: (i) the absence of certain functions or aspects of the mind which should be present in a normal individual – sometimes called 'negative symptoms'; and (ii) the presence of certain phenomena which are not present in a normal individual, and which probably represent a response of the healthy part of the schizophrenic's mind to the absent functions – sometimes called 'positive symptoms'. Some schizophrenics display only the latter, some only the former, but most display a combination of both.

For practical purposes the descriptive psychopathology of schizophrenia can be treated in three sections:

1 purely positive symptoms – *hallucinations and other abnormal experiences*, *delusions* and *catatonia*;

2 traditional psychopathological groupings containing positive and negative symptoms – *thought disorder* and *disturbances of emotions*; and

3 what used to be referred to as *psychological deficit*, purely negative symptoms – *impaired attention, intelligence, memory, perception* and *will*.

Neither the positive symptoms (or phenomena) nor the negative symptoms (or signs, because strictly speaking they are things we observe rather than what a patient complains about) exhaust the entire gamut of a schizophrenic's subjective experience or entirely account for all the possible behaviour. The condition has such a pervasive effect on the mind that all aspects are affected, including, for example, an individual's sense of time and appreciation of space. Moreover, schizophrenics may engage in bizarre behaviour which cannot be explained in terms of the categories of negative symptoms listed above. (see also Chapter 3.)

Hallucinations and other abnormal experiences

Definitions and classification

There are four categories of experience within this group of phenomena: anomalous experiences, illusions, hallucinations and pseudohallucinations.

Anomalous experiences, or distortions of a real perceptual experience, are those where a real perception of an object (i.e. the object actually perceived is really there) does not accord with its normal quality. Its colour may be different from usual, its shape may be strange, its size may be smaller or larger than realistically possible or it may be altered in a very subtle way – less or more familiar, less or more distant (or louder or softer in the auditory modality), less or more real or even less or more accentuated relative to the rest of the perceptual environment. None of these experiences is a hallucination, illusion or pseudohallucination (see below) because a real object is there, it is recognized as such, but it is merely registered as different from hitherto. Some of the experiences have attracted a specific label, e.g. *déjà vu* for an increase in familiarity, derealization for a loss of the sense of reality and micropsia if the perceived object looks smaller than normal.

Illusions are false perceptual experiences where an object that really exists 'out there' is completely misrecognized as an entirely different class of object, e.g. a moving curtain for a burglar or a rubber band for a snake. It is not an anomalous experience, because it is not a qualitative alteration in the perception of a correctly recognized object, but rather the complete misrecognition of something – the new 'something' looking exactly like a real example of what it would in fact look like. Illusions are mentioned here for completeness, but are not specific or indicative of schizophrenia.

A hallucination is a perception of something when in fact nothing exists in the perceptual field, a perception without an object, in short.

Table 2.1 Subtypes of hallucinations.

Modality
Visual
Auditory
Olfactory
Gustatory
Tactile, somatic, kinaesthetic

Timing with respect to sleep
Hypnagogic: just before falling asleep
Hypnopompic: on just waking up

Precipitation by sensory stimulus
Synaesthetic: precipitation by sensation in a different modality from
   hallucination (e.g. voice after seeing flashing light)
Functional (or reflex): precipitation by sensation in same modality (e.g.
   voice after hearing dripping tap. NB This is not an illusion because
   the dripping tap and the voice are *both* heard)

Content
e.g. Musical
Autoscopic
   Of self
Lilliputian
   Smaller than realistic
Teichopsia
   Geometrical shapes, particularly of battlements
   Characteristic of migraine

Table 2.2 Examples of anomalous experiences in schizophrenia.

Colour
'Colours meant a lot to me . . . stood out, not meant a lot, especially traffic lights.'

'All bright colours were ones that frightened me most – orange and red.'

Faces/people
'All I could see were people in a car and they looked like ghosts. They looked different, like statues or monuments, dead, as if cremated.'

'The right side [in his left field] of my mother's and sister's faces went completely black. When I looked in the mirror the right half of my own face [really the left half as it was a mirror image] also looked black.'

Environment
'I couldn't recognize any of my surroundings – people, places. I could recognize certain things. I could recognize qualities of a place, of surfaces. It was the organization of things which was different.'

'It was like being in one of my paintings [patient was an art student]. I used to go out and see the houses with fascination. I would stare out of the window for hours.'

A pseudohallucination is variously defined in the psychopathological literature. One school of thought (Hare 1973) considers it to be a hallucination with preserved insight. In other words, I might perceive an elephant in front of me (when none actually exists), and at the same time be aware of the falseness of my perceptual experience, i.e. I know that no elephant is there even though I see it. Another school of thought (Jaspers 1913) regards it as a hallucination, but one where the hallucinated object lacks the reality of a perception of the same object if it were really there – less vivid, less 'real', etc. This latter school of thought is perhaps a more philosophically correct perspective, because the distinction between a hallucination and a pseudohallucination may be more one of degree, as a careful analysis of most hallucinations (Merleau-Ponty 1962) will reveal that the apparent object is rarely experienced as 'realistically' as the comparable real object.

Hallucinations themselves are further divided into various types, according to modality, timing with respect to sleep, their occasional precipitation by a sensory stimulus and their content (Table 2.1). There are numerous causes of hallucinations besides schizophrenia (Cutting 1996).

Incidence and variety in schizophrenia

The incidence of all types of anomalous experiences in schizophrenia is about 50% (Cutting & Dunne 1989), and of all types of hallucinations about 50%. Visual hallucinations occur in 15% of all subjects, auditory in 50% of all subjects and tactile in 5% of all subjects (Cutting 1990).

The pattern of the anomalous experiences is very varied. Some examples are shown in Table 2.2. Colours and faces are often the focus of the anomalous experience, but there may be a complete alteration in the quality of the entire environment. This understandably induces a feeling of perplexity in the sufferer, and constitutes what is called delusional mood, because the experiences later solidify as beliefs about what was going on then, e.g. people looking at me in a funny way, etc. The anomalous experiences usually occur at the onset of an episode, and are often forgotten or become delusionally elaborated by the time the patient is interviewed.

The pattern of the hallucinations, on the other hand, is quite specific. The most common hallucination is a voice – not just any auditory hallucination, but a voice. Moreover, this voice has certain characteristics that make it even more specific for the condition: it is usually heard in a grammatical form that is different from how we experience our own thoughts (e.g. instead of 'I wonder what I'm going to have for supper tonight', the voice says, '*he* is wondering what to have for supper') and the sex of the voice (male or female) is nearly always identified, but the owner of the voice is usually not someone who is known to the subject. Added to all this is the fact that schizophrenic voices diminish if there is meaningful conversation going on around, and intensify if there is no background auditory noise or if the background noise is devoid of meaning (Margo *et al.* 1981). Moreover, schizophrenics with voices do not differ from schizophrenics without voices on measures of auditory acuity

(Collicutt & Hemsley 1981) or imagery (Starker & Jolin 1982). Typical examples of schizophrenic voices are: 'He's getting things the wrong way' (presumably referring to how he thought about himself), 'You're not going to smoke the cigarette the way you want to but the way we want you to.'

Schneider (1958) was so impressed with the regular occurrence of such 'voices' in schizophrenic patients that he elevated three types to the rank of first-rank symptoms of the condition:

1 voices speaking thoughts aloud;
2 voices arguing (two or more hallucinatory voices discussing the person in the third person); and
3 voices commenting on the subject's actions.

Other characteristics of the 'voices' are that they may be experienced outside the head, but they are usually poorly localized, and some patients do not distinguish them completely from their thoughts, i.e. they fulfil certain criteria for a pseudohallucination.

Finally, consider this example of ethological research: Green and Preston (1981) applied a throat microphone to one hallucinating schizophrenic, by means of which they picked up the following conversation (supporting the view that 'voices' are subvocalizations of real thoughts experienced by a subject rather than incorrect perceptual accounts of auditory stimuli in their environment). *Voice*, 'Mind your own business darling; I don't want him [referring to the experimenter] to know what I was doing.' When the experimenter asked the subject what was going on, he replied 'See that, I spoke to ask her [the owner of the voice] what she was doing, and she said, mind your own business.'

The pattern of a schizophrenic's visual hallucinations is less well established. Although infrequent, visual hallucinations do occur in a substantial minority of schizophrenics (Guttmann & Maclay 1937; Feinberg 1962; Cutting 1996). They appear to be of things which do not actually exist in the real world, or of part-objects, e.g. leg on a bedroom wall, 'a big animal like an octopus', 'something like a mouse running across the floor', 'mirages of a desert' or 'rat tail coming out of own anus'.

Illusions, in general, are rare, as are pseudohallucinations (barring the problem of establishing the strict phenomenological status of schizophrenic 'voices'). Olfactory (Rubert *et al.* 1961) and gustatory (De Morsier 1938) hallucinations are also rare. Somatic hallucinations are less rare (Cutting 1990).

Delusions

Definitions and classification

Various definitions of delusion exist (Schmidt 1940). Possibly the three best ones are Jaspers' (1913), that of the DSM-IIIR (American Psychiatric Association 1987) and Spitzer's (1990).

Jaspers' definition proposed three criteria: (i) it is a belief held with extraordinary conviction, with an incomparable subjective certainty; (ii) there is an imperviousness to other experiences and to compelling counterargument; and (iii) the content is impossible.

That in DSM-IIIR is:

A false personal belief based on incorrect inference about external reality and firmly sustained in spite of what almost everyone else believes and in spite of what constitutes incontrovertible and obvious proof or evidence to the contrary. The belief is not one ordinarily accepted by other members of the person's culture or sub-culture (i.e. it is not an article of religious faith). When a false belief involves an extreme value judgement, it is regarded as a delusion only when the judgement is so extreme as to defy credibility.

Spitzer defines delusion as follows:

X's statement is a delusion if it concerns the world, and is not an analytic statement (i.e. a linguistic tautology), and it is held with a subjective certainty only appropriate for statements about the mind.

The main differences between these definitions are Jaspers' emphasis on the inappropriate conviction, DSM-IIIR's mapping of the social context in which the delusion has to be placed, and Spitzer's restriction to a concern with the world (rather than self, body or mind). Given the complexity of the topic, all three definitions should be taken into account for their respective insights.

Delusions are currently classified according to four independent principles:

1 degree of inexplicability, e.g. primary;
2 nature of subverted mental function, e.g. delusional perception;
3 nosological significance, i.e. the extent to which the delusional state has been accorded independent status from the three major psychoses, e.g. sensitive delusion of reference; and
4 thematic content, e.g. jealousy.

These four classificatory systems are summarized in Table 2.3, along with a fifth system (Cutting 1996) which groups the themes in a more logical way.

Incidence and variety in schizophrenia

Delusions occur at some stage of the condition in more than 90% of schizophrenics.

Concerning the various types of delusions categorized in Table 2.3, some are more common than others and some have been elevated to the status of diagnostic criteria for schizophrenia.

Jaspers (1913) believed that primary delusions were pathognomonic of schizophrenia. In addition to the three properties that he believed belonged to any delusion – conviction, imperviousness to other experiences and impossibility of content – primary delusions possessed the further properties of 'ununderstandability', 'being unmediated by thought' and 'involvement of the whole personality' (Walker 1991).

Schneider (1958) was unhappy with this general formulation because of the practical problems of establishing whether a delusion fulfilled these latter three criteria. Only in the case of delusional perception, according to Schneider, could the

Table 2.3 Classification of delusions.

According to degree of inexplicability
Primary, pure, true
Secondary, delusion-like ideas
Overvalued idea

According to subverted mental function
Delusional perception
Delusional notion
Delusional memory
Delusional awareness
Delusional atmosphere/mood

According to degree of independent nosological status, e.g.
Paranoia
Delusional loving (de Clérambault's syndrome)
Monosymptomatic hypochondriacal psychosis

According to thematic content (traditional), e.g.
Lycanthropy (transformation into an animal)
Jealousy
Grandiosity
Influence/control

According to thematic content (logical, comprehensive, mutually
  exclusive)
Concerning the world
  Altered identity/class of things, e.g. Capgras' syndrome
  Altered quality, e.g. spouse unfaithful
  Altered chronicle of events, e.g. world going to blow up
  Altered evaluation, e.g. persecutory
  Altered self-reference, e.g. reference
  Nihilism, e.g. spouse dead
Concerning the mind
  Altered boundaries, e.g. thought broadcasting
  Altered function, e.g. cannot think
  Altered autonomy, e.g. thought insertion
Concerning the self
  Altered identity, e.g. X = Napoleon
  Altered ability, e.g. X is spiritual healer
  Altered autonomy, e.g. someone taken X over
  Altered evaluation, e.g. guilt
Concerning the body
  Altered structure, e.g. no brain
  Altered function, e.g. bowels do not work
  Altered autonomy, e.g. X's sensations are not X's

Table 2.4 Characteristic schizophrenic delusions.

Delusional perception	Normal perception has private and illogical meaning
Thought withdrawal	Thoughts cease and are simultaneously experienced as removed by external force
Thought insertion	Thoughts have a quality of not being own and are ascribed to external agency
Thought broadcasting	Thoughts escape into outside world where they are experienced by others
Made feelings	Feelings do not seem to be own, but are attributable to external force
Made impulses	Drive or impulse seems to be alien and external
Made volitional acts	Actions and movements felt to be under outside control
Somatic passivity	Experience of bodily sensations imposed by external agency
Bizarre delusions	e.g. parents exist in another time and place
Multiple delusions	e.g. nurses are Japanese, mirrors reflect the wrong way, haloperidol is made from shark's pancreas
Widespread delusions	e.g. husband acted in a sexually indiscrete way at a party, earthquake happening, grandson seriously ill

psychiatrist be sure that 'some abnormal significance . . . were attached . . . without any comprehensible rational or emotional justification'. This, according to Schneider, was because a two-stage process was involved: a normal perception and then an 'irrational and emotionally incomprehensible . . . delusional course'.

As well as delusional perception, Schneider also elevated certain delusional themes to the status of first-rank symptoms – the common denominator of which is a loss of autonomy or

boundaries in the spheres of body, self or mind. These are usually regarded as seven in number (Table 2.4). More recent formulations (e.g. Research Diagnostic Criteria (RDC); Carpenter *et al.* 1973; Spitzer *et al.* 1975; DSM-IIIR) recognize the fact that deluded schizophrenics *may not have* such first-rank symptoms but manics *may have* them, and give the following categories of delusion equal diagnostic significance – bizarre, multiple or widespread (involving more than one area of life). Of the themes listed in Table 2.3, the most diagnosis-specific in schizophrenia, relative to manics and psychotic depressives (all diagnosed by non-delusional criteria), were (McGilchrist & Cutting 1995; Cutting 1996) altered bodily structure, altered bodily autonomy, altered boundaries of mind, altered autonomy of mind and altered identity of the world.

Catatonia

Definition and classification

Catatonia refers to a set of complex movements, postures and actions whose common denominator is their involuntariness (Table 2.5). Not all involuntary movements fall within the

Table 2.5 Catatonic phenomena.

Stupor	Virtual absence of movement and speech in the presence of full consciousness
Catalepsy	Maintenance of unusual postures for long periods of time and no sense of discomfort, often accompanied by waxy flexibility (external manipulation of limb as though made of wax)
Automatism	Automatic obedience to commands, regardless of consequence
Mannerisms	Peculiar social habits, e.g. style of dress, handshake, writing or speech, at variance with social setting
Stereotypies	Repetitive movements of a single part of the body, divorced from mainstream of bodily activities
Posturing and grimacing	Peculiar positions of body (posturing) or face (grimacing) inappropriate to mainstream activity and social situation
Negativism	Behaviour which is consistently in opposition to social and apparent individual demands of a situation
Echopraxia	Automatic repetition of visually perceived actions of others

Table 2.6 Components of thought disorder.

Disorder of content, i.e. delusion including delusions about the autonomy of a subject's own thought processes, e.g. thought insertion

Disorder of form, i.e. formal thought disorder
Disorder of the mechanisms of thinking as characterized descriptively (intrinsic thinking disturbance, dyslogia)
    Concrete thinking
    Loosening of associations
    Overinclusion
    Illogicality
Disorder of language and speech
    Derailment, tangentiality, knight's move thinking
    Neologisms
    Poverty of speech (alogia)
    Poverty of content of speech
    Incoherence
    Pressure of speech
    Flight of ideas
    Retarded speech, mutism

category of catatonia; tics, chorea, dyskinesia, athetosis and ballismus are involuntary but not catatonic. It is partly convention and partly complexity that allocates certain movements or postures to the category. They are a heterogeneous bunch, ranging from a peculiar way of holding the head (posturing) to the entire annihilation of free will (as in negativism).

Incidence and variety in schizophrenia

According to the International Pilot Study of Schizophrenia (World Health Organization 1973), 7% of 811 schizophrenics exhibited one or other phenomenon. Other estimates (Morrison 1973; Guggenheim & Barbigian 1974) also gave a figure of between 5% and 10%. According to Abrams and Taylor (1976), mannerisms are the most common, followed, in descending order of frequency, by stereotypies, stupor, negativism, automatism and echopraxia.

Mannerisms, stereotype, negativism, catalepsy, automatism and posturing or grimacing are most specifically linked with schizophrenia. Stupor is more commonly linked with depressive psychosis or brainstem lesions (Johnson 1984; Barnes *et al.* 1986). Echopraxia is also seen in cases with frontal lobe lesions (Lhermitte *et al.* 1986). Abrams and Taylor (1976) claimed that all varieties of catatonia could occur in mania, but this is not my experience.

There is evidence that catatonic phenomena have diminished in frequency since Kraepelin's turn-of-the-century estimate of 20% in his series of patients with dementia praecox. There is also evidence that they are more common in schizophrenics from developing countries (World Health Organization 1973).

Nowadays, there is a tendency to lump catatonic phenomena with other involuntary movements such as tics, dyskinesia and chorea, and to deny them special status in schizophrenics (Rogers 1985).

Thought disorder

Definitions and classification

The term thought disorder covers a variety of positive *and* negative symptoms of schizophrenia, and is largely a misnomer because much of what is traditionally referred to as thought disorder is a disorder of spoken language.

The various components are set out in Table 2.6. The first distinction, identified by Schilder (1920), is between *disordered content* and *disordered form*. The former is synonymous with delusion. The latter comprises two categories (Andreasen 1982a; Cutting & Murphy 1988); (i) an intrinsic disturbance of thinking itself; and (ii) disordered language and speech.

The intrinsic disturbance of thinking includes such inferred and hypothetical descriptive notions as concrete thinking, overinclusion, illogicality and loosening of associations.

Concrete thinking is a tendency to select one aspect of a thing or concept, usually a physical quality or a personal association, at the expense of its overall meaning. It is traditionally tested by proverb interpretation, a concrete response being one which fails to take proper account of the metaphorical nature of proverbs.

Overinclusion is the tendency to include false or irrelevant items in a concept or category, in other words, to inappropriately widen the boundaries of a concept or category. It is sometimes assessed in the course of an object-sorting task, an overinclusive response being one which incorporates too many or inappropriate items within a category.

Illogicality is a tendency to offer bizarre explanations for things and events, explanations which not only grossly contravene the laws of logic, but also the 'way of the world'. It is traditionally tested by inviting a subject to complete a syllogism (e.g. if all alligators are reptiles, and some reptiles are green, then are all alligators green? True or false?)

Loosening of associations is sometimes used as a synonym for derailment (see below), in which case it refers to a disorder in the form of spoken speech. In the present context it carries the meaning of a disordered conceptual structure, as illustrated by the reply of a schizophrenic subject to one of the questions in the similarities subscale of the Wechsler Adult Intelligence Scale: in what way are an orange and a banana alike? They are Nature's produce! This is not wrong, just loose. Note that the traditional tests for these thinking disorders are not good at discriminating schizophrenics from normal subjects, with significant numbers of the latter overlapping with the former.

Disordered language and speech are usually held to contain the following main varieties. First, there is *derailment* or tangentiality or knight's move thinking – a failure to conform to the social rules of conversation and the needs of a listener by picking up on personal or idiosyncratic aspects of a word or phrase and not sticking to the overall theme of the discourse. Next there is *neologism*, the creation of new words, subsuming an allied phenomenon, word approximations or paraphasia, where recognized words are given a new meaning. Then there is *poverty of speech*, which is a grossly reduced output of speech, and *poverty of content of speech* where, despite an adequate fluency, the number of ideas expressed is substantially reduced. *Incoherence* refers to a breakdown in the grammatical structure of what is expressed, sometimes to such an extent that the speech resembles aphasia – hence schizophasia or 'word salad'. *Pressure of speech* is a speeding-up of the flow of speech; *flight of ideas* is a combination of pressure of speech and derailment; and *retardation*, of which *mutism* is an extreme form, is self-explanatory.

Two alternative classifications are in use, one theoretical (Chaika 1990) and one practical (Andreasen 1979a). Chaika proposes four levels in the breakdown of language, each responsible for some of the traditional clinical varieties. Level 1, the subtlest disorder, affects the richness of expression of ideas, of which poverty of content of speech is an example. At level 2, there is an internal lack of coherence in the construction of sentences, illustrated by derailment. By level 3, the conventionally agreed shared meanings of words is dispensed with, hence neologisms. Finally, at level 4, even the conventional rules of grammar disappear, and the utterance becomes an unintelligible jumble – incoherence.

Some items of thought disorder are regarded as positive symptoms of schizophrenia, e.g. derailment and illogicality; others are regarded as negative symptoms, e.g. poverty of speech. Several schedules for the assessment of the various types exist and the most useful of these are reviewed in Cutting (1994).

Incidence and variety in schizophrenia

Andreasen's (1979a) study on the incidence of 18 varieties of thought disorder in schizophrenics and manics still provides the best picture of its incidence and specificity in schizophrenia. Cutting and Murphy (1988) studied the incidence of four types of intrinsic thinking disturbance, and had neurotic controls, not manics.

In Andreasen's study, derailment (56%) was the most common variety in schizophrenia, but did not significantly distinguish this group from manics, whereas poverty of content of speech (40% schizophrenics, 19% manics) did discriminate the two diagnostic groups. Pressure of speech (27% schizophrenics, 72% manics) was another significant discriminator. Neologisms (2% schizophrenics) were rare.

Cutting and Murphy found that a loosening of associations (based on impaired ability to appreciate conceptual similarities)

Table 2.7 Examples of thought disorder in schizophrenia.

Derailment
'Mum loves God. She always compares me with God.
I want to know if there are any eggs in my ovaries.'

'They were frightening me about wishes and when I was 20 I blew out a candle and I was frightened of my mother.'

Incoherence
'That is when God pardoned the GP at 9.30 this morning, the catching of an instant philosophically speaking into time that only occurs at both at death turkeys in the freezer.'

'To do to ask is at the behest of my parents which seems a fairly inappropriate reason to me.'

Neologisms/word approximations

'Oumana'	God's love beyond me
'Cytic'	Extrasensory perception
'I froze people out'	Made them older
'Medetary'	Smoked cannabis because it was good for him
'Criton'	Something which expresses sexual identity
'Psycasm'	Like a Lucky Strike cigarette

Poverty of content of speech
'I asked for pudding. I wanted to get a pudding. I accepted the pudding. I brought the pudding to the room. I ate the pudding. I am an affair of certain self-fermenting proteins catalysing their own growth. I am certainly not going to accept a continuous adjustment of internal to external relations.'

'I need to see the appropriateness of today.'

Illogicality
'I went through the colour black in quite an easy task.'

'In my mind the kissing and cuddling in 1960 makes it rain in 1980.'

'I want to have a haircut because there's no oxygen on the ward.'

occurred in 5% of schizophrenics; overinclusion (based on the number of category inclusions of items ranging from appropriate to inappropriate) occurred in 25% of schizophrenics; concrete thinking (rated as concreteness in proverb interpretation) occurred in none of 20 schizophrenics; and illogicality (false conclusions in syllogisms) occurred in 10% of schizophrenics. All figures refer to the proportion of subjects falling outside of 2 SD from the control mean.

Examples of the main varieties encountered in schizophrenia are shown in Table 2.7. Four of the five examples given – loosening of associations, incoherence, poverty of content of speech and illogicality – are the only varieties of thought disorder considered to have diagnostic specificity in DSM-IIIR.

Disturbance of emotion

Definitions and classification

Emotion is a general term covering *feelings* ('individual unique and radical commotions of the psyche'; Jaspers 1913), *affect* ('a momentary and complex emotional process of great intensity with conspicuous bodily accompaniment and sequelae'; Jaspers 1913) and *mood* ('states of feeling or frames of mind that come about with prolonged emotion'; Jaspers 1913). Philosophers such as Jaspers and Wittgenstein (1980) emphasize the fact that emotion is an experience. Other philosophers (e.g. Ryle 1949) and behaviourist psychologists (e.g. Izard & Buechler 1980) emphasize the *motivational* aspect of emotion.

Feelings, affect, mood and motivation all have their psychopathological counterparts (Table 2.8), and examples from all four categories can be encountered in schizophrenia. Only one type – inappropriate affect – is generally held to be a positive symptom of schizophrenia, whereas several – blunting (or flattening) of affect, anhedonia (loss of feeling) and apathy (loss of motivation) – are regarded as negative symptoms.

Incidence and variety in schizophrenia

Anhedonia (loss of feeling) is sometimes divided into social, e.g. loss of pleasure from being with friends, and physical, e.g. loss of pleasure from seeing a beautiful sunset, being massaged, drinking, etc. It can be rated using a questionnaire (Chapman *et al.* 1980) or at interview (Harrow *et al.* 1977). Using the questionnaire of Chapman *et al.*, Watson *et al.* (1979) found that 45% of 312 schizophrenics fell outside the 90th percentile of alcoholic controls, although Cook and Simukonda (1981), who used the same questionnaire, found that only 34% of 52 schizophrenics fell outside 1 SD of nurses; social anhedonia accounted for most of this. Schuck *et al.* (1984) also found that physical anhedonia was no more prevalent in schizophrenics than in depressives. Harrow *et al.* (1977) found that only chronic, not acute, schizophrenics were significantly anhedonic.

Intensification of feelings is reported at the onset of schizo-

Table 2.8   Disturbances of emotion.

Normal aspects	Main psychopathological varieties
Feeling	Loss of feeling – anhedonia
	Heightened feeling
Affect	Inappropriate affect
	Flattened, blunting of, affect
Mood	Depression
	Elation
	Anxiety
Motivation	Apathy

phrenia, but there are no adequate studies of the topic. A patient of McGhie and Chapman (1961), for example, recalled:

> You have no idea what it's like doctor. You would have to experience it yourself. When you feel yourself going into a sort of coma you get really scared. It's like waiting on a landing craft going into D-Day. You tremble and panic. It's like no other fear on earth.

Inappropriate affect or parathymia is the display of an emotion considered inappropriate to the situation. It is usually an outburst of empty giggling and occurs in about 20% of acutely ill schizophrenics (Andreasen 1979b).

Flattening of affect or blunted affect can be observed in about 50% of acute (Andreasen 1979b) or chronic schizophrenics (McCreadie 1982). According to Andreasen, it is a composite rating by an observer of the following elements, in descending order of weighted significance: paucity of expressive gestures (57%); unchanging facial expression (53%); lack of vocal inflection (53%); decreased spontaneous movement (37%); poor eye contact (37%); affective non-responsivity (30%); slowed speech (17%); and increased latency of response (10%).

Depression is a non-specific accompaniment of schizophrenia. It is much more frequent in acute schizophrenia (70% – neurotic depression in CATEGO (Wing *et al.* 1974) – Knights & Hirsch 1981) than expected, although probably not much higher in chronic schizophrenia (clinical depression (10%) Barnes *et al.* 1989) than in the normal population. The relationship between depression and schizophrenia is more complicated than these bare figures indicate. There is the diagnostic dilemma to consider: do you exclude patients with 'first-rank symptoms of schizophrenia' from the category of depressive psychosis even if they fulfil all other criteria for this? According to Hirsch (1982), depression and schizophrenia both arise from a 'shared pathophysiological mechanism', and depression is 'revealed' as an integral part of schizophrenia in so far as it does not become obvious until after the acute phase has subsided, although the symptoms of depression are indeed most prevalent in the acute phase if systematically rated (Knights & Hirsch 1981). According to Crow (1986), who revives Griesinger's (1845) unitary psychosis theory, depression and schizophrenia are only far ends of the same spectrum. According to Galdi (1983), depression is increased by the use of neuroleptics. According to McGlashan and Carpenter (1976), remitted schizophrenics experience more depression as part of a recovery of insight into what they have been through.

Elation is also a non-specific accompaniment of schizophrenia, but may complicate the diagnostic issue in the same way as depression, as discussed above.

Anxiety is particularly marked at the outset, but is pathologically absent in the chronic stages.

Apathy is the most troublesome negative symptom of all (at least for carers of the sufferer). Although regarded as the psychopathological counterpart of the motivational component of emotion, it is, in my view, better regarded as a manifestation of impaired will in the condition, and will be discussed below. Its mention here is justified because most psychologists and many psychiatrists regard motivation as an aspect of emotion.

Psychological deficit

The terms dementia praecox, deterioration, defect state and pseudodementia have all been applied to the combination of impaired attention, apparent decline in intelligence, failures in memory, perceptual impoverishment and lack of will. The individual components are also referred to as psychological deficits or negative symptoms.

Attentional impairment

There is a large body of literature demonstrating that attention, particularly maintenance of attention, is impaired in schizophrenia (e.g. Asarnow & MacCrimmon 1978; Van den Bosch 1982). The various components of attention – maintenance, selectivity, span, shifting of focus – are not equally affected, and the brunt is borne by maintenance, shifting, span and selectivity in that order of severity.

Intellectual decline

Numerous studies have shown a decline in formally measured intelligence from a prepsychotic state to psychosis (Rappaport & Webb 1950) and, further, from acute to chronic psychosis (Trapp & James 1937). The intellectual decline affects all subtests of the Wechsler Adult Intelligence Scale, but particularly the performance subtests, and particularly digit symbol and picture arrangement (Cutting 1990). There is growing evidence, and some controversy, that schizophrenics have a particular profile of intellectual decline, relative to Alzheimer's disease (see Chapter 10).

Memory failures

Although amnesia is traditionally regarded as a symptom of organic psychosis and should not, according to this view, be prominent in a functional psychosis such as schizophrenia, there is increasing evidence that chronic schizophrenics do have a pervasive disturbance of memory. McKenna *et al.* (1990) demonstrated that the memory impairment in chronic schizophrenics was equivalent to a group of patients with definite brain injury (see Chapter 10).

Perceptual impoverishment

Schizophrenics turn away from the outside world and become preoccupied with their own subjective state (Sass 1992), and it is difficult to assess the patency of the actual perceptual processes. There is ample evidence that their perception of the world differs qualitatively from that of a normal person (Cutting 1990); this, in consequence, leads to an impoverishment in their appreciation of the outside world.

Lack of will

Chronic schizophrenics suffer from a profound apathy, sometimes known as abulia, and this stems from a fundamental deficiency in the mainspring of their life. Kraepelin (1913/1919) considered this their essential psychological problem. Unfortunately, the term 'will' has fallen into disuse for most of this century and there have been no experimental studies to assess the significance of Kraepelin's views.

Clustering of phenomena/symptoms

There is no shortage of attempts to classify the above psychopathological features of schizophrenia.

Bleuler (1911/1950) proposed a distinction between 'fundamental symptoms', those which were virtually pathognomonic, and 'accessory symptoms', those which occurred in other conditions as well. The former comprised disturbances of association and affectivity, ambivalence and autism. The latter included delusions, alterations in personality, speech and writing disorders and catatonia.

Schneider (1958) proposed a distinction between first-rank symptoms (see Table 2.4) and other symptoms, regarding the former as atheoretical diagnostic aids.

Andreasen (1982b) and Crow (1980) adapted Jackson's formulation of positive and negative symptoms as applied to neurological disorders to schizophrenia, and this has proved, in my view, one of the most useful classifications of phenomena. Andreasen recognizes five categories of negative symptoms: affective flattening, attentional impairment, alogia (poverty of speech), avolition (apathy) and anhedonia (asociality). Hallucinations, delusions, bizarre behaviour and certain instances of thought disorder (derailment, flight of ideas, illogicality) are the positive symptoms.

Liddle (1987) identified three statistical clusters of symptoms, calling them the psychomotor poverty syndrome (poverty of speech, flattened affect and decreased spontaneous movement), the disorganization syndrome (formal thought disorder and inappropriate affect) and the reality distortion syndrome (delusions and hallucinations).

Huber *et al.* (1980) divided symptoms into 'characteristic schizophrenic deficiency' types and 'non-characteristic'. The former included what he called '*coanaesthetic* symptoms', body hallucinations and the latter such complaints as 'reduced capacity for adaptation'.

All such classifications can be criticized on the grounds of either reliability or validity, and their usefulness will almost certainly be undermined or corroborated by neurobiological advances over the next decade or so.

Explanatory theories

Explanatory theories for schizophrenic phenomena abound (Cutting 1985). It may be that all these are so closely attached to a psychological theory of the mind that subsequent generations, who eschew that particular theory, will have to grasp the schizophrenic experience afresh. The best modern account is actually given in a book that relates schizophrenia to the artistic history of the last century – *Madness and Modernism* (Sass 1992) – emphasizing that the 'descriptive' psychopathology of schizophrenia is still a powerful source of information for all those interested in the workings of the mind in 'normals', as well as for those endeavouring to understand the nature and cause of schizophrenia.

References

Abrams, R. & Taylor, M.A. (1976) Catatonia. *Archives of General Psychiatry* **33**, 579–581.

American Psychiatric Association (1987) *Diagnostic and Statistical Manual of Mental Disorders*, 3rd edn. American Psychiatric Association, Washington DC.

Andreasen, N.C. (1979a) Thought, language and communication disorders. *Archives of General Psychiatry* **36**, 1315–1330.

Andreasen, N.C. (1979b) Affective flattening and the criteria for schizophrenia. *American Journal of Psychiatry* **136**, 944–947.

Andreasen, N.C. (1982a) Should the term 'thought disorder' be revised? *Comprehensive Psychiatry* **23**, 291–299.

Andreasen, N.C. (1982b) Negative symptoms in schizophrenia. *Archives of General Psychiatry* **39**, 784–788.

Asarnow, R.F. & MacCrimmon, D.J. (1978) Residual performance deficit in clinically remitted schizophrenics: a marker of schizophrenia? *Journal of Abnormal Psychology* **87**, 597–608.

Barnes, M.P., Saunders, M., Walls, T.J., Saunders, I. & Kirk, C.A. (1986) The syndrome of Karl Ludwig Kahlbaum. *Journal of Neurology, Neurosurgery and Psychiatry* **49**, 991–996.

Barnes, T.R.E., Curson, D.A., Liddle, P.F. & Patel, M. (1989) The nature and prevalence of depression in chronic schizophrenic in-patients. *British Journal of Psychiatry* **154**, 486–491.

Bleuler, E. (1911/1950) *Dementia Praecox.* International University Press, New York. Translated by J. Zinkin, from *Dementia Praecox oder die Gruppe der Schizophrenien.* Deuticke, Leipzig.

Carpenter, W.T., Strauss, J.S. & Bartko, J.J. (1973) Flexible system for the diagnosis of schizophrenia. *Science* **182**, 1275–1278.

Chaika, E. (1990) *Understanding Psychotic Speech: Beyond Freud and Chomsky.* Charles C. Thomas, Springfield.

Chapman, L.J., Chapman, J.P. & Raulin, M.L. (1980) Scales for physical and social anhedonia. *Journal of Abnormal Psychology* **85**, 374–382.

Collicutt, J.R. & Hemsley, D.R. (1981) A psychophysical investigation of auditory functioning in schizophrenia. *British Journal of Social and Clinical Psychology* **20**, 199–204.

Cook, M. & Simukonda, F. (1981) Anhedonia and schizophrenia. *British Journal of Psychiatry* **139**, 523–525.

Crow, T.J. (1980) Molecular pathology of schizophrenia: more than one disease process? *British Medical Journal* i, 66–68.

Crow, T.J. (1986) The continuum of psychosis and its implications for the structure of the gene. *British Journal of Psychiatry* **149**, 419–429.

Cutting, J. (1985) *The Psychology of Schizophrenia.* Churchill Livingstone, Edinburgh.

Cutting, J. (1990) *The Right Cerebral Hemisphere and Psychiatric Disorders.* Oxford University Press, Oxford.

Cutting, J. (1994) The assessment of thought disorder. In: *Assessment of Psychosis: A Practical Handbook* (eds T. Barnes & H. Nelson), pp. 41–50. Farrand Press, London.

Cutting, J. (1996) *Two Worlds, Two Minds, Two Hemispheres: A Reinterpretation of Psychopathology.* Oxford University Press, Oxford.

Cutting, J. & Dunne, F. (1989) Subjective experience of schizophrenia. *Schizophrenia Bulletin* **15**, 217–231.

Cutting J. & Murphy, D. (1988) Schizophrenia thought disorder. *British Journal of Psychiatry* **152**, 310–319.

De Morsier, G. (1938) Les hallucinations. *Revue d'Oto'neuro-ophthalmologie* **16**, 241–252.

Feinberg, I. (1962) A comparison of the visual hallucinations in schizophrenia with those induced by mescaline and LSD-25. In: *Hallucinations* (ed. L.J. West), pp. 64–76. Grune & Stratton, New York.

Galdi, J. (1983) The causality of depression in schizophrenia. *British Journal of Psychiatry* **142**, 621–625.

Green, P. & Preston, M. (1981) Reinforcement of vocal correlates of auditory hallucinations by auditory feedback. *British Journal of Psychiatry* **139**, 204–208.

Griesinger, W. (1845) *Mental Pathology and Therapeutics.* New Sydenham Society, London. Translated (1867) from *Die Pathologie und Therapie der Psychischen Krankheiten.* Krabbe, Stuttgart.

Guggenheim, F.G. & Barbigian, H.M. (1974) Catatonic schizophrenia: epidemiology and clinical course. *Journal of Nervous and Mental Diseases* **158**, 291–305.

Guttmann, E. & Maclay, W.S. (1937) Clinical observations on schizophrenic drawings. *British Journal of Medical Psychology* **16**, 184–205.

Hare, E.H. (1973) A short note on pseudohallucinations. *British Journal of Psychiatry* **122**, 469–476.

Harrow, M., Grinker, R.R., Holzman, P.S. & Kayton, L. (1977) Anhedonia and schizophrenia. *American Journal of Psychiatry* **134**, 794–797.

Hirsch, S.R. (1982) Depression 'revealed' in schizophrenia. *British Journal of Psychiatry* **140**, 421–424.

Huber, G., Gross, G., Schuttler, R. & Linz, M. (1980) Longitudinal studies of schizophrenic patients. *Schizophrenia Bulletin* **6**, 592–605.

Izard, C.E. & Buechler, S. (1980) Aspects of consciousness and personality in terms of differential emotions theory. In: *Emotion; Theory, Research and Experience* (eds R. Plutchik & H. Kellerman), Vol. 1, pp. 165–187. Academic Press, New York.

Jaspers, K. (1913/1963) *General Psychopathology.* Manchester

University Press, Manchester. Translated by J. Hoenig & M.W. Hamilton from *Allgemeine Psychopathologie*. Springer Verlag, Berlin.

Johnson, J. (1984) Stupor and akinetic mutism. In: *Contemporary Neurology* (ed. M.J.G. Harrison), pp. 96–102. Butterworths, London.

Knights, A. & Hirsch, S.R. (1981) 'Revealed' depression and drug treatment of schizophrenia. *Archives of General Psychiatry* 38, 806–811.

Kraepelin, E. (1913/1919) *Psychiatrie*, 8th edn, Vol. 3, Part 2. Churchill Livingstone, Edinburgh. Translated by R.M. Barclay as *Dementia Praecox and Paraphrenia*.

Lhermitte, F., Pillon, B. & Serdaru, M. (1986) Human autonomy and the frontal lobes. I. Imitation and utilization behaviour, a neuropsychological study of 75 patients. *Annals of Neurology* 19, 326–334.

Liddle, P.F. (1987) Schizophrenic syndromes, cognitive performance and neurological dysfunction. *Psychological Medicine* 17, 49–57.

McCreadie, R.G. (1982) The Nithsdale schizophrenia survey. I. Psychiatric and social handicaps. *British Journal of Psychiatry* 140, 582–586.

McGhie, A. & Chapman, J. (1961) Disorders of attention and perception in early schizophrenia. *British Journal of Medical Psychology* 34, 103–115.

McGilchrist, I. & Cutting, J. (1995) Somatic delusions in schizophrenia and the affective psychoses. *British Journal of Psychiatry* 167, 350–361.

McGlashan, T.H. & Carpenter, W.T. (1976) Postpsychotic depression in schizophrenia. *Archives of General Psychiatry* 33, 231–239.

McKenna, P.J., Tamlyn, D., Lund, C.E. *et al.* (1990) Amnesic syndrome in schizophrenia. *Psychological Medicine* 20, 967–972.

Margo, A., Hemsley, D.R. & Slade, P.D. (1981) The effects of varying auditory input on schizophrenic hallucinations. *British Journal of Psychiatry* 139, 122–127.

Merleau-Ponty, M. (1962) *Phenomenology of Perception*. Routledge & Kegal Paul, London.

Morrison, J.R. (1973) Catatonia: retarded and excited types. *Archives of General Psychiatry* 28, 39–41.

Rappaport, S.R. & Webb, W.B. (1950) An attempt to study intellectual deterioration by premorbid and psychotic testing. *Journal of Consulting Psychology* 14, 95–98.

Rogers, D. (1985) The motor disorders of severe psychiatric illness: a conflict of paradigms. *British Journal of Psychiatry* 147, 221–232.

Rubert, S.L., Hollender, M.H. & Mehrhof, E.G. (1961) Olfactory hallucinations. *Archives of General Psychiatry* 5, 313–318.

Ryle, G. (1949) *The Concept of Mind*. Penguin, Harmondsworth.

Sass, L.A. (1992) *Madness and Modernism*. Basic Books, New York.

Schilder, P. (1920) On the development of thoughts. In: *Organisation and Pathology of Thought* (ed. D. Rappaport), pp. 497–518. Columbia University Press, New York. Translated by Rappaport, D. (1951).

Schmidt, G. (1940) A review of the German literature on delusion between 1914 and 1939. In: *The Clinical Roots of the Schizophrenia Concept* (eds J. Cutting & M. Shepherd), pp. 104–134. Cambridge University Press, Cambridge. Translated by H. Marshall (1987) from Der Wahn in deutschsprachigen Schriftum der letzten 24 Jahre (1914–1939). *Zentrulblatt für die gesamte Neurologie und Psychiatrie* 97, 113–143.

Schneider, K. (1958) *Clinical Psychopathology*. Translated by M.W. Hamilton (1959). Grune & Stratton, New York.

Schuck, J., Leventhal, D., Rothstein, H. & Irizarry, V. (1984) Physical anhedonia and schizophrenia. *Journal of Abnormal Psychology* 93, 342–344.

Spitzer, M. (1990) On defining delusions. *Comprehensive Psychiatry* 31, 377–397.

Spitzer, R.L., Endicott, J. & Robins, E. (1975) *Research Diagnostic Criteria*. New York State Psychiatric Institute, New York.

Starker, S. & Jolin, A. (1982) Imagery and hallucinations in schizophrenic patients. *Journal of Nervous and Mental Diseases* 170, 448–451.

Trapp, C.E. & James, E.B. (1937) Comparative intelligence ratings on the four types of dementia praecox. *Journal of Nervous and Mental Diseases* 86, 399–404.

Van den Bosch, R.J. (1982) *Attentional Correlates of Schizophrenia and Related Disorders*. Lisse, Swets & Zeitlinger.

Walker, C. (1991) Delusion: What did Jaspers really say? *British Journal of Psychiatry* 159, (Suppl. 14), 94–103.

Watson, C.G., Jacobs, L. & Kucala, T. (1979) A note on the pathology of anhedonia. *Journal of Clinical Psychology* 35, 740–743.

Wing, J.K., Cooper, J.E. & Sartorius, N. (1974) *Measurement and Classification of Psychiatric Symptoms*. Cambridge University Press, Cambridge.

Wittgenstein, L. (1980) *Remarks on the Philosophy of Psychology*. Basil Blackwell, Oxford.

World Health Organization (1973) *Report of the International Pilot Study of Schizophrenia*, Vol. 1. World Health Organization, Geneva.

3 | The symptoms of schizophrenia

R.L.M. Fuller, S.K. Schultz and N.C. Andreasen

Schizophrenia is characterized by a multiplicity of symptoms arising from almost all domains of mental function, e.g. language, emotion, reasoning, motor activity and perception. These symptoms vary between patients, creating very diverse symptom profiles. The symptoms can include experiencing false perceptions (hallucinations), having false beliefs of control or danger (delusions), expressing disorganized speech and behaviour (positive formal thought disorder, bizarre behaviour), having impaired goal-directed behaviour (avolition), exhibiting blunted affect, being unable to find pleasure in activities or in the company of others (anhedonia/asociality), poverty of speech and thought (alogia) and impaired attention. The symptoms are often divided into positive and negative. Positive symptoms reflect an excess or distortion of normal function (e.g. hallucinations and delusions), while negative symptoms reflect a diminution or loss of normal function (e.g. flattening of affect and poverty of speech). (See also Chapter 2.)

History of positive and negative symptoms

The nineteenth century English physicians John Russell Reynolds and John Hughlings Jackson first used the terms 'positive' and 'negative'. Reynolds (1858, 1861) discussed positive and negative symptoms within the context of epilepsy in a descriptive and theoretical way. Jackson (1931) suggested that they should be understood in terms of inhibitory processes. (The temporal relationship of these publications is misleading because Jackson was Reynolds' contemporary, but his works were published posthumously.)

> Disease is said to 'cause' the symptoms of insanity. I submit that disease only produces negative mental symptoms, answering to the dissolution, and that all elaborate positive mental symptoms (illusions, hallucinations, delusions, and extravagant conduct) are the outcome of activity of nervous elements untouched by any pathological process; that they arise during activity on the lower level of evolution remaining.

Jackson (1931) believed that the florid positive symptoms were a release phenomenon, occurring when underlying brain processes become disinhibited as a result of a pathological insult to a higher level of brain functioning, while negative symptoms represented a more generalized loss of functions.

While many of the pioneers of psychiatric phenomenology recognized the importance of negative symptoms, they did not use this term. For example, Emil Kraepelin wrote extensively about avolition and affective flattening as central and defining features of 'dementia praecox'.

> There are apparently two principal groups of disorders that characterize the malady. On the one hand we observe a weakening of those emotional activities which permanently form the mainsprings of volition. . . . Mental activity and instinct for occupation become mute. The result of this highly morbid process is emotional dullness, failure of mental activities, loss of mastery over volition, of endeavour, and ability for independent action. . . . The second group of disorders consists in the *loss of the inner unity* of activities of intellect, emotion, and volition in themselves and among one another. . . . The near connection between thinking and feeling, between deliberation and emotional activity on the one hand, and practical work on the other is more or less lost. Emotions do not correspond to ideas. The patient laughs and weeps without recognizable cause, without any relation to their circumstances and their experiences, smile as they narrate a tale of their attempted suicide. (Kraepelin 1919, pp. 74–75)

Eugen Bleuler (1911/1950) spoke of the 'group of schizophrenias', but argued that a single defining feature was present in all people suffering from the illness. This feature, a disturbance in the ability to formulate coherent thought and language (often referred to as 'thought disorder' or 'loose associations'), was the most important of the 'fundamental symptoms'. Bleuler considered these 'fundamental symptoms' to be present in all patients: loss of continuity of associations, loss of affective responsiveness, loss of attention, loss of volition, ambivalence and autism. Bleuler held that these symptoms reflect underlying abnormalities in basic cognitive and emotive processes, while he relegated hallucinations and delusions to the status of 'accessory' or secondary symptoms.

Certain symptoms of schizophrenia are present in every case and in every period of the illness even though, as with every other disease symptom, they must have attained a certain degree of intensity before they can be recognized with any certainty. . . . Besides the specific permanent or fundamental symptoms, we can find a host of other, more accessory manifestations such as delusions, hallucinations, or catatonic symptoms. . . . As far as we know, the fundamental symptoms are characteristic of schizophrenia, while the accessory symptoms may also appear in other types of illness. (Bleuler 1911/1950, p. 13)

Kurt Schneider (1959) changed the focus of schizophrenia symptomatology with his assertion that the fundamental symptoms of schizophrenia reflect an inability to define the boundaries between self and non-self, resulting in experiences such as voices conversing or commenting, delusions of control or passivity, and thought withdrawal or insertion. He posited that these easily identifiable florid positive symptoms, which he called 'first rank symptoms', were the defining characteristics of schizophrenia (Schneider 1959). The clinical definition of schizophrenia shifted at this point to an emphasis on these positive or Schneiderian first-rank symptoms. A series of diagnostic tools were developed, such as the Present State Examination (Wing 1970), the Schedule for Affective Disorders and Schizophrenia (Endicott & Spitzer 1978), Research Diagnostic Criteria (Spitzer et al. 1978) and the DSM-III (American Psychiatric Association 1980), which defined schizophrenia according to a narrow band of positive symptoms.

However, clinical realties relatively quickly led to a corrective return to Bleulerian and Kraepelinian ideas, reintroduced as an emphasis on the importance of negative symptoms as central to the concept of schizophrenia. With this realization came three types of explanatory models attempting to account for the heterogeneity of the symptom profile in schizophrenia. These models include categorical, dimensional and unitary approaches to schizophrenia. Each model will be described in detail below.

Models of schizophrenia

Categorical models

Interest in negative symptoms re-emerged in the 1970s, as exemplified by Strauss and Carpenter (1974) and Andreasen (1979a,b,c). The turning point came perhaps from the works of Crow who, in 1980, proposed a new typology for schizophrenia, which integrated clinical presentation, pathophysiology and treatment response in a single model (Crow 1980; Crow et al. 1981). Patients with type I schizophrenia presented clinically with positive symptoms such as delusions and hallucinations; Crow posited that the underlying pathophysiological mechanism for this subtype was a biochemical imbalance, such as an excess of dopamine D_2 receptors. Therefore, he hypothe-

sized that the resulting clinical manifestations would be more likely to respond favourably to antipsychotic medication, to be characterized by exacerbations and remissions, and to have a more favourable outcome. Conversely, patients with type II schizophrenia, presenting with symptoms such as affective flattening and poverty of speech, were said to be manifestating an underlying structural/anatomical abnormality reflected by ventricular enlargement and cortical atrophy in neuroimaging studies. These symptoms therefore would tend to be poorly responsive to somatic treatment, follow a chronic course, and predict poor outcome.

Crow's original model did not specify which of the various descriptors of type I vs. type II should be used in studies designed to disconfirm or verify the hypothesized dichotomy; that is, clinical presentation, pathophysiology or treatment response. Therefore the model was difficult to test. Andreasen developed two detailed standardized rating scales, the Scale for the Assessment of Negative Symptoms (SANS) (Andreasen 1983) and the Scale for the Assessment of Positive Symptoms (SAPS) (Andreasen 1984), for reliably assessing symptoms and exploring other aspects of the relationships between positive symptoms, negative symptoms and cognitive, psychosocial and neurobiological correlates of schizophrenia. One result from validation studies of these scales was Andreasen's proposal of three subtypes of patients with schizophrenia: negative, positive and mixed (Andreasen & Olsen 1982). Both Crow (1980) and Andreasen et al. (1982) proposed that the negative symptoms of schizophrenia were indicators of a single 'subtype'.

Dividing patients into mutually exclusive subgroups is firmly rooted in the 'disease model' in medicine. Symptomatology is the measure used to identify a category, and at this point the categories are referred to as 'syndromes' (literally, a running together), because they constitute an identifiable clinical pattern that makes sense in the context of observed relationships of the symptoms. Once a specific pathophysiology or aetiology is identified, syndromes are elevated to the status of recognized diseases. In the 'categorical approach' it is assumed that the subtypes identified will differ from one another (and that this will eventually be discovered and documented) in terms of their pathophysiological mechanisms or aetiology, which may be reflected in differing responses to treatment, course of morbidity and underlying neurobiology.

The typology of schizophrenia proposed by Crow was inherently categorical, with subjects classified as either type I or II. The expansion of this conceptualization by Andreasen to include a mixed type was also categorical. The research produced from the categorical approach was prolific throughout the 1980s, but eventually the need for a new type of explanatory model arose. Dividing patients into mutually exclusive groups based on positive and negative symptoms was eventually abandoned, for several reasons. First, most patients were of a 'mixed' subtype, and many fewer were purely 'positive' or 'negative' (Andreasen 1985). Secondly, longitudinal studies revealed that the symptoms of patients varied over time (Breier et al. 1987; Marneros et al. 1991).

One of the most difficult problems in the investigation and assessment of negative symptoms in schizophrenia involves the recognition that their measurement may be confounded by a variety of other factors. The four most commonly implicated factors are:

1 neuroleptic side-effects, such as akinesia;
2 depression, which has been reported to be present in schizophrenia in the early course of the illness (Knights & Hirsch 1981; Wassink *et al.* 1999), not to decrease in severity as the psychotic symptoms abate with medication (Knights & Hirsch 1981) and to be frequent during the residual phase (Siris 1991);
3 a response to positive symptoms, for example avoiding social interactions because of paranoia; and
4 environmental understimulation resulting from chronic institutionalization (Carpenter *et al.* 1985).

Carpenter and his group have been most active in their attempts to disentangle 'primary' and 'secondary' negative symptoms (Carpenter & Kirkpatrick 1988). Carpenter defines primary, or 'deficit', symptoms as enduring core-negative symptoms of schizophrenia such as anhedonia and blunted affect. The secondary symptoms, however, are those negative symptoms that may be considered consequential to other symptoms or treatment of schizophrenia. Carpenter's deficit symptoms include flattened affect, anhedonia, poverty of speech, curbing of interest and decrease in curiosity, lack of sense of purpose and diminished social drive. By definition, these symptoms must not be fully accounted for by depression, anxiety, medication effects or environmental deprivation. The non-deficit syndrome is defined by an absence of these deficit symptoms with the presence of any other schizophrenia symptoms, such as disorganized thought or hallucinations.

Dimensional models

A more recent strategy for addressing the heterogeneity of the phenotype in schizophrenia is the dimensional approach. While 'categories' traditionally arise from disease models, 'dimensions' are often derived from the study of normal psychology; therefore, students of dimensional approaches have shown less concern about identifying brain–behaviour relationships. Dimensions define groups of symptoms that co-occur, but the co-occurrence is noted through statistical techniques such as factor analysis. While categories classify individuals, dimensions classify symptoms. Therefore, dimensions can overlap within a given individual and be additive.

Bilder *et al.* (1985) identified three distinct clusters of symptoms using correlative analysis of symptom ratings and neuropsychological data, providing the first validating evidence for the distinction between symptom dimensions.

1 The disorganization cluster included alogia, attentional impairment, positive formal thought disorder and bizarre behaviour.
2 The blunted affect and volition cluster included affective flattening, avolition/apathy and anhedonia.

3 The florid psychotic cluster included delusions, hallucinations and 'breadth of psychosis'.

Impaired neuropsychological performance was strongly association with the disorganized symptoms and, to a lesser extent, was associated with the blunted affect symptoms but was not associated with the psychotic symptoms. Andreasen and Grove (1986) replicated this finding in the second study, validating this distinction of three symptom dimensions, and subsequently many others have had similar findings (Kulhara *et al.* 1986; Liddle 1987a,b; Arndt *et al.* 1991; Gur *et al.* 1991; Brown & White 1992; Minas *et al.* 1992; Miller *et al.* 1993). Arndt *et al.* (1995) found that the negative symptoms, unlike the psychotic or disorganized symptoms, are stable over time. Liddle (1987b) used factor analysis to examine the relationship between symptoms in a group of patients with schizophrenia and began using the often cited dimension names of 'disorganization', 'psychomotor poverty' and 'reality distortion'. He also provided further validating evidence for these dimensions with imaging data (Liddle *et al.* 1992; see Chapter 22 for further discussion).

Later studies have further validated the finding that the negative and disorganized dimensions are associated with impairments in cognitive functioning (Liddle 1987a,b; Liddle & Morris 1991). O'Leary *et al.* (2000) further specified the nature of the impairment by investigating a large sample (134) of patients with schizophrenia. Negative symptoms were related to generalized brain dysfunction, the disorganized symptoms were related to verbal processing abnormalities and the psychotic symptoms showed no relationship to cognitive impairment.

One potential drawback of the dimensional approach is its disregard for the boundaries of the classical disease model which searches for the underlying construct of an illness. A comparable approach would be to search for the principal basis of a feature existing both in schizophrenia and other diseases, e.g. hallucinations, as they are found in schizophrenia, mania and epilepsy. The consequence of many investigations has been to treat dimensions as categories, resulting in attempts to localize specific symptoms.

Unitary models

A newer alternative, the unitary model, draws from the tradition of Bleuler (1911/1950), who attempted to identify what he considered to be the single fundamental abnormality in schizophrenia. Bleuler defined the fundamental symptoms of schizophrenia as those caused by a 'loosening of associations', which were present in all patients, tended to occur only in schizophrenia and therefore were pathognomonic of the illness. Thus, the unitary model stresses that there is a single unifying construct which explains the heterogeneity of the phenotype of schizophrenia. This model proposes that schizophrenia has one fundamental problem in a basic cognitive process.

One recent unitary model suggests that the fundamental deficit is a disruption of the fluid co-ordination of mental activity, called 'cognitive dysmetria' (Andreasen *et al.* 1996, 1998, 1999; Andreasen 1997, 1999). Synchrony refers to the normal

Neuropsychology and cognitive impairment

There have been reports of cognitive impairment in schizophrenia since the illness was first described by Kraepelin (1919) and Bleuler (1911/1950). A remarkably consistent pattern emerges; cognitive impairment is associated with negative (Andreasen & Olsen 1982; Cornblatt *et al.* 1985; Gaebel *et al.* 1987; Keilp *et al.* 1988; Braff 1989; Andreasen *et al.* 1990; Merriam *et al.* 1990) and disorganized symptoms (Bilder *et al.* 1985; Frith *et al.* 1991), but is not associated with psychotic symptoms (Bilder *et al.* 1985; Cuesta & Peralta 1995; O'Leary *et al.* 2000). Further validating evidence exists. Negative symptoms have been found to be associated with impaired conceptual thinking, object naming and long-term memory (Liddle 1987a,b), a slowing of mental activity (Liddle & Morris 1991) and poor performance on tests of verbal learning and memory, verbal fluency, visual memory and visual–motor sequencing (O'Leary *et al.* 2000). Disorganized symptoms are associated with poor performance on tests of concentration, immediate recall and list learning (Liddle 1987a,b), an inability to inhibit inappropriate responses (Liddle & Morris 1991), lower verbal IQ and poor concept attainment (see Chapter 10; O'Leary *et al.* 2000).

Genetic studies

It has been recognized for many decades that schizophrenia aggregates among relatives of schizophrenic patients to a greater degree than in the general population. However, very little information exists on the correlation of genetics and the symptoms of schizophrenia. It has been proposed that the negative dimension of schizophrenia may represent a genetic subtype of the illness. In support of this hypothesis, some studies (Kay *et al.* 1986; McGuffin & Owen 1991), but not all (Pearlson *et al.* 1985; Alda *et al.* 1991), showed that first-degree relatives of patients with schizophrenia and high levels of negative symptoms have a higher morbid risk than the relatives of patients with schizophrenia and predominantly positive symptoms. Patients with a family history of schizophrenia are reported to have more treatment-resistant negative symptoms, which are related to poor psychosocial functioning, than those patients with no family history (Malaspina *et al.* 2000). Moreover, a reanalysis of previously published twin studies showed that negative symptoms in one twin predicts a higher concordance rate (Dworkin *et al.* 1988).

Kendler *et al.* (2000) attempted to provide evidence for linkage between families with schizophrenia-related disorders and chromosomal regions based on major symptoms of the illness. They found that families with positive evidence for linkage on the genomic region 8p (D8S283–D8S552) were likely to include probands with symptom profiles of thought disorder, affective deterioration, chronic course, poor outcome and minimal depressive symptoms.

Population-based association studies typically use the psychiatric diagnosis, i.e. the symptoms, as the phenotypic expression of illness. However, it is possible to use biological traits correlated with the illness as other indicators of phenotypic expression. For example, a specific pathological indicator such as the p50 auditory sensory gating deficit in schizophrenia may be used to identify susceptibility loci (Freedman 1998). Other examples include impaired prepulse inhibition, impaired habituation to the startle reflex, as well as eye-tracking and eye-blinking abnormalities. Such approaches may identify useful phenotypes for schizophrenia that are not based solely on diagnostic categories. Strategies like these are continuing to evolve at a rapid pace, each offering the potential for new insights into the genetic factors involved in the expression of schizophrenia (see Chapters 14 and 15).

Response to treatment

Medication is effective in reducing both positive and, to some extent, negative symptoms, but this is covered in detail in other chapters (see Chapters 8, 10 and 24–26).

Conclusions

The last two or three decades have been a rich era for the conceptualization and study of the role of symptoms in schizophrenia. The concepts of symptom dimensions have been carefully investigated, providing knowledge of cognitive impairment, structural and functional neuroanatomy and genetic bases for schizophrenia. The new horizon involves investigating the construct of an underlying cognitive dysfunction (e.g. cognitive dysmetria, working memory, a disturbance in consciousness, impaired information processing) that contributes to all the symptoms, both positive and negative.

References

Addington, J. & Addington, D. (1991) Positive and negative symptoms of schizophrenia: their course and relationship over time. *Schizophrenia Research* 5, 51–59.

Alda, M., Zvolsky, P. & Dvorakova, M. (1991) Study of chronic schizophrenics with positive and negative family histories of psychosis. *Acta Psychiatrica Scandinavica* 83, 334–337.

American Psychiatric Association (1980) *Diagnostic and Statistical Manual of Mental Disorders (DSM-III)*, 3rd edn. American Psychiatric Association, Washington DC.

Andreasen, N.C. (1979a) Affective flattening and the criteria for schizophrenia. *American Journal of Psychiatry* **136**, 944–947.

Andreasen, N.C. (1979b) Thought, language, and communication disorders. I. Clinical assessment, definition of terms, and evaluation of their reliability. *Archives of General Psychiatry* 36, 1315–1321.

Andreasen, N.C. (1979c) Thought, language, and communication disorders. II. Diagnostic significance. *Archives of General Psychiatry* 36, 1325–1330.

Andreasen, N.C. (1983) *The Scale for the Assessment of Negative Symptoms (SANS)*. University of Iowa, Iowa City, IA.

Andreasen, N.C. (1984) *The Scale for the Assessment of Positive Symptoms (SAPS)*. University of Iowa, Iowa City, IA.

Andreasen, N.C. (1985) Positive vs. negative schizophrenia: a critical evaluation. *Schizophrenia Bulletin* **11**, 380–389.

Andreasen, N.C. (1997) Linking mind and brain in the study of mental illnesses: a project for a scientific psychopathology. *Science* **275**, 1586–1593.

Andreasen, N.C. (1999) A unitary model of schizophrenia: Bleuler's 'fragmented phrene' as schizencephaly. *Archives of General Psychiatry* **56**, 781–787.

Andreasen, N.C. & Grove, W.M. (1986) Evaluation of positive and negative symptoms in schizophrenia. *Psychiatrie and Psychobiologie* **1**, 108–121.

Andreasen, N.C. & Olsen, S. (1982) Negative versus positive schizophrenia: definition and validation. *Archives of General Psychiatry* **39**, 789–794.

Andreasen, N.C., Olsen, S.A., Smith, M.R., Dennert, J.W. & Smith, M.R. (1982) Ventricular enlargement in schizophrenia: definition and prevalence. *American Journal of Psychiatry* **139**, 297–302.

Andreasen, N.C., Ehrhardt, J.C., Swayze, V.W. II *et al.* (1990) Magnetic resonance imaging of the brain in schizophrenia: the pathophysiologic significance of structural abnormalities. *Archives of General Psychiatry* **47**, 35–44.

Andreasen, N.C., Flaum, M., Arndt, S. *et al.* (1991) Positive and negative symptoms: assessment and validity. *Negative Versus Positive Schizophrenia* (eds A. Marneros, N.C. Andreasen & M.T. Tsuang), pp. 28–51. Springer-Verlag Berlin, Heidelberg.

Andreasen, N.C., Rezai, K., Alliger, R. *et al.* (1992) Hypofrontality in neuroleptic-naive and in patients with chronic schizophrenia: assessment with xenon-133 single-photon emission computed tomography and the Tower of London. *Archives of General Psychiatry* **49**, 943–958.

Andreasen, N.C., Flashman, L., Flaum, M. *et al.* (1994) Regional brain abnormalities in schizophrenia measured with magnetic resonance imaging. *Journal of the American Medical Association* **272**, 1763–1769.

Andreasen, N.C., O'Leary, D.S., Cizadlo, T. *et al.* (1996) Schizophrenia and cognitive dysmetria: a positron-emission tomography study of dysfunctional prefrontal–thalamic–cerebellar circuitry. *Procedures of the National Academy of Sciences of the USA* **93**, 9985–9990.

Andreasen, N.C., Paradiso, S. & O'Leary, D.S. (1998) 'Cognitive dysmetria' as an integrative theory of schizophrenia: a dysfunction in cortical–subcortical–cerebellar circuitry? *Schizophrenia Bulletin* **24** (2), 203–218.

Andreasen, N.C., Nopoulos, P., O'Leary, D.S. *et al.* (1999) Defining the phenotype of schizophrenia: cognitive dysmetria and its neural mechanisms. *Biological Psychiatry* **46**, 908–920.

Arndt, S., Alliger, R.J. & Andreasen, N.C. (1991) The distinction of positive and negative symptoms: the failure of a two-dimensional model. *British Journal of Psychiatry* **158**, 317–322.

Arndt, S., Andreasen, N.C., Flaum, M., Miller, D. & Nopoulos, P. (1995) A longitudinal study of symptom dimensions in schizophrenia: prediction and patterns of change. *Archives of General Psychiatry* **52** (5), 352–360.

Barnes, T.R., Hutton, S.B., Chapman, M.J. *et al.* (2000) West London first-episode study of schizophrenia: clinical correlates of duration of untreated psychosis. *British Journal of Psychiatry* **177** (3), 207–211.

Barta, P.E., Pearlson, G.D. & Powers, R.E. (1990) Auditory hallucinations and smaller superior temporal gyrus volume in schizophrenia. *American Journal of Psychiatry* **147**, 1457–1462.

Barta, P.E., Powers, R.E., Aylward, E.H. *et al.* (1997) Quantitative MRI volume changes in late onset schizophrenia and Alzheimer's disease compared to normal controls. *Psychiatry Research* **68**, 65–75.

Biehl, H., Maurer, K. & Schubart, C. (1986) Prediction of outcome and utilization of medical services in a prospective study of first onset schizophrenics: results of a prospective 5-year follow-up study. *European Archives of Psychiatry and Neurological Sciences* **236**, 139–147.

Bilder, R.M., Mukherjee, S. & Rieder, R.O. (1985) Symptomatic and neuropsychological components of defect states. *Schizophrenia Bulletin* **11**, 409–491.

Bleuler, E. (1911/1950) *Dementia Praecox or the Group of Schizophrenias*. Translated by J. Zinkin. International Universities Press, New York.

Braff, D.L. (1989) Sensory input deficits and negative symptoms in schizophrenic patients. *American Journal of Psychiatry* **146**, 1006–1011.

Braff, D.L. (1993) Information processing and attention dysfunctions in schizophrenia. *Schizophrenia Bulletin* **19**, 233–259.

Breier, A., Wolkowitz, O.M., Doran, A.R. *et al.* (1987) Neuroleptic responsivity of negative and positive symptoms in schizophrenia. *American Journal of Psychiatry* **144** (12), 1549–1555.

Breier, A., Schreiber, J. & Dyer, J. (1991) National Institute of Mental Health longitudinal study of chronic schizophrenia: prognosis and predictors of outcome. *Archives of General Psychiatry* **48**, 239–246.

Brown, K. & White, T. (1992) Syndromes of chronic schizophrenia and some clinical correlates. *British Journal of Psychiatry* **161**, 317–322.

Buchsbaum, M.S., Yang, S., Hazlett, E. *et al.* (1997) Ventricular volume and asymmetry in schizotypal personality disorder and schizophrenia assessed with magnetic resonance imaging. *Schizophrenia Research* **27**, 45–53.

Carpenter, W.T. & Kirkpatrick, B. (1988) The heterogeneity of the long-term course of schizophrenia. *Schizophrenia Bulletin* **14**, 645–659.

Carpenter, W.T., Strauss, J.S. & Bartko, J.J. (1985) On the heterogeneity of schizophrenia. In: *Controversies in Schizophrenia* (ed. M. Alpert), pp. 25–37. Guildford Press, New York.

Cohen, M.B., Lake, R.R., Graham, L.S. *et al.* (1989) Quantitative iodine-123 IMP imaging of brain perfusion in schizophrenia. *Journal of Nuclear Medicine* **30** (10), 1616–1620.

Cornblatt, B.A., Lenzenweger, M.F. & Dworkin, R.H. (1985) Positive and negative schizophrenic symptoms: attention and information processing. *Schizophrenia Bulletin* **11**, 397–407.

Craig, T.J., Bromet Fennig, E.J., Tanenberg-Karant, S., Lavelle, M. & Galambos, J. (2000) Is there an association between duration of untreated psychosis and 24-month clinical outcome in a first-admission series? *American Journal of Psychiatry* **157**, 60–66.

Crow, T.J. (1980) Molecular pathology of schizophrenia: more than one disease process? *British Medical Journal* **280**, 66–68.

Crow, T.J., Corsellis, J.A.N., Cross, A.J. *et al.* (1981) The search for changes underlying the type II syndrome. In: *Biological Psychiatry* (eds C. Perris, G. Struwe & B. Jansson), pp. 727–731. Elsevier North-Holland Biomedical Press, Amsterdam,

Cuesta, M. & Peralta, V. (1995) Cognitive disorders in the positive, negative and disordered syndromes of schizophrenia. *Psychiatry Research* **58**, 227–235.

Dewan, M.J., Pandurangi, A.K., Lee, S.H. *et al.* (1983) Central brain morphology in chronic schizophrenic patients: a controlled CT study. *Biological Psychiatry* **18** (10), 1133–1140.

Dworkin, R.H., Lenzenweger, M.F. & Moldin, S.O. (1988) A multidimensional approach to the genetics of schizophrenia. *American Journal of Psychiatry* **145**, 1077–1083.

Endicott, J. & Spitzer, R.L. (1978) A diagnostic interview: the Schedule for Affective Disorders and Schizophrenia (SADS). *Archives of General Psychiatry* **35**, 837–844.

Developmental maturation can also affect the localization of hallucinations in space. Internal localization of hallucinations is more common in younger children and makes these experiences more difficult to differentiate subjectively from inner speech or thoughts (Garralda 1984). Formal thought disorder may also appear very similar to the pattern of illogical thinking and loose associations seen in children with immature language development. Negative symptoms can appear very similar to non-psychotic language and social impairments and can also be easily confused with anhedonia and depression.

Differential diagnosis

Psychotic symptoms in children and adolescents are diagnostically non-specific, occurring in a wide range of functional psychiatric, neurodevelopmental and organic brain disorders. The differential diagnosis of schizophrenia in childhood and adolescence is summarized in Table 4.1. A summary of physical investigations in children and adolescents with suspected schizophrenia is listed in Table 4.2.

Affective, schizoaffective and 'atypical' psychoses

The high rate of positive psychotic symptoms found in adolescent onset major depression and mania can lead to diagnostic confusion (Joyce 1984). Affective psychoses are most likely to be misdiagnosed as schizophrenia if a rigid Schneiderian concept of schizophrenia is applied with its emphasis on first-rank symptoms. Because significant affective symptoms also occur in about one-third of first-episode patients with schizophrenia, it may be impossible to make a definitive diagnosis on the basis of a single cross-sectional assessment. In DSM-IV the distinction between schizophrenia, schizoaffective disorder and affective psychoses is determined by the relative predominance and temporal overlap of psychotic symptoms (hallucinations and delusions) and affective symptoms (elevated or depressed mood). Given the difficulty in applying these rules

with any precision, there is a need to identify other features to distinguish between schizophrenia and affective psychoses. Irrespective of the presence of affective symptoms, the most discriminating symptoms of schizophrenia are an insidious onset and the presence of negative symptoms (Hollis 1999). Similarly, complete remission from a first psychotic episode within 6 months of onset is the best predictor of a diagnosis of affective psychosis (Hollis 1999). Schizoaffective and atypical psychoses are unsatisfactory diagnostic categories with low predictive validity and little longitudinal stability (Hollis 2000).

Autistic spectrum and developmental language disorders

Kolvin (1971), in a landmark study, clearly distinguished the symptoms and correlates of core autism with onset before age 3 from adult-type schizophrenia beginning in late childhood and early adolescence. However, some children on the autistic spectrum (usually with atypical autism or Asperger syndrome) have social and cognitive impairments that overlap closely with the premorbid phenotype described in schizophrenia. Furthermore, children on the autistic spectrum may also develop psychotic symptoms in adolescence (Volkmar & Cohen 1991). Towbin et al. (1993) have labelled another group of children who seem to belong within the autistic spectrum as having 'multiplex developmental disorder'. An increased risk for psychosis has also been noted in developmental language disorders (Rutter & Mawhood 1991). While some children on the autistic spectrum can show a clear progression into classic schizophrenia, others show a more episodic pattern of psychotic symptoms without the progressive decline in social functioning and negative symptoms characteristic of child and adolescent onset schizophrenia.

Often it is only possible to distinguish between schizophrenia and disorders on the autistic spectrum by taking a careful developmental history that details the age of onset and pattern of autistic impairments in communication, social reciprocity and interests/behaviours. According to DSM-IV, schizophrenia

Table 4.2 Physical investigations in child and adolescent onset psychoses.

Investigation	Target disorder
Urine drug screen	Drug-related psychosis (amphetamines, ecstasy, cocaine, LSD and other psychoactive compounds)
EEG	Complex partial seizures/TLE
MRI brain scan	Ventricular enlargement, structural brain anomalies (e.g. cavum septum pellucidum)
	Enlarged caudate (typical antipsychotics)
	Demyelination (metachromatic leucodystrophy)
	Hypodense basal ganglia (Wilson's disease)
Serum copper and caeruloplasmin	Wilson's disease
Urinary copper	
Arylsulphatase A (white blood cell)	Metachromatic leucodystrophy
Karyotype/cytogenetics (FISH)	Sex chromosome aneuploidies, velocardiofacial syndrome (22q11 microdeletion)

FISH, fluorescence in situ hybridization; MRI, magnetic resonance imaging; TLE, temporal lobe apilepsy.

cannot be diagnosed in a child with autism/pervasive developmental disorder (PDD) unless hallucinations/delusions are present for at least 1 month. DSM-IV does not rank the active phase symptoms of thought disorder, disorganization or negative symptoms as sufficient to make a diagnosis of schizophrenia in the presence of autism. In contrast, ICD-10 does not include evidence of autism/PDD as an exclusion criteria for the diagnosis of schizophrenia.

'Multidimensionally impaired syndrome' and schizotypal personality disorder

'Multidimensionally impaired syndrome' (MDI) is a term coined to describe children who have brief transient psychotic symptoms, emotional lability, poor interpersonal skills, normal social skills and multiple deficits in information processing (Gordon et al. 1994). The diagnostic status of this group remains to be resolved. Short-term follow-up suggests that they do not develop full-blown schizophrenic psychosis. However, they have an increased risk of schizophrenia-spectrum disorders among first-degree relatives and the neurobiological findings (e.g. brain morphology) are similar to those in childhood onset schizophrenia (Kumra et al. 1998c). This group may possibly represent a genetically high-risk phenotype for schizophrenia rather than a prodromal state.

Children with schizotypal personality disorder (SPD) lie on a phenotypic continuum with schizophrenia and have similar cognitive and social impairments and are prone to magical thinking, mood disturbances and non-psychotic perceptual disturbances. Distinction from the prodromal phase of schizophrenia is particularly difficult when there is a history of social and academic decline without clear-cut or persisting psychotic symptoms. It has been reported that negative symptoms and attention in SPD improve with a low dose of risperidone (0.25–2.0 mg) (Rossi et al. 1997).

Epilepsy

Psychotic symptoms can occur in temporal and frontal lobe partial seizures. A careful history is usually sufficient to reveal an aura followed by clouding of consciousness and the sudden onset of brief ictal psychotic phenomena often accompanied by anxiety, fear, derealization or depersonalization. However, longer lasting psychoses associated with epilepsy can occur in clear consciousness during postictal or interictal periods (Sachdev 1998). In epileptic psychoses, hallucinations, disorganized behaviour and persecutory delusions predominate, while negative symptoms are rare. Children with complex partial seizures also have increased illogical thinking and use fewer linguistic-cohesive devices which can resemble formal thought disorder (Caplan et al. 1992). A positron emission tomography (PET) study has shown hypoperfusion in the frontal, temporal and basal ganglia in psychotic patients with epilepsy compared with non-psychotic epileptic patients (Gallhofer et al. 1985).

Epilepsy and schizophrenia may co-occur in the same individual, so that the diagnoses are not mutually exclusive. The onset of epilepsy almost always precedes psychosis unless seizures are secondary to antipsychotic medication. In a long-term follow-up of 100 children with temporal lobe epilepsy, 10% developed schizophrenia in adult life (Lindsay et al. 1979).

An EEG should be performed if a seizure disorder is considered in the differential diagnosis or arises as a side-effect of antipsychotic treatment. Ambulatory EEG monitoring and telemetry with event recording may be required if the diagnosis remains in doubt.

Neurodegenerative disorders

Rare neurodegenerative disorders occurring in late childhood and adolescence can mimic schizophrenia. The most important examples are Wilson's disease (hepatolenticular degeneration) and metachromatic leucodystrophy. These disorders usually involve significant extrapyramidal symptoms (e.g. tremor, dystonia and bradykinesia) or other motor abnormalities (e.g. unsteady gait) and a progressive loss of skills (dementia) that can aid the distinction from schizophrenia. Suspicion of a neurodegenerative disorder is one of the clearest indications for brain magnetic resonance imaging (MRI) in child and adolescent onset psychoses. Children and adolescents with schizophrenia show relative grey matter reduction with white matter sparing. In contrast, metachromatic leucodystrophy is characterized by frontal and occipital white matter destruction and demyelination. In Wilson's disease hypodense areas are seen in the basal ganglia, together with cortical atrophy and ventricular dilatation. The pathognomonic Kayser–Fleischer ring in Wilson's disease begins as a greenish-brown crescent-shaped deposit in the cornea above the pupil (this is most easily seen during slit lamp examination). In Wilson's disease there is increased urinary copper excretion, and reduced serum copper and serum caeruloplasmin levels. The biochemical marker for metachromatic leucodystrophy is reduced arylsulphatase-A (ASA) activity in white blood cells. This enzyme deficiency results in a deposition of excess sulphatides in many tissues including the central nervous system.

Drug psychoses

Recreational drug use is increasingly common among young people, so the co-occurrence of drug use and psychosis is to be expected. What is less certain is the nature of any causal connection. Psychotic symptoms can occur as a direct pharmacological effect of intoxication with stimulants (amphetamines, ecstasy and cocaine), hallucinogens (lysergic acid diethylamide 'LSD', psilocybin 'magic mushrooms' and mescaline) and cannabis (Poole & Brabbins 1996). The psychotic symptoms associated with drug intoxication are usually short-lived and resolve within a few days of abstinence from the drug. These drugs can have surprisingly long half-lives, with cannaboids still measurable up to 6 weeks after a single dose. Psychotic symptoms in the form of 'flashbacks' can also occur after cessation from chronic cannabis and LSD abuse. These phenomena are similar to alcoholic hallucinosis and typically involve transient vivid auditory hallucinations occurring in clear consciousness.

It is often assumed that there is a simple causal relationship between drug use and psychosis, with any evidence of drug use excluding the diagnosis of a functional psychosis. However, drug use can also be a consequence of psychosis with patients using drugs to 'treat' their symptoms in the early stages of a psychotic relapse. Overall, there is very little evidence to invoke a separate entity of 'drug-induced' psychosis in cases where psychotic symptoms arise during intoxication but then persist after the drug is withdrawn (Poole & Brabbins 1996). Patients whose so-called 'drug-induced' psychoses last for more than 6 months appear to have more clear-cut schizophrenic symptoms, a greater familial risk for psychosis and greater premorbid dysfunction (Tsuang et al. 1982). DSM-IV takes the sensible position that a functional psychosis should not be excluded unless there is compelling evidence that symptoms are entirely a result of drug use.

Other investigations

Whether any physical investigations should be viewed as 'routine' is debatable. However, it is usual to obtain a full blood count and biochemistry including liver and thyroid function and a drug screen (urine or hair analysis). The high yield of cytogenetic abnormalities reported in childhood onset schizophrenia (Kumra et al. 1998d; Nicholson et al. 1999) suggests the value of cytogenetic testing including karyotyping for sex chromosome aneuploidies and fluorescent in situ hybridization (FISH) for chromosome 22q11 deletions (velocardiofacial syndrome). The evidence of progressive structural brain changes (Rapoport et al. 1999) indicates the value of obtaining a baseline and annual follow-up brain MRI scans, although this is not a diagnostic test.

Epidemiology

Incidence and prevalence

Good population-based incidence figures for child and adolescent onset schizophrenia are notably lacking. What data do exist describe broader categories of psychosis, with diagnoses made without the benefit of standardized assessments. Gillberg et al. (1986) calculated age-specific prevalence for all psychoses (including schizophrenia, schizophreniform, affective psychosis, atypical psychosis and drug psychoses) in the age range 13–18 years using case-register data from Goteborg, Sweden. Of the cases, 41% had a diagnosis of schizophrenia. At age 13 years, the prevalence for all psychoses was 0.9/10 000, showing a steady increase during adolescence and reaching a prevalence of 17.6/10 000 at age 18 years.

Sex ratio

Males are over-represented in many clinical studies of childhood onset schizophrenia (Russell et al. 1989; Green et al. 1992; Russell 1994; Spencer & Campbell 1994). However, other studies of predominantly adolescent onset schizophrenia have described an equal sex ratio (Gordon et al. 1994; Werry et al. 1994; Hollis 2000). The interpretation of these studies is complicated by the possibility of referral biases to clinical centres. In an epidemiological study of first admissions for schizophrenia and paranoia in children and adolescents there was an equal sex ratio for patients under the age of 15 (Galdos et al. 1993; Lewine 1994). The finding of an equal sex distribution with adolescent onset is intriguing as it differs from the consistent male predominance (ratio 2:1) reported in incident samples of early adult onset schizophrenia (Castle & Murray 1991). Clearly, future studies require population-based incident samples free from potential referral biases.

Aetiology and risk factors

Pregnancy and birth complications

Pregnancy and birth complications (PBCs) have been implicated as a risk factor in schizophrenia (see Chapter 13). In a meta-analysis of 20 case–control studies, subjects who developed schizophrenia were more than twice as likely to have been exposed to PBCs as controls (Geddes & Lawrie 1995). However, the findings from two other large case–control studies suggest that the link between schizophrenia and PBCs may be much weaker than previously assumed (Kendall et al. 2000). In one case–control study of childhood onset schizophrenia, Matsumoto et al. (1999) reported an odds ratio of 3.5 for PBCs, suggesting a greater risk in very early onset cases. However, in the NIMH study of childhood onset schizophrenia, PBCs were no more common in cases than in sibling controls (Nicholson et al. 1999). Even if there is a significant association, it remains unclear whether there is any causal connection between PBCs and schizophrenia. There is a strong argument that PBCs are *consequences* rather than *causes* of abnormal neurodevelopment (Goodman 1988). This view is supported by the finding that schizophrenics have smaller head size at birth than controls (McGrath & Murray 1995), which is likely to be a consequence of either defects in genetic control of neurodevelopment or earlier environmental factors, such as viral exposure.

Puberty

The close temporal association between the onset of puberty and a marked increase in the incidence of schizophrenia suggests that biological (or social) events around puberty may be related to the expression of psychotic symptoms. Galdos et al. (1993) reported an association between the timing of menarche and onset of psychosis in girls. However, this finding has not been supported by subsequent studies. Frazier *et al.* (1997) found no relationship between the onset of psychosis and indices of puberty in cases recruited to the NIMH study of childhood onset schizophrenia. For both boys and girls the timing of pubertal events were similar for cases and controls.

Psychosocial risks

One possible explanation for an atypically early onset of schizophrenia could be differential exposure to psychosocial adversity, such as higher levels of parental hostility and criticism ('high EE'). High levels of expressed emotion (EE) among relatives of adult schizophrenics has been shown to be a predictor of psychotic relapse and poor outcome (Leff & Vaughn 1985). Although the role of high EE in precipitating the onset of schizophrenia has not been established, it is theoretically plausible that high EE might act to 'bring forward' the onset of the disorder in a vulnerable individual. Goldstein (1987) reported that parental EE measures of criticism and overinvolvement taken during adolescence were associated with an increased risk of schizophrenia spectrum disorders in young adulthood. However, a causal link is not proven, and the association may reflect either an expression of some common underlying trait or a parental response to premorbid disturbance in the preschizophrenic adolescent. Similarly, high EE in the parents of schizophrenic patients may be a reaction to the illness rather than a cause. There is no evidence that the parents of childhood onset patients show higher levels of EE than do parents of adult onset patients – in fact the reverse may be true. J.R. Asarnow *et al.* (1994) used the Five Minute Speech Sample to measure parental EE and found that childhood onset schizophrenics were no more likely to have 'high EE' parents than normal controls. Overall, there seems little evidence to suggest that the onset of schizophrenia in childhood can be explained by exposure to higher levels of parental criticism and hostility than that experienced by adult onset patients. Indeed, it appears that, on average, the parents of childhood onset schizophrenics generally express *lower* levels of criticism and hostility than parents of adult onset patients because of a greater tendency to attribute their childrens' behaviour to an illness which is beyond their control (Hooley 1987).

Neurobiology of schizophrenia

Neurodevelopmental models of schizophrenia

Over the last decade the concept of schizophrenia as a neurodevelopmental disorder has taken a strong hold, although 'neurodevelopmental' is often used with a wide range of meanings. It is possible to distinguish 'early' and 'late' neurodevelopmental models, with a third 'risk' model incorporating ideas from developmental psychopathology (Hollis & Taylor 1997).

The 'early' neurodevelopmental model emerged from the ideas of Fish (1957) who proposed that the neuropathology in schizophrenia was of perinatal origin. The 'early' neurodevelopmental model views the primary cause of schizophrenia as a static 'lesion' occurring during fetal brain development (Murray & Lewis 1987; Weinberger 1987). The putative 'lesion' could be of either neurogenetic or environmental origin (e.g. virus infection or fetal hypoxia). Two main lines of evidence support the 'early' neurodevelopmental model. First, there is an absence of gliosis in the postmortem brains of schizophrenic patients, which suggests a neurodevelopmental rather than a neurodegenerative pathology (see Chapter 17). Secondly, a more indirect line of evidence includes the association of schizophrenia with premorbid social and cognitive impairments (Foerster *et al.* 1991; Done *et al.* 1994; Jones *et al.* 1994), pregnancy and birth complications (Lewis & Murray 1987; McNeil 1995) and minor physical anomalies (Gualtieri *et al.* 1982; Guy *et al.* 1983). According to this 'early' model, during childhood the 'lesion' is relatively silent giving rise only to subtle behavioural symptoms (premorbid social and cognitive impairments). However, in adolescence, or early adult life, the 'lesion' interacts with the process of *normal* brain maturation (e.g. myelination of corticolimbic circuits and/or synaptic pruning and remodelling) to manifest itself in the form of psychotic symptoms.

There are several weaknesses in the 'early' neurodevelopmental model. First, it fails to provide a satisfactory account of the long latency between the putative perinatal damage/lesion and the typical onset of symptoms in late adolescence or early adult life. Secondly, an early neurodevelopmental insult on its own cannot account for the finding of increased extracerebral (sulcal) cerebrospinal fluid (CSF) space in schizophrenia. Diffuse loss of brain tissue limited to the pre- or perinatal periods would result in enlargement of the lateral ventricles but not increased extracerebral CSF space (Woods 1998).

The 'late' neurodevelopmental model, first proposed by Feinberg (1983, 1997), argues that the key neuropathological events in schizophrenia occur as a result of *abnormal* brain development during adolescence. The current formulation of the 'late' neurodevelopmental model proposes that *excessive* synaptic and/or dentritic elimination occurs during adolescence producing aberrant neural connectivity and psychotic symptoms (Woods 1998; McGlashen & Hoffman 2000). This 'late' model characterizes schizophrenia as a *progressive* late onset neurodevelopmental disorder in contrast to the 'early' model that proposes a *static* lesion during the perinatal period. The 'late' model predicts that progressive structural brain changes and cognitive decline will be seen in adolescence around the onset of psychosis. The excessive synaptic pruning during adolescence proposed in the 'late' model is simply an amplification of the normal process of neuronal remodelling with progressive pruning and elimination of synapses that begins in early childhood and extends through late adolescence (Huttenlocher 1979; Purves & Lichtmen 1980). These major regressive changes in adolescence with remodelling of neural connections are likely to be under genetic control with synaptic elimination in schizophrenia representing an extreme of normal variation (Feinberg 1983). In the 'late' model, premorbid abnormalities in early childhood are viewed as non-specific risk factors rather than early manifestations of an underlying schizophrenic neuropathology.

Both the 'early' and 'late' models suppose that there is a direct and specific expression of the eventual brain pathology as schizophrenic disorder. A third viewpoint, the 'risk' model, proposes that early and/or late brain pathology acts as a risk factor rather than a sufficient cause so that its effects can only be understood in the light of an individual's exposure to other risk and protective factors (Hollis & Taylor 1997). This latter formulation provides a probabilistic model of the onset of schizophrenia in which aberrant brain development is expressed as neurocognitive impairments that interact with the environment to produce psychotic symptoms. The following sections examine how well current neurobiological research evidence supports these competing neurodevelopmental models of schizophrenia (for further discussion of these theories see Chapters 13 and 15).

Neuropathology

In the postmortem brains of schizophrenic patients there is an absence of gliosis which is the necessary hallmark of neurodegeneration (Roberts et al. 1986). The prominent neuropathology in schizophrenia is not the classic form involving neuronal cell death, but instead a loss or reduction in dendritic spines and synapses which are the elements of neural connectivity (Garey et al. 1998; Glantz & Lewis 2000). As a result, the brain in schizophrenia is characterized by increased neuronal density, decreased intraneuronal space and reduced overall brain volume. Furthermore, the decrease in dentritic spine density appears to be both region and disease specific. A reduction in dendritic spine density has been reported on pyramidal cells in layer III of the temporal cortex (Garey et al. 1998) and the dorsolateral prefrontal cortex (Glantz & Lewis 2000) but not on pyramidal cells in the visual cortex of schizophrenic patients (Glantz & Lewis 2000). These findings are compatible with the hypothesis of reduced cortical and/or thalamic excitatory glutaminergic inputs to the dorsolateral prefrontal cortex in schizophrenia (see Chapter 17 for other perspectives on neuropathology).

Structural brain abnormalities

Neuroimaging and postmortem studies have shown that the brain as a whole and the frontal and temporal cortices in particular are smaller than in normal subjects (Andreasen et al. 1990; Nopoulos et al. 1995). Brain volume reductions in schizophrenia are specific to grey matter (Gur et al. 2000a) which supports neuropathological findings of increased neuronal density and reduced intraneuronal neurophil rather than neuronal loss (Selemon et al. 1995).

Across a range of neuroimaging studies, the volume of the hippocampus and amygdala is reduced bilaterally by 4.5–10% (Nelson et al. 1998; Gur et al. 2000a). Prefrontal grey matter volume is reduced by about 10% (Gur et al. 2000b). Enlargement of the third and lateral ventricles is a consistent finding,

with ventricular volume increased by about 40% bilaterally (Lawrie & Abukmeil 1998). Ventricular enlargement is associated with neuropsychological impairment and negative symptoms (Vita et al. 1991). Studies of the basal ganglia have produced more inconsistent results, possibly as a function of the increase in basal ganglia volume associated with the use of traditional antipsychotics. Interestingly, when patients are switched to the atypical antipsychotic clozapine there is a reduction of basal ganglia volume (Chakos et al. 1995).

The brain changes reported in child and adolescent onset schizophrenia appear to be very similar to those described in adult onset schizophrenia, supporting the idea of an underlying neurobiological continuity. In the NIMH study of childhood onset schizophrenia (onset less than 12 years of age), subjects had smaller brains than normal subjects, with larger lateral ventricles and reduced prefrontal lobe volume (Jacobsen & Rapoport 1998). Similar to findings from adult studies, reduced total cerebral volume is associated with negative symptoms (Alaghband-Rad et al. 1997). The midsagittal thalamic area is decreased while the midsagittal area of the corpus callosum is increased (Giedd et al. 1996), suggesting that the reduction in total cerebral volume in childhood onset schizophrenia is brought about by a relative reduction in grey matter with sparing of white matter. Childhood onset patients have a higher rate of developmental brain abnormalities than controls, including an increased frequency of an enlarged cavum septum pelucidum (Nopoulos et al. 1998). Abnormalities of the cerebellum have also been found including reduced volume of the vermis, midsagittal area and inferior posterior lobe (Jacobsen et al. 1997a).

Progressive brain changes

Two different types of progressive brain change have been described in schizophrenia. First, treatment with traditional antipsychotics appears to cause progressive enlargement of the basal ganglia, with these structures returning to their original size when patients are transferred to the atypical antipsychotic clozapine (Frazier et al. 1996). Secondly, there is evidence of progressive volume reductions in the temporal and frontal lobes during the first 2–3 years after the onset of schizophrenia (Gur et al. 1998). In the NIMH study of childhood onset schizophrenia, longitudinal repeated MRI scans through adolescence have revealed a progressive increase in ventricular volume and progressive decrease in cortical volume with frontal (11% decrease) and temporal lobes (7% decrease) disproportionately affected (Rapoport et al. 1997, 1999). Both patients and controls showed progressive reductions in frontal and parietal lobe volumes, with schizophrenic subjects showing a relatively greater loss of temporal lobe volume than controls (Jacobsen et al. 1998). The reduction seen in temporal lobe structures may occur rather later in the illness course than the reduction in frontal lobe and midsagittal thalamic structures. Progressive changes appear to be time limited to adolescence with the rate of volume reduction in frontal and temporal structures declining as subjects reach adult life.

Because progressive brain changes have been described *after* the onset of psychosis, it is possible that they are a consequence of neurotoxic effects of psychosis or, possibly, antipsychotic medication. Evidence that progressive brain changes precede the onset of psychosis is very limited. Pantelis *et al.* (2000) have provided a preliminary report of brain MRI findings in high-risk subjects scanned before and after the transition into psychosis. For those subjects who developed psychosis there were longitudinal volume reductions in the medial temporal region (hippocampus, entorhinal cortex, inferior frontal and fusiform gyrus). There were no significant longitudinal changes in cases that remained non-psychotic. These are potentially important findings which, if replicated, would provide strong support for the idea that excessive developmental reductions in temporal lobe volume have a key role in the onset of psychosis.

Functional brain imaging

The emergence of functional brain imaging technology has provided a unique opportunity to link symptoms and cognitive deficits in schizophrenia to underlying brain activity. Liddle *et al.* (1992) studied the relationship between symptom dimensions (negative, positive and disorganization) in adult schizophrenic subjects and regional cerebral blood flow (rCBF) using PET. Negative symptoms (e.g. affective blunting, avolition and alogia) were associated with reduced rCBF in the dorsolateral prefrontal cortex (DLPFC). Disorganization (e.g. formal thought disorder and bizarre behaviour) was associated with reduced rCBF in the right ventrolateral prefrontal cortex and increased rCBF in the anterior cingulate. Positive symptoms (e.g. hallucinations and delusions) were associated with increased rCBF in the left medial temporal lobe, and reduced rCBF in the posterior cingulate and left lateral temporal lobe. The most consistent association in the literature, across a variety of imaging methods, has been between negative symptoms and reduced frontal activity.

However, a simple description of 'hypofrontality' in schizophrenia does not capture the complex pattern of changes involving interconnected frontal areas and changes across time. In a PET study in childhood onset schizophrenia using the Continuous Performance Test (CPT), Jacobsen *et al.* (1997b) reported reduced activation compared with healthy controls in the mid and superior frontal gyrus, and increased activation in the inferior frontal, supramarginal gyrus and insula. The finding of hypofrontality in schizophrenia is a dynamic state-related phenomenon with evidence of remission of hypofrontality in asymptomatic patients (Spence *et al.* 1998). Localizationist models based on focal cerebral dysfunction in schizophrenia have tended to give way to more dynamic models of cerebral 'disconnectivity' based on dysfunctional neural networks or systems. Models of cerebral connectivity view normal higher brain function as depending on the integrated activity of widely distributed neurocognitive networks, rather than the activity of discrete brain areas in isolation (Bullmore *et al.* 1997). In normal individuals, the functional anatomy of a verbal fluency task

(generation of words beginning with a given letter) can be examined using PET and has consistently shown activation of the left DLPFC and reciprocal deactivation of the superior temporal gyrus (STG). A number of investigators have reported a failure of normal STG deactivation (disconnectivity) in schizophrenic patients during a verbal fluency task (Friston *et al.* 1995; Dolan *et al.* 1996). However, left DLPFC–STG disconnectivity appears to be a state-related marker of psychosis as it is not found in asymptomatic schizophrenic patients (Dye *et al.* 1999; Spence *et al.* 2000) and may possibly be associated with active auditory hallucinations (Spence *et al.* 2000). In contrast, schizophrenic patients in remission do show reduced connectivity between the left DLPFC and anterior cingulate cortex relative to normal controls (Spence *et al.* 2000).

In summary, models of cerebral disconnectivity fit well with both neuropathological and functional neuroimaging data. What is becoming clear is that functional disconnectivity may both identify state-related changes associated with current symptomatology as well as more stable trait-related markers of neurocognitive vulnerability to psychosis.

Magnetic resonance spectroscopy: abnormal neuronal metabolism

Magnetic resonance spectroscopy (MRS) is an imaging technique that can be used to extract *in vivo* information on dynamic biochemical processes at a neuronal level. Proton (^{1}H) MRS focuses on changes in the neuronal marker N-acetylaspartate (NAA). Studies in adult schizophrenic patients have shown reductions in NAA in the hippocampal area and DLPFC. Similar reductions in NAA ratios specific to the hippocampus and DLPFC (Bertolino *et al.* 1998) and frontal grey matter (Thomas *et al.* 1998) have been reported in childhood onset schizophrenia, suggesting neuronal damage or malfunction in these regions.

Pettegrew *et al.* (1991) used phosphorus-31 (^{31}P) MRS in first-episode non-medicated schizophrenics and found reduced phosphomonoester (PME) resonance and increased phosphodiester (PDE) resonance in the prefrontal cortex. This result is compatible with reduced synthesis and increased breakdown of connective processes in the prefrontal cortex. A similar finding of reduced PME and increased PDE resonance has been reported in autistic adults, although they showed increased prefrontal metabolic activity, which was not seen in schizophrenic subjects (Pettegrew *et al.* 1991). It is possible that excessive synaptic elimination is not specific to schizophrenia, but its timing, location and extent may have crucial implications for the development of executive functions, and the risk of psychosis, in late childhood and adolescence.

Implications for neurodevelopmental models of schizophrenia

Taken together, the neuropathological and brain imaging findings provide considerable support for the idea of progressive neurodevelopmental changes in schizophrenia including excessive synaptic elimination resulting in aberrant neural connectivity. The 'early' neurodevelopmental model involving a static pre- or perinatal brain insult fails to account for the progressive nature of brain volume reductions in adolescence, and the fact that reduced brain volume is not accompanied by reduced intracranial volume. While early random events in fetal neurodevelopment (e.g. hypoxia, viruses) may affect baseline synaptic density, genetically determined excessive synaptic elimination as proposed by the 'late' neurodevelopmental model may be the neurobiological process underlying disorders in the schizophrenia spectrum (McGlashen & Hoffman 2000). What is unclear is whether excessive synaptic elimination in the prefrontal cortex (and possibly other brain regions) is a sufficient cause for psychosis to occur or whether it simply provides a vulnerable neurocognitive substrate that must interact with environmental stressors (e.g. cognitive or social demands) to produce psychotic symptoms.

Genetics

Genetic risk and early onset schizophrenia

If there is a continuum of transmitted liability for schizophrenia then, as with other disorders of presumed multifactorial origin, early onset cases of schizophrenia should be associated with a greater genetic loading (Childs & Scriver 1986). Pulver *et al.* (1990) found an increased morbid risk of schizophrenia in relatives of male probands under the age of 17. Meanwhile, Sham *et al.* (1994) found an increased morbid risk in females under age 21 compared with males or later onset females. While both of these studies suggest an inverse relationship between age at onset and transmitted liability, albeit with different gender-specific effects and age cut-offs, it would be dangerous to simply extrapolate these age trends to a younger childhood onset population. Unfortunately, there is a dearth of genetic studies of childhood onset schizophrenia that have used adequate methodology. In the only major twin study of childhood onset schizophrenia, Kallman and Roth (1956) reported an uncorrected MZ concordance rate of 88.2% and a DZ concordance rate of 22.9%. Adult onset schizophrenia clustered in the families of childhood onset probands, providing support for a similar genetic aetiology. Data from family studies suggest that child and adolescent onset schizophrenia carries a greater familial risk of psychosis than adult onset schizophrenia. In the Maudsley study, Hollis (1999) found that 20% of child and adolescent onset schizophrenia cases had at least one first-degree relative with schizophrenia, and 50% had a first-degree relative with psychosis. These rates are somewhat higher than those reported by Sham *et al.* (1994) for adult schizophrenic probands (13% of adult probands had a first-degree relative with schizophrenia and 23% had a first-degree relative with any psychosis). Data from the Maudsley study (Hollis 1999) also show that the presence of negative symptoms in the proband predicts a family history of schizophrenia. This provides further support for the idea that negative symptoms may represent the genetically transmitted phenotype in schizophrenia (Tsuang 1993).

Cytogenetic abnormalities

The association between schizophrenia and chromosomal deletions offers another possible clue to the location of candidate genes. The velocardiofacial syndrome (VCFS) microdeletion on chromosome 22q11 is associated with learning difficulties, short stature, palate abnormalities, cardiac anomalies and parkinsonism. VCFS has also been associated with schizophrenia, occurring at a rate of 2% compared with 0.02% in the normal population (Karayiorgou *et al.* 1995). VCFS appears to be associated with an earlier age of onset of schizophrenia in adults (Bassett *et al.* 1999). In the NIMH study of childhood onset schizophrenia, five cases out of 47 (10.6%) had previously undetected cytogenetic abnormalities (Nicholson *et al.* 1999). These included 3/47 (6.3%) with VCFS, one with Turner syndrome (deletion of a long arm of one X chromosome) and one with a balanced translocation of chromosomes 1 and 7. One study has reported an association, found only in males, between childhood onset schizophrenia and an excess of CAG/CTG trinucleotide expansions (Burgess *et al.* 1998). These findings point to possibly greater genetic heterogeneity in child and adolescent onset forms of schizophrenia.

Neuropsychology

Pattern of cognitive deficits

There is growing awareness that cognitive deficits in schizophrenia represent a core feature of the disorder and cannot simply be dismissed as secondary consequences of psychotic symptoms (Breier 1999). The degree of cognitive impairment is greater in child and adolescent onset than in adult onset patients. A consistent finding in child and adolescent onset patients is a mean IQ of between 80 and 85 (1 SD below the population mean), with about one-third of cases having an IQ below 70 (Jacobsen & Rapoport 1998; Hollis 1999). This represents a mean IQ score about 10 points lower than the mean IQ in adult schizophrenia. These findings raise several important questions. First, are the cognitive deficits specific or generalized: are some aspects of cognitive functioning affected more than others? Secondly, which deficits precede the onset of psychosis and could be causal, and which are consequences of psychosis? Thirdly, is the pattern of deficits specific to schizophrenia or shared with other developmental and psychotic disorders? Fourthly, are cognitive impairments progressive or static after the onset of psychosis?

Recent research (R. Asarnow *et al.* 1994, 1995) suggests that children with schizophrenia have specific difficulties with cognitive tasks that make demands on short-term working memory and selective and sustained attention and speed of processing.

These deficits are similar to the deficits reported in adult schizophrenia (Nuechterlain & Dawson 1984; Saykin *et al.* 1994). Deficits of attention, short-term and recent long-term memory have also been reported in adolescents with schizophrenia (Friedman *et al.* 1996). In contrast, well-established 'overlearned' rote language and simple perceptual skills are unimpaired in child and adolescent onset schizophrenia. Asarnow *et al.* (1991, 1995) have shown that children with schizophrenia have impairments on the span of apprehension task (a target stimulus has to be identified from an array of other figures when displayed for 50 ms). Performance on the task deteriorates markedly when increasing demands are made on information processing capacity (e.g. increasing the number of letters in the display from three to 10). Furthermore, event-related potentials on the span of apprehension task in both children and adults with schizophrenia, compared with age-matched controls, show less negative endogenous activity measured between 100 and 300 ms after the stimulus. Similar findings of reduced event-related potentials have been found during the CPT in both childhood and adult onset schizophrenia (Strandburg *et al.* 1999). These findings indicate a deficit in the allocation of attentional resources to a stimulus (Strandburg *et al.* 1994; Asarnow *et al.* 1995). As with adults, children and adolescents with schizophrenia show high basal autonomic activity and less autonomic responsivity than controls (Gordon *et al.* 1994), with attenuated increases in skin conductance following the presentation of neutral sounds (Zahn *et al.* 1997). Childhood onset patients, like adults, show increased reaction times with a loss of ipsimodal advantage compared with healthy controls (Zahn *et al.* 1998). Abnormalities in smooth pursuit eye movements (SPEM) have also been found in adolescent schizophrenics (mean age 14.5), which suggests continuity with the finding of abnormal SPEM in adult schizophrenics (Iacono & Koenig 1983). Children with schizophrenia also show similar impairments to adult patients on tests of frontal lobe executive function such as the Wisconsin Card Sorting Test (WCST; R. Asarnow *et al.* 1994).

In summary, while basic sensorimotor skills, associative memory and simple language abilities tend to be preserved in children with schizophrenia, deficits are most marked on tasks which require focused and sustained attention, flexible switching of cognitive set, high information processing speed and suppression of prepotent responses (Asarnow *et al.* 1995). Similar deficits affecting attention, memory and motor skills have been found in children genetically at 'high risk' for schizophrenia (Erlenmeyer-Kimling *et al.* 2000) and non-psychotic relatives of schizophrenic probands (Park *et al.* 1995). This adds further weight to the argument that cognitive deficits cannot be simply dismissed as non-specific consequences of schizophrenic symptoms, but rather are likely to be indicators of underlying genetic and neurobiological risk.

Executive functions and onset of schizophrenia

A diverse array of cognitive processes has been integrated under the cognitive domain of 'executive functions' which are presumed to be mediated by the prefrontal cortical system. Executive function skills are necessary to generate and execute goal-directed behaviour, especially in novel situations. Goal-orientated actions require that information in the form of plans and expectations are held 'on-line' in working memory and flexibly changed in response to feedback. Much of social behaviour and social development would appear to depend on these capacities as they involve integration of multiple sources of information, appreciation of others' mental states, inhibition of inappropriate prepotent responses and rapid shifting of attention.

Any cognitive theory of schizophrenia needs to explain the timing of onset which usually occurs during adolescence or early adulthood. Deficits in executive function and social cognition could be the developmental abnormality that predisposes to schizophrenia as executive function deficits impinge on social skills that usually emerge in early adolescence. This period is associated with a rapid growth in abstract analytical skills, together with the development of the sophisticated social and communication abilities that underlie successful social relationships. It is during this period of development (approximately age 8–15 years) that preschizophrenic social impairments become most apparent (Done *et al.* 1994) and there is also a relative decline in cognitive abilities in preschizophrenic subjects (Jones *et al.* 1994).

According to this 'risk' model of executive function deficit, the onset of psychosis depends on the interaction between social and cognitive capacities and the demands of the environment. During adolescence, increasing academic and social demands may act as stressors on a 'high-risk' subject, pushing them over the threshold for psychosis. The greater the premorbid impairment, the earlier the age that a critical liability threshold will be passed and symptoms emerge. This model predicts that similar executive function deficits are found in non-psychotic genetically 'high-risk' relatives. However, executive function deficits are probably not a primary cause of schizophrenia given that they also occur in other neurodevelopmental disorders including autism (Ozonoff *et al.* 1991; Hughes & Russell 1993) and attention deficit hyperactivity disorder (ADHD) (Welsh *et al.* 1991; Pennington *et al.* 1993; Karatekin & Asarnow 1998).

Course of cognitive deficits

Kraepelin's term 'dementia praecox' implied a progressive cognitive decline as part of the disease process. Jones *et al.* (1994) described how academic performance becomes progressively more deviant during adolescence in those individuals destined to develop schizophrenia in adult life. There is also some tentative evidence for a decline in IQ following the onset of psychosis in childhood onset schizophrenia. In the NIMH study (Alaghband-Rad *et al.* 1995), the mean postpsychotic IQ was 83.7 (SD 17.3) compared with a mean prepsychotic IQ of 87.7 (SD 25.4). Although a decline in IQ during the early phase of psychosis has been reported in adults with schizophrenia (Bilder *et al.* 1992), in the NIHM study the decline was in both raw and scaled IQ scores and continued for up to 24–48 months after onset (Jacobsen & Rapoport 1998). There was no evidence for a decline in postpsychotic IQ raw scores repeated after 2 years, although scaled (age-adjusted) IQ scores did still decline (Bedwell *et al.* 1999). Russell *et al.* (1997) found a small non-significant IQ decline, of only 2–3 points, in a 20-year longitudinal follow-up study of IQ in schizophrenia (about one-third of these cases had first onset of psychosis in adolescence).

In summary, when raw scores, rather than scaled scores, are analysed, there is little evidence for an absolute loss in cognitive ability in the early postpsychotic phase of schizophrenia. If a true decline does occur it is during, or before, the transition to psychosis. The small drop in IQ after the onset of psychosis could possibly be caused by the effect of psychotic symptoms on performance. Overall, the evidence points more to a premature arrest, or slowing, of normal cognitive development in child and adolescent onset schizophrenia rather than to a dementia.

Course and outcome

Short-term course

Child and adolescent onset schizophrenia characteristically runs a chronic course, with only a small minority of cases making a full symptomatic recovery from the first psychotic episode. In the Maudsley study of child and adolescent onset psychoses (Hollis 2000), only 12% of schizophrenic cases were in full remission at discharge, compared with 50% of cases with affective psychoses. The short-term outcome for schizophrenia presenting in early life appears to be worse than that of first-episode adult patients (Robinson *et al.* 1999). If full recovery does occur then it is most likely within the first 3 months of onset of psychosis. In the Maudsley study, those adolescent onset patients who were still psychotic after 6 months had only a 15% chance of achieving full remission, while over half of all patients who made a full recovery had active psychotic symptoms for less than 3 months (Hollis 1999). The clinical implication is that the early course over the first 6 months is the best predictor of remission and that longer observation over 6 months adds relatively little new information.

Long-term outcome

A number of long-term follow-up studies of child and adolescent onset schizophrenia all describe a typically chronic unremitting long-term course with severely impaired functioning in adult life (Eggers 1978; Werry *et al.* 1991; Schmidt *et al.* 1995; Eggers & Bunk 1997; Hollis 2000). Several common themes emerge from these studies. First, the generally poor outcome of early onset schizophrenia conceals considerable heterogeneity. About one-fifth of patients in most studies have a good outcome with only mild impairment, while at the other extreme about one-third of patients are severely impaired requiring intensive social and psychiatric support. Hence, for an individual patient diagnosis alone is a relatively crude prognostic indicator. Secondly, after the first few years of illness there is little evidence of further progressive decline. This suggests that in the first 10–15 years of illness, at least, the course is relatively stable, although further progression may occur later in life. Thirdly, child and adolescent onset schizophrenia has a worse outcome than either adolescent onset affective psychoses or adult onset schizophrenia. This suggests that outcome and clinical severity are related to both diagnosis and the age at onset. Fourthly, social functioning, in particular the ability to form friendships and love relationships, appears to be very impaired in early onset schizophrenia. Taken together, these findings confirm that schizophrenia presenting in childhood and adolescence lies at the extreme end of a continuum of phenotypic severity.

Mortality

The risk of premature death is increased in child and adolescent onset psychoses. In the Maudsley study (Hollis 1999), there were nine deaths out of the 106 cases followed up (8.5%). The standardized mortality ratio (SMR) was 1250 (95% CI 170–5500), which represents a 12-fold increase in the risk of death compared with an age- and sex-matched general UK population over the same period. Of the nine deaths in the cohort, seven were male and seven had a diagnosis of schizophrenia. Three subjects suffered violent deaths, two died from self-poisoning, and three had unexpected deaths resulting from previously undetected physical causes (cardiomyopathy and status epilepticus) which were possibly associated with high-dose antipsychotic medication.

The death rate in child and adolescent onset schizophrenia and other psychoses appears to be significantly higher than in the adult form of the disorder. In adults, the 'all cause' SMR for schizophrenia has been reported as 157 (95% CI 153–160) (Harris & Barraclough 1997). In a Norwegian study of adolescent psychiatric inpatients, Kjelsberg (2000) reported an SMR for psychosis of 390 in males and 1130 in females.

Prognosis

The predictors of poor outcome in adolescent onset affective psychoses include premorbid social and cognitive impairments (Werry & McClellan 1992; Hollis 1999), a prolonged first psychotic episode (Schmidt *et al.* 1995), extended duration of untreated psychosis (Hollis 1999) and the presence of negative symptoms (Hollis 1999). Premorbid functioning and negative symptoms at onset provide better prediction of long-term outcome than categorical diagnosis (Hollis 1999). This finding suggests that premorbid social and cognitive impairments and negative symptoms lie at the core of a valid clinical concept of schizophrenia.

Treatment approaches

General principles

While antipsychotic drugs remain the cornerstone of treatment in child and adolescent onset schizophrenia, all young patients with schizophrenia require a multimodal treatment package that includes pharmacotherapy, family and individual counselling, education about the illness and provision to meet social and educational needs (Clark & Lewis 1998).

Primary prevention and early detection

In theory at least, the onset of schizophrenia could be prevented if an intervention reduced the premorbid 'risk' status. However, the difficulty with the premorbid phenotype as currently conceived (subtle social and developmental impairments) is its extremely low specificity and positive predictive value for schizophrenia in the general population, assuming that these premorbid features are a causal risk factor (Erlenmeyer-Kimling et al. 2000). Future refinement of the premorbid phenotype is likely to include genetic and neurocognitive markers in order to achieve acceptable sensitivity and specificity. At present, primary prevention remains on the distant horizon.

In contrast to primary prevention, the aims of early detection are to identify the onset of deterioration in vulnerable individuals with a high predictive validity. Predictive power increases markedly in adolescence around the onset of the prodrome (Davidson et al. 1999). Recent work has attempted to identify 'high-risk' or early prodromal states with the aim of intervening to prevent the active phase of schizophrenia (McGrorry & Sing 1995; Yung et al. 1996). However, only about one-fifth of these 'high-risk' cases go on to develop frank psychosis and it has proved impossible to distinguish these 'high-risk' cases from others who remain non-psychotic. Clearly, interventions directed at 'high-risk' or prodromal states need to benefit the whole population at risk, the majority of whom will not develop schizophrenia. A pragmatic stance would be to monitor children and adolescents with a strong family history and/or suggestive prodromal symptoms to ensure prompt treatment of psychosis.

Strong claims have been made that early recognition and treatment of psychotic symptoms in schizophrenia improves outcome. The association between a long duration of untreated psychosis (DUP) and poor long-term outcome in schizophrenia (Loebel et al. 1992; Wyatt 1995; Birchwood et al. 1997) supports this view. A similar association has been found in child and adolescent onset psychoses (Hollis 1999). While the association between DUP and poor outcome seems secure, the causal connection is far less certain. DUP is also associated with insidious onset and negative symptoms which could confound links with poor outcome. While there are good a priori clinical reasons for the early treatment of symptoms to relieve distress and prevent secondary impairments, as yet it remains unproven whether early intervention actually alters the long-term course of schizophrenia.

Pharmacological treatments

Because of the very small number of trials of antipsychotics conducted with child and adolescent patients, it is necessary to extrapolate most evidence on drug efficacy from studies in adults. This seems a reasonable approach given that schizophrenia is essentially the same disorder whether it has onset in childhood or adult life. However, age-specific factors such as the greater risk of extrapyramidal side-effects (EPSs) and treatment resistance to traditional antipsychotics in younger patients (Kumra et al. 1998b) should also influence drug choice.

The typical antipsychotic haloperidol has been shown to be superior to placebo in two double-blind controlled trials of children and adolescents with schizophrenia (Pool et al. 1976; Spencer & Campbell 1994). It is estimated that about 70% of patients show good or partial response to antipsychotic treatment, although this may take 6–8 weeks to be apparent (Clark & Lewis 1998). The main drawbacks concerning the use of high-potency typical antipsychotics such as haloperidol in children and adolescents is the high risk of EPSs (produced by D_2 blockade of the nigrostriatal pathway), tardive dyskinesia and the lack of effect against negative symptoms and cognitive impairment. Treatment with typical antipsychotics is also associated with enlargement of the caudate nucleus which can be reversed with clozapine (Frazier et al. 1996). Clozapine (the prototypic atypical) has been shown to be superior to haloperidol in a double-blind trial of 21 cases of childhood onset schizophrenia (Kumra et al. 1996). Large open clinical trials of clozapine confirm its effectiveness in child and adolescent onset schizophrenia (Siefen & Remschmidt 1986; Remschmidt et al. 1994). Similar, although less marked, benefits of olanzepine over typical antipsychotics in childhood onset schizophrenia have been reported (Kumra et al. 1998a).

Drawing this evidence together, a strong case can be made for the first-line use of atypicals in child and adolescent schizophrenia (clozapine is only licensed in the UK for treatment-resistant schizophrenia). Treatment resistance in child and adolescent patients should be defined as follows:

1 non-response with at least two conventional antipsychotics (from different chemical classes) each used for at least 4–6 weeks; and/or
2 significant adverse effects with conventional antipsychotics.

While atypicals reduce the risk of EPSs, they can produce other troublesome side-effects (usually dose-related) including weight gain (olanzapine), sedation, hypersalivation and seizures (clozapine). The risk of blood dyscrasias on clozapine is effectively managed by mandatory routine blood monitoring. However, knowledge about potential adverse reactions with the newest atypicals is very limited in child and adolescent patients. A further consideration is the cost of newer atypicals compared with traditional antipsychotics. In the UK, a 1-month supply of haloperidol costs less than £2, compared with £100–120 for the newer atypicals and £200 for clozapine. Although economic studies of cost-effectiveness have suggested that the costs of the atypicals are recouped in reduced inpatient stays and indirect social costs (Aitchison & Kerwin 1997), the availability of these drugs, particularly in developing countries, may well be limited because of their high cost. In the late 1990s, the use of atypical antipsychotics by UK child psychiatrists was still low. Over a 2-year period, only 10% of child and adolescent psychiatrists who prescribed antipsychotics in the Trent Health Region had used an atypical drug (Slaveska *et al.* 1998).

Currently, there is no clear consensus about the choice of antipsychotics in children and adolescents with schizophrenia. Some authorities suggest starting with a trial of a traditional antipsychotic (e.g. haloperidol) with substitution of an atypical if the traditional antipsychotic is either not tolerated or ineffective after 6–8 weeks (Clark & Lewis 1998). However, clinical trial evidence suggests that clozapine is the most effective antipsychotic in child and adolescent onset schizophrenia, although its use is restricted to treatment-resistant cases.

A very powerful case can be made for using atypicals such as olanzapine, quetiapine or risperidone as a first-line treatment, given that child and adolescent onset schizophrenia is characterized by negative symptoms, cognitive impairments, sensitivity to EPSs and relative resistance to traditional antipsychotics.

Psychosocial and family interventions

The rationale for psychosocial family interventions follows from the association between high EE and the risk of relapse in schizophrenia (Leff & Vaughn 1985; Dixon & Lehman 1995). The overall aim is to prevent relapse (secondary prevention) and improve the patient's level of functioning by modifying the family atmosphere. Lam (1991) conducted a systematic review of published trials of psychoeducation and more intensive family interventions in schizophrenia and drew the following conclusions. First, education packages on their own increase knowledge about the illness but do not reduce the risk of relapse. Secondly, more intensive family intervention studies with high EE relatives have shown a reduction in relapse rates linked to a lowering of EE. Thirdly, family interventions tend to be costly and time-consuming with most clinical trials employing highly skilled research teams. Whether these interventions can be transferred into routine clinical practice is uncertain. Fourthly, interventions have focused on the reduction of EE in 'high-risk' families. Whether low EE families would also benefit from these interventions is less clear. This is particularly relevant to the families of children and adolescents with schizophrenia as, on average, these parents express *lower* levels of criticism and hostility than parents of adult onset patients (J.R. Asarnow *et al.* 1994). Hence, routine family interventions aiming to reduce high EE may be well-intentioned but misguided in their focus.

Cognitive–behaviour therapy

In adult patients, cognitive therapy has been used to reduce the impact of treatment-resistant positive symptoms (Tarrier *et al.* 1993). Cognitive–behaviour therapy (CBT) has been shown to be effective in treating negative as well as positive symptoms in schizophrenia resistant to standard antipsychotic drugs, with efficacy sustained over 9 months of follow-up (Sensky *et al.* 2000; see Chapter 33). Whether CBT is equally effective with younger patients, or those with predominant negative symptoms, remains to be established.

Cognitive remediation

Cognitive remediation is a relatively new psychological treatment which aims to arrest or reverse the cognitive impairments in attention, concentration and working memory seen in schizophrenia (Hayes & McGrath 2000; Wykes *et al.* 2000). The results of an early controlled trial in adults are promising, with gains found in the areas of memory and social functioning (Wykes *et al.* 2000). The relatively greater severity of cognitive impairments in child and adolescent patients suggests that early remediation strategies may be particularly important in these younger patients. Helpful advice can also be offered to parents, teachers and professionals, such as breaking down information and tasks into small manageable parts to reduce demands on working memory and speed of processing.

Organization of treatment services

It is a paradox that patients with very early onset schizophrenia have the most severe form of the disorder yet they often receive inadequate and poorly co-ordinated services. One reason for this state of affairs may be that the core responsibility for schizophrenia is seen to lie within adult psychiatric services. In the UK, community-based child and adolescent mental health services (CAMHS) provide the first-line assessment and care for child and young adolescent psychoses, with only about half of these cases referred to specialist inpatient units (Slaveska *et al.* 1998). While inpatient admission is often unnecessary, generic CAMHS services are usually not well placed to provide a comprehensive assessment and treatment service for very early onset psychoses. First, the very low population prevalence of psychosis reduces the predictive value of diagnosis outside specialist centres. Secondly, community-based services often lack familiarity with newer therapies for psychoses including atypical antipsychotics.

One possible model would be to establish specialist regional very early onset psychosis teams serving a population of about 5 million, akin to specialist cancer centres. These expert teams would be primarily outpatient-based but with access to inpatient facilities if required. Hence, the focus would be quite different from the more traditional general purpose adolescent inpatient unit. The teams could offer early diagnostic assessments for children and younger adolescents with suspected psychotic disorders and set up treatment plans in collaboration with more local child and adult psychiatric services. Ideally, these teams would be linked to a university academic centre with an interest in psychosis research and treatment evaluation.

Conclusions

The last decade has seen a dramatic growth in our understanding of the clinical course and neurobiological correlates of schizophrenia presenting in childhood and adolescence. It is now clear that adult-based diagnostic criteria have validity in this age group and the disorder has clinical and neurobiological continuity with schizophrenia in adults. Child and adolescent onset schizophrenia is a severe variant of the adult disorder associated with greater premorbid impairment, a higher familial risk, more severe clinical course and poorer outcome. The poor outcome of children and adolescents with schizophrenia has highlighted the need to target early and effective treatments and develop specialist services for this high-risk group. The last decade has witnessed the introduction of new atypical antipsychotics with improved side-effect profiles and efficacy, and these drugs are likely to replace the traditional antipsychotics as first-line drug therapy for child and adolescent onset schizophrenia.

However, a fundamental understanding of the underlying genetic and neurobiological basis of schizophrenia is still to be achieved. The finding of a progressive reduction in brain volume in very early onset patients and reduced synaptic density in the prefrontal cortex suggests the possibility that excessive synaptic elimination during adolescence may underlie the aetiology of schizophrenia. While significant advances in the next decade are likely to flow from technical developments in molecular genetics and neuroimaging, advance is limited by the defining diagnostic paradigm of schizophrenia. It is widely recognized that the clinical syndrome of schizophrenia contains considerable aetiological and clinical heterogeneity. Therefore, the challenge will be to identify the genetic, neurobiological and cognitive basis of this heterogeneity. Real advance in the field will depend on a more sophisticated understanding of the interplay between genetics, neurodevelopment and environment. This will involve identifying the molecular genetic basis of neurocognitive susceptibility traits for schizophrenia. The developmental mechanisms that translate neurocognitive risks into disorder will need to be understood. Unravelling neurocognitive and clinical heterogeneity should lead to improvements in our ability to deliver individually targeted treatments, as well as the ability to identify 'at risk' children and adolescents in order to prevent the onset of psychosis.

References

Aitchison, K.J. & Kerwin, R.W. (1997) The cost effectiveness of clozapine. *British Journal of Psychiatry* **171**, 125–130.

Alaghband-Rad, J., McKenna, K., Gordon, C.T. *et al.* (1995) Childhood onset schizophrenia: the severity of premorbid course. *Journal of the American Academy of Child and Adolescent Psychiatry* **34**, 1273–1283.

Alaghband-Rad, J., Hamburger, S.D., Giedd, J., Frazier, J.A. & Rapoport, J.L. (1997) Childhood onset schizophrenia: biological markers in relation to clinical characteristics. *American Journal of Psychiatry* **154**, 64–68.

American Psychiatric Association (1980) *Diagnostic and Statistical Manual of Mental Disorders*, 3rd edn. American Psychiatric Association, Washington, DC.

American Psychiatric Association (1994) *Diagnostic and Statistical Manual of Mental Disorders*, 4th edn. American Psychiatric Association, Washington, DC.

Andreasen, N., Ehrhardt, J.C., Swazye, V.W. *et al.* (1990) Magnetic resonance imaging of the brain in schizophrenia. *Archives of General Psychiatry* **47**, 35–44.

Asarnow, J.R. & Ben-Meir, S. (1988) Children with schizophrenia spectrum and depressive disorders: a comparative study of premorbid adjustment, onset pattern and severity of impairment. *Journal of Child Psychology and Psychiatry* **29**, 477–488.

Asarnow, J.R., Thompson, M.C., Hamilton, E.B., Goldstein, M.J. & Guthrie, D. (1994) Family expressed emotion, childhood onset depression, and childhood onset schizophrenic spectrum disorders: is expressed emotion a non-specific correlate of psychopathology or a specific risk factor for depression? *Journal of Abnormal Psychology* **22**, 129–146.

Asarnow, R., Granholm, E. & Sherman, T. (1991) Span of apprehension in schizophrenia. In: *Handbook of Schizophrenia*, Vol. 5. *Neuropsychology, Psychophysiology and Information Processing* (eds S.R. Steinhauer, J.H. Gruzelier & J. Zubin), pp. 335–370. Elsevier, Amsterdam.

Asarnow, R., Asamen, J., Granholm, E. *et al.* (1994) Cognitive/neuropsychological studies of children with schizophrenic disorder. *Schizophrenia Bulletin* **20**, 647–669.

Asarnow, R., Brown, W. & Stranberg, R. (1995) Children with schizophrenic disorder: neurobehavioural studies. *European Archives of Psychiatry and Clinical Neuroscience* **245**, 70–79.

Bassett, A.S., Chow, E., Scutt, L., Hodkinson, K. & Weksberg, R. (1999) Psychiatric phenotype of a genetic subtype of schizophrenia [Abstract]. *Schizophrenia Research* **36**, 87.

Bedwell, J.S., Keller, B., Smith, A.K. *et al.* (1999) Why does postpsychotic IQ decline in childhood onset schizophrenia? *American Journal of Psychiatry* **156**, 1996–1997.

Beratis, S., Gabriel, J. & Hoidas, S. (1994) Age at onset in subtypes of schizophrenic disorders. *Schizophrenia Bulletin* **20**, 287–296.

Bertolino, A., Kumra, S., Callicott, J.H. *et al.* (1998) Common pattern of cortical pathology in childhood onset and adult onset schizophrenia as identified by proton magnetic resonance spectroscopic imaging. *American Journal of Psychiatry* **155**, 1376–1383.

Bilder, R.M., Lipschutz-Broch, L., Reiter, G. *et al.* (1992) Intellectual deficits in first-episode schizophrenia: evidence for progressive deterioration. *Schizophrenia Bulletin* **18**, 437–448.

Birchwood, M., McGorry, P. & Jackson, H. (1997) Early intervention in schizophrenia. *British Journal of Psychiatry* **170**, 2–5.

Bleuler, E. (1911/1950) Dementia praecox. In: *The Group of Schizophrenias*. Translated by J. Zinkin. International Universities Press, New York.

Breier, A. (1999) Cognitive deficit in schizophrenia and its neurochemical basis. *British Journal of Psychiatry* **174** (Suppl. 37), 16–18.

Bullmore, E.T., O'Connell, P., Frangou, S. & Murray, R.M. (1997) Schizophrenia as a developmental disorder or neural network integrity: the dysplastic net hypothesis. In: *Neurodevelopment and Adult Psychopathology* (eds M.S. Kesheravan & R.M. Murray), pp. 253–266. Cambridge University Press, Cambridge.

Burgess, C.E., Lindblad, K., Sidransky, E. *et al.* (1998) Large CAG/CTG repeats are associated with childhood onset schizophrenia. *Molecular Psychiatry* **3**, 321–327.

Caplan, R., Guthrie, D., Shields, W.D. & Mori, L. (1992) Formal thought disorder in paediatric complex partial seizure disorder. *Journal of Child Psychology and Psychiatry* **33**, 1399–1412.

Castle, D. & Murray, R. (1991) The neurodevelopmental basis of sex differences in schizophrenia. *Psychological Medicine* **21**, 565–575.

Chakos, M.H., Lieberman, J.A., Alvir, J. *et al.* (1995) Caudate nuclei volumes in schizophrenic patients treated with typical antipsychotics or clozapine. *Lancet* **345**, 456–457.

Childs, B. & Scriver, C.R. (1986) Age at onset and causes of disease. *Perspectives in Biology and Medicine* **29**, 437–460.

Clark, A. & Lewis, S. (1998) Treatment of schizophrenia in childhood and adolescence. *Journal of Child Psychology and Psychiatry* **39**, 1071–1081.

Davidson, M., Reichenberg, M.A., Rabinowitz, J. *et al.* (1999) Behavioral and intellectual markers for schizophrenia in apparently healthy male adolescents. *American Journal of Psychiatry* **156**, 1328–1335.

De Sanctis, S. (1906) On some varieties of dementia praecox. In: *Rivista Sperimentale de Freniatria e Medicina Legale Delle Alienazioni Mentale* (ed. J.G. Howell), pp. 141–165. Translated by M.L. Osbourn. Brunner Mazel, New York.

Dixon, L.B. & Lehman, A.F. (1995) Family interventions for schizophrenia. *Schizophrenia Bulletin* **21**, 631–643.

Dolan, R.J., Fletcher, P., Frith, C.D. *et al.* (1996) Dopaminergic modulation of impaired cognitive activation in the anterior cingulate cortex in schizophrenia. *Nature* **378**, 180–182.

Done, J.D., Crow, T.J., Johnstone, E. & Sacker, A. (1994) Child-hood antecedents of schizophrenia and affective illness: social adjustment at ages 7 and 11. *British Medical Journal* **309**, 699–703.

Dye, S.M., Spence, S.A., Bench, C.J. *et al.* (1999) No evidence for left superior temporal dysfunction in asymptomatic schizophrenia and bipolar disorder: PET study of verbal fluency. *British Journal of Psychiatry* **175**, 367–374.

Eggers, C. (1978) Course and prognosis in childhood schizophrenia. *Journal of Autism and Childhood Schizophrenia* **8**, 21–36.

Eggers, C. & Bunk, D. (1997) The long-term course of childhood onset schizophrenia: a 42-year follow-up. *Schizophrenia Bulletin* **23**, 105–117.

Erlenmeyer-Kimling, L., Rock, D., Roberts, S.A. *et al.* (2000) Attention, memory and motor skills as childhood predictors of schizophrenia-related psychoses: the New York High Risk Project. *Archives of General Psychiatry* **157**, 1416–1422.

Feinberg, I. (1983) Schizophrenia: caused by a fault in programmed synaptic elimination during adolescence. *Journal of Psychiatric Research* **17**, 319–344.

Feinberg, I. (1997) Schizophrenia as an emergent disorder of late brain maturation. In: *Neuorodevelopment and Adult Psychopathology* (eds M.S. Keshervan & R.M. Murray), pp. 237–252. Cambridge University Press, Cambridge.

Fish, B. (1957) The detection of schizophrenia in infancy. *Journal of Nervous and Mental Diseases* **125**, 1–24.

Fish, B. & Rivito, E.R. (1979) Psychoses of childhood. In: *Basic Handbook of Child Psychiatry*, Vol. 2 (ed. J.D. Noshpitz), pp. 249–304. Basic Books, New York.

Foerster, A., Lewis, S., Owen, M. & Murray, R.M. (1991) Pre-morbid adjustment and personality in psychosis. *British Journal of Psychiatry* **158**, 171–176.

Frazier, J.A., Giedd, J.N., Kaysen, D. *et al.* (1996) Childhood onset schizophrenia: brain magnetic resonance imaging rescan after 2 years of clozapine maintenance. *American Journal of Psychiatry* **153**, 564–566.

Frazier, J.A., Alaghband-Rad, J., Jacobsen, L. *et al.* (1997) Pubertal de-velopment and the onset of psychosis in childhood onset schizophrenia. *Psychiatry Research* **70**, 1–7.

Friedman, L., Finding, R.L., Buch, J. *et al.* (1996) Structural MRI and neuropsychological assessments in adolescent patients with either schizophrenia or affective disorders. *Schizophrenia Research* **18**, 189–190.

Friston, K.J., Herold, S., Fletcher, P. *et al.* (1995) Abnormal fronto-temporal interactions in schizophrenia. In: *Biology of Schizophrenia and Affective Diseases* (ed. S.J. Watson), pp. 449–481. Raven, New York.

Frith, C.D. (1994) Theory of mind in schizophrenia. In: *The Neuropsychology of Schizophrenia* (eds A. David & J.S. Cutting), pp. 147–161. Lawrence Erlbaum, Hove.

Galdos, P.M., van Os, J. & Murray, R. (1993) Puberty and the onset of psychosis. *Schizophrenia Research* **10**, 7–14.

Gallhofer, B., Trimble, M.R., Frackowiak, R., Gibbs, J. & Jones, T. (1985) A study of cerebral blood flow and metabolism in epileptic psychosis using positron emission tomography and oxygen. *Journal of Neurology, Neurosurgery and Psychiatry* **48**, 201–206.

Garey, L.J., Ong, W.Y., Patel, T.S. *et al.* (1998) Reduced dendritic spine density on cerebral cortical pyramidal neurons in schizophrenia. *Journal of Neurology, Neurosurgery and Psychiatry* **65** (4), 446–453.

Garralda, M.E. (1984) Hallucinations in children with conduct and emotional disorders. I. The clinical phenomena. *Psychological Medicine* **14**, 589–596.

Geddes, J.R. & Lawrie, S.M. (1995) Obstetric complications and schizophrenia: a meta-analysis. *British Journal of Psychiatry* **167**, 786–793.

Giedd, J.N., Castellanos, F.X., Rajapaske, J.C. *et al.* (1996) Quantitative analysis of grey matter volumes in childhood onset schizophrenia and attention deficit/hyperactivity disorder. *Society for Neuroscience Abstracts* **22**, 1166.

Gillberg, C., Wahlstrom, J., Forsman, A., Hellgren, L. & Gillberg, J.C. (1986) Teenage psychoses: epidemiology, classification and reduced optimality in the pre-, peri- and neonatal periods. *Journal of Child Psychology and Psychiatry* **27**, 87–98.

Glantz, L.A. & Lewis, D.A. (2000) Decreased dendritic spine density on prefrontal cortical pyramidal neurones in schizophrenia. *Archives of General Psychiatry* **57**, 65–73.

Goldstein, M.J. (1987) The UCLA High Risk Project. *Schizophrenia Bulletin* **13**, 505–514.

Goodman, R. (1988) Are complications of pregnancy and birth causes of schizophrenia? *Developmental Medicine and Child Neurology* **30**, 391–406.

Gordon, C.T., Frazier, J.A., McKenna, K. *et al.* (1994) Childhood onset schizophrenia: a NIMH study in progress. *Schizophrenia Bulletin* **20**, 697–712.

Green, W., Campbell, M., Hardesty, A. *et al.* (1984) A comparison of schizophrenic and autistic children. *Journal of the American Academy of Child Psychiatry* **23**, 399–409.

Green, W., Padron-Gayol, M., Hardesty, A. & Bassiri, M. (1992) Schizophrenia with childhood onset: a phenomenological study of 38 cases. *Journal of the American Academy of Child and Adolescent Psychiatry* **31**, 968–976.

Gualtieri, C.T., Adams, A. & Chen, C.D. (1982) Minor physical abnormalities in alcoholic and schizophrenic adults and hyperactive and autistic children. *American Journal of Psychiatry* **139**, 640–643.

Gur, R.E., Cowell, P., Turetsky, B.I. *et al.* (1998) A follow-up magnetic resonance imaging study of schizophrenia: relationship of neuroanatomical changes to clinical and neurobehavioural measures. *Archives of General Psychiatry* **55**, 145–152.

Gur, R.E., Turetsky, B.I., Cowell, P. *et al.* (2000a) Temporolimbic volume reductions in schizophrenia. *Archives of General Psychiatry* **57**, 769–775.

Gur, R.E., Cowell, P., Latshaw, A. *et al.* (2000b) Reduced dorsal and orbital prefrontal gray matter volumes in schizophrenia. *Archives of General Psychiatry* **57**, 761–768.

Guy, J.D., Majorski, L.V., Wallace, C.J. & Guy, M.P. (1983) The incidence of minor physical anomalies in adult schizophrenics. *Schizophrenia Bulletin* **9**, 571–582.

Hafner, H. & Nowotny, B. (1995) Epidemiology of early onset schizophrenia. *European Archives of Psychiatry and Clinical Neuroscience* **245**, 80–92.

Harris, E.C. & Barraclough, B. (1997) Excess mortality of mental disorder. *British Journal of Psychiatry* **173**, 11–53.

Hayes, R.L. & McGrath, J.J. (2000) Cognitive rehabilitation for people with schizophrenia and related conditions: a systemic review and meta-analysis [Abstract]. *Schizophrenia Research* **41**, 221–222.

Hollis, C. (1995) Child and adolescent (juvenile onset) schizophrenia: a case–control study of premorbid developmental impairments. *British Journal of Psychiatry* **166**, 489–495.

Hollis, C. (1999) *A study of the course and adult outcomes of child and adolescent onset psychoses.* PhD thesis, University of London.

Hollis, C. (2000) The adult outcomes of child and adolescent onset schizophrenia: diagnostic stability and predictive validity. *American Journal of Psychiatry* **157**, 1652–1659.

Hollis, C. & Taylor, E. (1997) Schizophrenia: a critique from the developmental psychopathology perspective. In: *Neuorodevelopment and Adult Psychopathology* (eds M.S. Keshervan & R.M. Murray), pp. 213–233. Cambridge University Press, Cambridge.

Hooley, J.M. (1987) The nature and origins of expressed emotion. In: *Understanding Major Mental Disorder: the Contribution of Family Interaction Research* (eds K. Hahlweg & M.J. Goldstein), pp. 176–194. Family Process, New York.

Hughes, C. & Russell, J. (1993) Autistic children's difficulty with mental disengagement with an object: its implications for theories of autism. *Developmental Psychology* **29**, 498–510.

Huttenlocher, P.R. (1979) Synaptic density in human prefrontal cortex: developmental changes and effects of aging. *Brain Research* **163**, 195–205.

Iacono, W.G. & Koenig, W.G.R. (1983) Features that distinguish smooth pursuit eye tracking performance in schizophrenic, affective disordered and normal individuals. *Journal of Abnormal Psychology* **92**, 29–41.

Jacobsen, L. & Rapoport, J. (1998) Research update: childhood onset schizophrenia – implications for clinical and neurobiological research. *Journal of Child Psychology and Psychiatry* **39**, 101–113.

Jacobsen, L., Giedd, J.N., Berquin, P.C. *et al.* (1997a) Quantitative morphology of the cerebellum and fourth ventricle in childhood onset schizophrenia. *American Journal of Psychiatry* **154**, 1663–1669.

Jacobsen, L., Hamburger, S.D., Van Horn, J.D. *et al.* (1997b) Cerebral glucose metabolism in childhood onset schizophrenia. *Psychiatry Research* **75**, 131–144.

Jacobsen, L., Giedd, J.N., Castellanos, F.X. *et al.* (1998) Progressive reductions in temporal lobe structures in childhood onset schizophrenia. *American Journal of Psychiatry* **155**, 678–685.

Jones, P. & Done, J. (1997) From birth to onset: a developmental perspective of schizophrenia in two national birth cohorts. In: *Neuorodevelopment and Adult Psychopathology* (eds M.S. Keshervan & R.M. Murray), pp. 119–136. Cambridge University Press, Cambridge.

Jones, P., Rogers, B., Murray, R. & Marmot, M. (1994) Child development risk factors for adult schizophrenia in the British 1946 birth cohort. *Lancet* **344**, 1398–1402.

Joyce, P.R. (1984) Age of onset in bipolar affective disorder and misdiagnosis of schizophrenia. *Psychological Medicine* **14**, 145–149.

Kallman, F.J. & Roth, B. (1956) Genetic aspects of preadolescent schizophrenia. *American Journal of Psychiatry* **112**, 599–606.

Karatekin, C. & Asarnow, R.F. (1998) Working memory in childhood onset schizophrenia and attention deficit/hyperactivity disorder. *Psychiatry Research* **80**, 165–176.

Karayiorgou, M., Morris, M.A., Morrow, B. *et al.* (1995) Schizophrenia susceptibility associated with interstitial deletions of chromosome 22q11. *Proceedings of the National Academy of Sciences of the USA* **92**, 7612–7616.

Kendall, R.E., McInneny, K., Juszczak, E. & Bain, M. (2000) Obstetric complications and schizophrenia: two case–control studies based on structured obstetric records. *British Journal of Psychiatry* **176**, 516–522.

Kjelsberg, E. (2000) Adolescent psychiatric in-patients: a high risk group for premature death. *British Journal of Psychiatry* **176**, 121–125.

Kolvin, I. (1971) Studies in the childhood psychoses. I. Diagnostic criteria and classification. *British Journal of Psychiatry* **118**, 381–384.

Kraepelin, E. (1919) *Dementia Praecox.* Translated by R. Barclay. Livingstone, Edinburgh.

Kumra, S., Frazier, J.A., Jacobsen, L.K. *et al.* (1996) Childhood onset schizophrenia: a double blind clozapine–haloperidol comparison. *Archives of General Psychiatry* **53**, 1090–1097.

Kumra, S., Jacobsen, L.K., Lenane, M. *et al.* (1998a) Childhood onset schizophrenia: an open-label study of olanzapine in adolescents. *Journal of the American Academy of Child and Adolescent Psychiatry* **37**, 360–363.

Kumra, S., Jacobsen, L.K., Lenane, M. *et al.* (1998b) Case series: spectrum of neuroleptic-induced movement disorders and extrapyramidal side-effects in childhood onset schizophrenia. *Journal of the American Academy of Child and Adolescent Psychiatry* **37**, 221–227.

Kumra, S., Jacobsen, L.K., Lenane, M. *et al.* (1998c) 'Multidimensionally impaired disorder': is it a variant of very early onset schizophrenia? *Journal of the American Academy of Child and Adolescent Psychiatry* **37**, 91–99.

Kumra, S., Wiggs, E., Krasnewich, D. *et al.* (1998d) Brief report: association of sex chromosome anomalies with childhood onset psychotic disorders. *Journal of the American Academy of Child and Adolescent Psychiatry* **37**, 292–296.

Lam, D.H. (1991) Psychosocial family intervention in schizophrenia: a review of empirical studies. *Psychological Medicine* **21**, 423–441.

Lawrie, S.M. & Abukmeil, S.S. (1998) Brain abnormalities in schizophrenia: a systematic and quantitative review of volumetric magnetic resonance imaging studies. *British Journal of Psychiatry* **172**, 110–120.

Leff, J. & Vaughn, C. (1985) *Expressed Emotion in Families: its Significance for Mental Illness.* Guilford Press, London.

Lewine, R.R.J. (1994) Comments on 'Puberty and the onset of psychosis' by P.M. Galdos *et al. Schizophrenia Research* **13**, 81–83.

Lewis, S.W. & Murray, R.M. (1987) Obstetric complications, neurodevelopmental deviance and risk of schizophrenia. *Journal of Psychiatric Research* **21**, 414–421.

Liddle, P., Friston, K.J., Frith, C.D. *et al.* (1992) Patterns of cerebral blood flow in schizophrenia. *British Journal of Psychiatry* **160**, 179–186.

Lindsay, J., Ounsted, C. & Richards, P. (1979) Long-term outcome of children with temporal lobe seizures. II. Marriage, parenthood and sexual indifference. *Developmental Medicine and Child Neurology* **21**, 433–440.

Loebel, A.D., Lieberman, J.A., Alvir, J.M.N. *et al.* (1992) Duration of psychosis and outcome in first episode schizophrenia. *American Journal of Psychiatry* **149**, 1183–1188.

McGlashen, T.H. & Hoffman, R.E. (2000) Schizophrenia as a disorder of developmentally reduced synaptic connectivity. *Archives of General Psychiatry* **57**, 637–648.

McGrath, J. & Murray, R. (1995) Risk factors for schizophrenia: from conception to birth. In: *Schizophrenia* (eds S.R. Hirsch & D.R. Weinberger), pp. 187–205. Blackwell Science, Oxford.

McGrorry, P. & Sing, B. (1995) Schizophrenia: risk and possibility. In: *Handbook of Studies on Preventative Psychiatry* (eds B. Raphael & G. Burrows), pp. 491–514. Elsvier Science, Amsterdam.

McNeil, T.F. (1995) Perinatal risk factors and schizophrenia: selective review and methodological concerns. *Epidemiology Review* **17**, 107–112.

Malmberg, A., Lewis, G., David, A. & Allebeck, P. (1998) Premorbid adjustment and personality in people with schizophrenia. *British Journal of Psychiatry* **172**, 308–313.

Matsumoto, H., Takei, N., Saito, H., Kachi, K. & Mori, N. (1999) Childhood onset schizophrenia and obstetric complications: a case–control study. *Schizophrenia Research* **38**, 93–99.

Maziade, M., Bouchard, S., Gingras, N. *et al.* (1996) Long-term stability of diagnosis and symptom dimensions in a systematic sample of patients with onset of schizophrenia in childhood and early adolescence. II. Positive/negative distinction and childhood predictors of adult outcome. *British Journal of Psychiatry* **169**, 371–378.

Murray, R.M. & Lewis, S.W. (1987) Is schizophrenia a neurodevelopmental disorder? *British Medical Journal* **295**, 681–682.

Nelson, M.D., Saykin, A.J., Flashman, L.A. & Riodan, H.J. (1998) Hippocampal volume reduction in schizophrenia assessed by magnetic resonance imaging: a meta-analytic study. *Archives of General Psychiatry* **55**, 433–440.

Nicholson, R.M., Giedd, J.N., Lenane, M. *et al.* (1999) Clinical and neurobiological correlates of cytogenetic abnormalities in childhood onset schizophrenia. *American Journal of Psychiatry* **156**, 1575–1579.

Nicholson, R.M., Lenane, M., Singaracharlu, S. *et al.* (2000) Premorbid speech and language impairments in childhood onset schizophrenia: association with risk factors. *Schizophrenia Research* **41**, 55.

Nopoulos, P., Torres, I., Flaum, M. *et al.* (1995) Brain morphology in first-episode schizophrenia. *American Journal of Psychiatry* **152**, 1721–1723.

Nopoulos, P.C., Giedd, J.N., Andreasen, N.C. & Rapoport, J.L. (1998) Frequency and severity of enlarged septi pellucidi in childhood onset schizophrenia. *American Journal of Psychiatry* **155**, 1074–1079.

Nuechterlain, K.H. & Dawson, M.E. (1984) Information processing and attentional functioning in the developmental course of schizophrenic disorders. *Schizophrenia Bulletin* **10**, 160–203.

van Os, J., Jones, P., Lewis, G. *et al.* (1997) Developmental precursors of affective illness in a general population birth cohort. *Archives of General Psychiatry* **54**, 625–631.

Ozonoff, S., Pennington, B.F. & Rogers, S.J. (1991) Executive function deficits in high-functioning autistic individuals: relationship to theory of mind. *Journal of Child Psychology and Psychiatry* **32**, 1081–1105.

Pantelis, C., Velakoulis, D., Suchling, P. *et al.* (2000) Left medial temporal volume reduction occurs during transition from high-risk to first-episode psychosis. *Schizophrenia Research* **41**, 35.

Park, S., Holzman, P.S. & Goldman-Rakic, P.S. (1995) Spatial working memory deficits in the relatives of schizophrenic patients. *Archives of General Psychiatry* **52**, 821–828.

Pennington, B.F., Groisser, D. & Welsh, M.C. (1993) Contrasting deficits in attention deficit hyperactivity disorder versus reading disability. *Developmental Psychology* **29**, 511–523.

Pettegrew, J.W., Keshavan, M.S., Panchalingam, K. *et al.* (1991) Alterations in brain high energy phosphate and membrane phospholipid metabolism in first episode, drug naive schizophrenics: a pilot study of the dorsal prefrontal cortex by *in vivo* phosphorous-31 nuclear magnetic resonance spectroscopy. *Archives of General Psychiatry* **48**, 563–568.

Pool, D., Bloom, W., Miekle, D.H., Roniger, J.J. & Gallant, D.M. (1976) A controlled trial of loxapine in 75 adolescent schizophrenic patients. *Current Therapeutic Research* **19**, 99–104.

Poole, R. & Brabbins, C. (1996) Drug-induced psychosis. *British Journal of Psychiatry* **168**, 135–138.

Potter, H.W. (1933) Schizophrenia in children. *American Journal of Psychiatry* **12**, 1253–1270.

Pulver, A., Brown, C.H., Wolyniec, P. *et al.* (1990) Schizophrenia: age at onset, gender and familial risk. *Acta Psychiatrica Scandinavica* **82**, 344–351.

Purves, D.L. & Lichtmen, J.W. (1980) Elimination of synapses in the developing nervous system. *Science* **210**, 153–157.

Rapoport, J.L., Giedd, J., Kumra, S. *et al.* (1997) Childhood onset schizophrenia: progressive ventricular change during adolescence. *Archives of General Psychiatry* **54**, 897–903.

Rapoport, J.L., Giedd, J., Blumenthal, J. *et al.* (1999) Progressive cortical change during adolescence in childhood onset schizophrenia: a longitudinal magnetic resonance imaging study. *Archives of General Psychiatry* **56**, 649–654.

Remschmidt, H., Schultz, E. & Martin, M. (1994) An open trial of clozapine with thirty-six adolescents with schizophrenia. *Journal of Child and Adolescent Psychopharmacology* **4**, 31–41.

Roberts, G.W., Colter, N., Lofthouse, R. *et al.* (1986) Gliosis in schizophrenia: a survey. *Biological Psychiatry* **21**, 1043–1050.

Robinson, D., Woerner, M.G., Alvir, J.M. *et al.* (1999) Predictors of relapse following a first episode of schizophrenia or schizoaffective disorder. *Archives of General Psychiatry* **56**, 241–247.

Rossi, A., Mancini, F., Stratta, P. *et al.* (1997) Risperidone, negative symptoms and cognitive deficit in schizophrenia: an open study. *Acta Psychiatrica Scandinavica* **95**, 40–43.

Russell, A.J., Monro, J.C., Jones, P.B., Hemsley, D.R. & Murray, R.M. (1997) Schizophrenia and the myth of intellectual decline. *American Journal of Psychiatry* **154**, 635–639.

Russell, A.T. (1994) The clinical presentation of childhood onset schizophrenia. *Schizophrenia Bulletin* **20**, 631–646.

Russell, A.T., Bott, L. & Sammons, C. (1989) The phenomena of schizophrenia occurring in childhood. *Journal of the American Academy of Child and Adolescent Psychiatry* **28**, 399–407.

Rutter, M. (1972) Childhood schizophrenia reconsidered. *Journal of Autism and Childhood Schizophrenia* **2**, 315–407.

Rutter, M. & Mawhood, L. (1991) The long-term psychosocial sequelae of specific developmental disorders of speech and language. In: *Biological Risk Factors for Psychosocial Disorders* (eds M. Rutter & P. Casaer), pp. 233–259. Cambridge University Press, Cambridge.

Sachdev, P. (1998) Schizophrenia-like psychosis and epilepsy: the status of the association. *American Journal of Psychiatry* **155**, 325–336.

Saykin, A.J., Shtasel, D.L., Gur, R.E. *et al.* (1994) Neuropsychological deficits in neuroleptic-naive patients with first episode schizophrenia. *Archives of General Psychiatry* **512**, 124–131.

Schmidt, M., Blanz, B., Dippe, A., Koppe, T. & Lay, B. (1995) Course of patients diagnosed as having schizophrenia during first episode occurring under age 18 years. *European Archives of Psychiatry and Clinical Neuroscience* **245**, 93–100.

Selemon, L.D., Rajkowska, G. & Goldman-Rakic, P.S. (1995) Abnormally high neuronal density in the schizophrenic cortex: a morphometric analysis of prefrontal area 9 and occipital area 17. *Archives of General Psychiatry* **52**, 805–818.

Sensky, T., Turkington, D., Kingdon, D. *et al.* (2000) A randomized controlled trial of cognitive–behavioral therapy for persistent symptoms in schizophrenia resistant to medication. *Archives of General Psychiatry* **57**, 165–172.

Sham, P.C., Jones, P.B., Russell, A. *et al.* (1994) Age at onset, sex, and familial psychiatric morbidity in schizophrenia. Report from the Camberwell Collaborative Psychosis Study. *British Journal of Psychiatry* **165**, 466–473.

Siefen, G. & Remschmidt, H. (1986) Behandlungsergebnisse mit Clozapin bei schizophrenen Jungendlichen. *Zeitschrift fur Kinder- und Jungendpsychiatrie* **14**, 245–257.

Sigurdsson, E., Fombonne, E., Sayal, K. & Checkley, S. (1999) Neurodevelopmental antecedents of early onset bipolar affective disorder. *British Journal of Psychiatry* **174**, 121–127.

Slaveska, K., Hollis. C.P. & Bramble, D. (1998) The use of antipsychotics by the child and adolescent psychiatrists of Trent region. *Psychiatric Bulletin* **22**, 685–687.

Spence, S.A., Hirsch, S.R., Brooks, D.J. *et al.* (1998) Prefrontal cortex activity in people with schizophrenia and control subjects: evidence from positron emission tomography for remission of 'hypofrontality' with recovery from acute schizophrenia. *British Journal of Psychiatry* **172**, 316–323. [Published erratum appears in *British Journal of Psychiatry* 1998; **172**, 543.]

Spence, S.A., Liddle, P.F., Stefan, M.D. *et al.* (2000) Functional anatomy of verbal fluency in people with schizophrenia and those at genetic risk: focal dysfunction and distributed disconnectivity reappraised. *British Journal of Psychiatry* **176**, 52–60.

Spencer, E.K. & Campbell, M. (1994) Children with schizophrenia: diagnosis, phenomenology and pharmacotherapy. *Schizophrenia Bulletin* **20**, 713–725.

Strandburg, R.J., Marsh, J.T., Brown, W.S., Asarnow, R.F. & Guthrie, D. (1994) Information processing deficits across childhood and adult onset schizophrenia. *Schizophrenia Bulletin* **20**, 685–696.

Strandburg, R.J., Marsh, J.T., Brown. W.S. *et al.* (1999) Continuous-processing ERPS in adult schizophrenia: continuity with childhood onset schizophrenia. *Biological Psychiatry* **45**, 1356–1369.

Tarrier, N., Beckett, R., Harwood, S. *et al.* (1993) A trial of two cognitive behavioural methods of treating drug resistant residual symptoms in schizophrenic patients. I. Outcome. *British Journal of Psychiatry* **162**, 524–532.

Thomas, M.A., Ke, Y., Levitt, J. *et al.* (1998) Preliminary study of frontal lobe ^{1}H MR spectroscopy in childhood onset schizophrenia. *Journal of Magnetic Resonance Imaging* **8**, 841–846.

Towbin, K.R., Dykens, E.M., Pearson, G.S. & Cohen, D.J. (1993) Conceptualising 'borderline syndrome of childhood' and 'childhood schizophrenia' as a developmental disorder. *Journal of the American Academy of Child and Adolescent Psychiatry* **32**, 775–782.

Tsuang, M.T. (1993) Genotypes, phenotypes and the brain: a search for connections in schizophrenia. *British Journal of Psychiatry* **163**, 299–307.

Tsuang, M.T., Simpson, J.C. & Kronfold, Z. (1982) Subtypes of drug abuse with psychosis. *Archives of General Psychiatry* **39**, 141–147.

Vita, A., Dieci, M., Giobbio, G.M. *et al.* (1991) CT scan abnormalities and outcome of chronic schizophrenia. *American Journal of Psychiatry* **148**, 1577–1579.

Volkmar, F.R. & Cohen, D.J. (1991) Comorbid association of autism and schizophrenia. *American Journal of Psychiatry* **148**, 1705–1707.

Weinberger, D.R. (1987) Implications of normal brain development for the pathogenesis of schizophrenia. *Archives of General Psychiatry* **44**, 660–669.

Welsh, M.C., Pennington, B.F. & Groisser, D.B. (1991) A normative-developmental study of executive function: a window on pre-frontal function in children? *Developmental Neuropsychology* **7**, 131–139.

Werry, J.S. (1992) Child and adolescent (early onset) schizophrenia: a review in light of DSM-IIIR. *Journal of Autism and Developmental Disorders* **22**, 601–624.

Werry, J.S. & McClellan, J.M. (1992) Predicting outcome in child and adolescent (early onset) schizophrenia and bipolar disorder. *Journal of the American Academy of Child and Adolescent Psychiatry* **31**, 147–150.

Werry, J.S., McClellan, J.M. & Chard, L. (1991) Childhood and adolescent schizophrenia, bipolar and schizoaffective disorders: a clinical and outcome study. *Journal of the American Academy of Child and Adolescent Psychiatry* **30**, 457–465.

Werry, J.S., McClellan, J.M., Andrews, L. & Ham, M. (1994) Clinical features and outcome of child and adolescent schizophrenia. *Schizophrenia Bulletin* **20**, 619–630.

Woods, B.T. (1998) Is schizophrenia a progressive neurodevelopmental disorder? Toward a unitary pathogeneic mechanism. *American Journal of Psychiatry* **155**, 1661–1670.

World Health Organization (1978) *International Classification of Diseases*, 9th edn (ICD-9). World Health Organization, Geneva.

World Health Organization (1992) *The ICD-10 Classification of Mental and Behavioural Disorders: Diagnostic Criteria for Research*. World Health Organization, Geneva.

Wyatt, R.J. (1995) Early intervention in schizophrenia: can the course be altered? *Biological Psychiatry* **38**, 1–3.

Wykes, T., Reeder, C., Williams, C. *et al.* (2000) Cognitive remediation: predictors of success and durability of improvements [Abstract]. *Schizophrenia Research* **41**, 221.

Yung, A.R., McGorry, P.D., McFarlane, C.A. *et al.* (1996) Monitoring and care of young people at incipient risk of psychosis. *Schizophrenia Bulletin* **22**, 283–303.

Zahn, T.P., Jacobson, L.K., Gordon, C.T. *et al.* (1997) Autonomic nervous system markers of pathophysiology in childhood onset schizophrenia. *Archives of General Psychiatry* **54**, 904–912.

Zahn, T.P., Jacobson, L.K., Gordon, C.T. *et al.* (1998) Attention deficits in childhood onset schizophrenia: reaction time studies. *Journal of Abnormal Psychology* **107**, 97–108.

5 Atypical psychotic disorders

C.B. Pull, J.M. Cloos and N.V. Murthy

Atypical psychotic disorders designate psychotic conditions that cannot be easily classified as either schizophrenia or a mood disorder with psychotic features. They form a heterogeneous and poorly understood collection of disorders that are regarded as probably unrelated to schizophrenia and affective disorder, but on which surprisingly little empirical research has been carried out up to now. The terminology used to designate the individual disorders in this group as well as the proportion of patients that are regarded as having one of these disorders varies from country to country.

Atypical psychotic disorders can conveniently be divided according to their typical duration into a group of chronic persistent delusional disorders and a group of acute and transient psychotic disorders.

Schizoaffective disorder is described in a separate chapter and will not be detailed again here.

Historical background

In the successive editions of his *Textbook of Psychiatry* Kraepelin gradually evolved a system of classification to which all subsequent systems have paid tribute. In describing those conditions known today as functional psychoses, Kraepelin leaned heavily on clinical course and prognosis. In the sixth edition of his textbook, Kraepelin (1899) distinguished three classes of psychoses: manic-depressive psychoses, dementia praecox and paranoia. In the eighth edition, Kraepelin (1909–15) introduced the concept of the paraphrenias that are separated from the paranoid form of dementia praecox.

Kraepelin described dementia praecox as a single disease progressing towards 'psychic enfeeblement' (*psychische Schwäche*) and presenting three forms: hebephrenia, catatonia and dementia paranoides. Paranoia was characterized by systematized delusions, without hallucinations and accompanied by perfect presentation of clear and orderly thinking. Paraphrenia shared many of the characteristics of paranoia and schizophrenia. The main difference from paranoia was that in paraphrenia the delusions were accompanied by prominent hallucinations, and the main difference from schizophrenia was that paraphrenia did not progress to a dementia-like state.

Although Kraepelin's nosology was gradually to establish its position, several aspects of his classification have been either neglected or opposed, to varying degrees, depending on national schools of psychiatry. This has led to either an extension or a narrowing of the concept of dementia praecox, and consequently of schizophrenia. In Britain and in the USA, terms such as paranoia and paraphrenia were rarely used in practice, and psychoses that were not organic were classified, up to a recent past, as either schizophrenic or affective (Kendell 1993). The French, Scandinavian and German schools of psychiatry have, on the contrary, excluded from schizophrenia different types of acute and transient psychoses as well as a number of chronic delusional disorders (for a further discussion see Chapter 1).

Transient psychotic disorders

A considerable number of labels have been proposed to designate transient psychotic disorders which are regarded as neither schizophrenic nor affective. Although the different eponyms seem to refer to the same group of patients, systematic clinical information that would give rise to concepts that can be clearly defined and separated from each other is not yet available. The incidence of these disorders seems to be more frequent in developing countries than in other parts of the world (Sartorius *et al.* 1986).

Prominent concepts in this field are the *bouffées délirantes* of the French, the 'reactive' or 'psychogenic' psychoses and the 'schizophreniform' psychoses of the Scandinavian and the 'cycloid psychoses' of the German tradition, as well as a number of so-called culture-bound psychoses.

Bouffées délirantes

The concept of *bouffée délirante polymorphe des dégénérés* was introduced by Magnan and Legrain (1895), at the end of the nineteenth century, as part of a complex classification of the delusional states of degeneracy. The classical description of *bouffée délirante*, as given by Magnan's pupil Legrain (1886), rests on the following criteria:

1 sudden onset, 'like a bolt from the blue';
2 polymorphous delusions and hallucinations of any kind;
3 clouded consciousness associated with emotional instability;
4 absence of physical signs, i.e. the disorder is not caused by any organic mental disorder;
5 rapid return to the premorbid level of functioning; and
6 relapses may occur, but individual episodes are separated by symptom-free intervals.

Whereas Magnan and Legrain stated that *bouffées délirantes* occur without any identifiable precipitating factor, the current consensus holds that there is a variant of the disorder occasioned by psychological stressors.

Using the results of a national enquiry, the present author (Pull *et al.* 1987) has developed explicit diagnostic inclusion and exclusion criteria for both genuine or Magnan type as well as for stress-related *bouffée délirante*. The striking outcome of this enquiry is that the concept of *bouffée délirante*, as used by present-day French psychiatrists, has not changed in 100 years, with the exception that the theory of degeneracy is no longer used.

In the past, the disorder was diagnosed by French psychiatrists nearly three times as frequently as acute schizophrenia (Pichot & Debray 1971). According to Pichot (1990), empirical studies indicate that when stringent diagnostic criteria are applied, the disorder is not commonly reported among new cases. However, the concept of *bouffée délirante polymorphe* remains popular in France, as proven by a recent study in which nearly one-third of acute admissions were diagnosed with this disorder (Ferrey & Zebdi 1999).

Psychogenic or reactive psychoses

The concept of psychogenic or reactive psychosis has been developed in Scandinavia. The first comprehensive survey of the concept of psychogenic psychosis is to be found in a monograph by the Danish psychiatrist Wimmer (1916). According to Wimmer, psychogenic psychoses are clinically independent of schizophrenia and manic-depressive psychosis, usually develop in a predisposed individual, are caused by psychosocial factors (which also determine the content and form of the disorder), have a great tendency to recover and seem never to end in deterioration.

The prognostic validity of psychogenic psychosis has been investigated by Faergeman (1963), who made a follow-up study of Wimmer's cases. Of the 113 original cases of psychogenic psychosis, 66 were confirmed by Faergeman, whereas one-third were rediagnosed as suffering from schizophrenia.

According to Strömgren (1974, 1989), 65% of psychogenic psychoses are emotional reactions, 15% are disorders of consciousness and 20% are paranoid types. The results of a dual mating study suggest that reactive psychoses do not contribute liability factors to the development of schizophrenia or manic-depressive psychosis and that major psychoses do not contribute liability factors to reactive psychosis (Gottesman & Bertelsen 1989).

Pitta and Blay (1997) investigated the concepts of reactive psychoses as they are classified in standardized diagnostic systems by retrospectively applying criteria from DSM-IIIR, DSM-IV, ICD-10 and Present State Examination (PSE) diagnostic systems on 26 cases of reactive psychosis and psychosis not otherwise specified, to evaluate their agreement with those obtained using ICD-9. They found that case-note diagnoses obtained using DSM-IIIR, DSM-IV, ICD-10 criteria and the PSE-CATEGO program show a low level of agreement with ICD-9 diagnoses and although DSM-IIIR provides criteria for brief reactive psychosis, and DSM-IV and ICD-10 provide such criteria for brief or acute psychotic disorder, these bear little relationship to the original concept of the disorder.

Schizophreniform psychoses

The concept of schizophreniform psychosis was described in Norway by Langfeldt (1939). Langfeldt differentiated between two groups of psychoses usually diagnosed as schizophrenia: a group with poor prognosis, labelled 'genuine' or 'process' schizophrenia, and a group with good prognosis, labelled 'schizophreniform' psychosis.

The following factors were considered by Langfeldt to be correlated with good prognosis: a well-adjusted premorbid personality, the presence of identifiable precipitating factors, sudden onset, the presence among an otherwise schizophrenic symptomatology of disturbance of mood, clouding of consciousness and the absence of blunted affect.

A great deal of research (Garmezy 1968; Brockington *et al.* 1978) has been focused on an objective separation between 'process' schizophrenia and 'schizophreniform' psychosis, but there is no decisive evidence that two types are of a qualitatively different nature. Two studies reclassified Langfeldt's 100 cases of schizophreniform psychoses according to ICD-9 and DSM-III (Bergem *et al.* 1990), and DSM-IIIR, respectively (Guldberg *et al.* 1991), and concluded that most of the 'schizophreniform psychoses' turned out to be affective disorders with psychotic features.

1987; Signer 1991a) and organic mental disorder (Signer & Cummings 1987).

De Clérambault's original description of erotomania as a syndrome of pathological emotions that follow an orderly evolution differs from Kraeplin's views on erotomania, who placed the disorder among the paranoias (Signer 1991b). The term has undergone a number of reformulations in recent times and is now included in contemporary definitions as a specific form of delusional disorder ('erotomanic type'), characterized by delusional beliefs of being loved. This restrictive modern definition has been questioned by professionals involved in the research on 'stalking', a form of human behaviour characterized by obsessional following and harassing of a specific individual which now constitutes a criminal offence in most English-speaking nations, and in which erotomania often plays an important part (Mullen *et al.* 2000).

Cotard syndrome

Under the name *délire de négation*, Cotard (1880, 1882) described patients who complained of having lost not only their possessions and social status, but also their hearts, blood, intestines or brains. Currently, the term is often confined to the belief of being dead, which is conceptually too restrictive (Berrios & Luque 1995a). It has become rarer in recent years, at least in its complete form, probably because the underlying disorder responds to pharmacotherapy before the psychopathological manifestations of the syndrome develop. The syndrome is usually associated with severe forms of depression and chronic forms of the syndrome may occur in organic mental disorders.

A review of 100 cases of Cotard syndrome reported since 1880 found differences between younger and older subjects, the latter showing more organic disorder, auditory hallucinations and delusions of non-existence (Berrios & Luque 1995b). The cases were classified into a 'type I' group, being closer to the delusional than the affective disorders, and a mixed 'type II' group showing anxiety, depression and auditory hallucinations (Berrios & Luque 1995b). Some support exists that right hemisphere dysfunction, such as perceptual impairment and abnormal perceptual experience as well as an incorrect interpretation of these, contributes to the development of the syndrome, thus showing similarities to the neuropsychological origins of Capgras syndrome (Young *et al.* 1994; Gerrans 2000).

Kretschmer's *sensitiver Beziehungswahn*

In a monograph published in 1918, Kretschmer described a type of paranoia which developed in sensitive personalities when a precipitating event, termed key experience (*Schlüsselerlebnis*), occurred at the correct time in the person's life. According to Kretschmer, the prognosis was good. In particular, patients with the disorder did not develop schizophrenia. According to Pichot (1983), Kretschmer's description was to have a major impact on psychiatric thinking. By setting forth that a particular delusional state could be 'understood', Kretschmer 'opened the path to the dissolution of process endogeny and the establishment of the psychogenic conception of the psychoses'.

Schizotypal (personality) disorder
(see also Chapter 7)

The term schizotypal was introduced to modern psychiatric nosology largely as the result of family studies in schizophrenia (Kety *et al.* 1978; Kendler *et al.* 1981). The disorder is more common among family members of individuals with schizophrenia and is part of the genetic 'spectrum' of disorders associated with schizophrenia. Schizotypal disorder is characterized by eccentric behaviour and anomalies of thinking and affect which resemble those seen in schizophrenia, and has been demonstrated to have phenomenological, biological, treatment and outcome characteristics similar to those of schizophrenia, although no definite and characteristic schizophrenic anomalies have occurred at any stage and no single feature is invariably present. Patients with schizotypal disorder show cognitive impairment as in schizophrenia, but the impairment appears to be more focal and involves mainly working memory, verbal learning and sustained attention rather than generalized intellectual deficits. Temporal lobe volume is reduced, as in schizophrenic patients, but the frontal lobe functions seem to be intact, thus preventing the more severe cognitive and social deteriorations seen in schizophrenia. A better capacity for compensatory buffering in lateral and subcortical brain regions may also explain the lower susceptibility of schizotypal patients to psychotic symptoms (Kirrane & Siever 2000).

The disorder is sometimes difficult to differentiate either from simple schizophrenia or from schizoid or paranoid personality disorders. It runs a chronic course with fluctuations of intensity. There is no definite onset and the evolution and course resemble those of a personality disorder. Schizotypal disorder is therefore listed among the personality disorders in DSM-IV, while ICD-10 places it under the atypical psychotic disorders.

Atypical psychotic disorders in DSM-IV
(for a further dicussion of classification issues and a comparison of DSM-IV and ICD-10 see Chapter 1)

In DSM-IV of the American Psychiatric Association (1994), atypical psychotic disorders (as defined here) are described under the heading 'Schizophrenia and Other Psychotic Disorders'. DSM-IV lists five major disorders in this section:
1 delusional disorder;
2 brief psychotic disorder;
3 schizophreniform disorder;
4 schizoaffective disorder;
5 induced or shared psychotic disorder (*folie à deux*).
Schizotypal disorder is listed among the personality disorders.

Table 5.3 DSM-IV classification of non-organic atypical psychotic disorders.

295.40	Schizophreniform disorder Specify if: without good prognostic features with good prognostic features
295.70	Schizoaffective disorder Specify type: bipolar depressive
297.1	Delusional disorder Specify type: erotomanic, grandiose jealous, persecutory somatic, mixed, unspecified
298.8	Brief psychotic disorder Specify type: with marked stressor(s) (brief reactive) without marked stressor(s) with postpartum onset
297.3	Shared psychotic disorder (*folie à deux*)
298.9	Psychotic disorder not otherwise specified

The DSM-IV classification of atypical psychotic disorders is presented in Table 5.3. Important changes have been made in the nomenclature and description of 'atypical' psychotic disorders from DSM-III (American Psychiatric Association 1981) to DSM-IIIR (American Psychiatric Association 1987; Kendler *et al.* 1989), and again from DSM-IIIR to DSM-IV (American Psychiatric Association 1994).

Delusional disorder

According to the DSM, current evidence from demographic, family and follow-up studies suggests that delusional disorder is probably distinct from both schizophrenia and mood disorders. In the three recent editions of the classification, the essential feature of the disorder is the presence of one or more persistent delusions that are not caused by any other mental disorder, such as schizophrenia, schizophreniform disorder, a mood disorder, an organic factor or the direct effects of a substance. Apart from the impact of the delusion(s) or its ramifications, functioning is not markedly impaired and behaviour is not obviously odd or bizarre.

The term 'paranoid', which was used in DSM-III to designate this type of disorder, has been changed to 'delusional' disorder in DSM-IIIR and DSM-IV. While the diagnosis of paranoid disorder could only be applied to people with delusions of persecution or jealousy, the inclusion criteria for delusional disorder are much broader in that they require only the presence of one or more 'non-bizarre' (non-schizophrenic) delusions, without further specification.

Two other important changes that were made in the criteria for delusional disorder in DSM-IIIR have been retained in DSM-IV. First, the minimum duration of the disorder has been increased from 1 week to 1 month and, secondly, persistent tactile and olfactory hallucinations are no longer excluded if related to the delusional theme (whereas auditory or visual hallucinations may not be present for more than a few hours).

Delusional disorder can be subdivided according to the predominant delusional theme in erotomanic type, grandiose type, jealous type, persecutory type, somatic type, mixed type (when delusions characteristic of more than one type are present but no one theme predominates) or unspecified type.

Although the prevalence is low, the disorder is not rare. Age of onset is usually middle or late adulthood; the older age being associated with the persecutory type, the younger with the somatic type (Yamada *et al.* 1998). The course is variable. Familial transmission is suspected and comorbid mood disorders may be present (Manschreck 1996). Cases seem to respond equally well to treatment whatever the specific delusional content and, when adequately treated, the prognosis is reasonably good (Munro & Mok 1995).

Campana *et al.* (1998) studied eye-tracking abnormalities in patients with delusional disorder and compared them with normal controls. They found abnormalities in smooth pursuit eye movements, which they concluded indicates a cerebral dysfunction similar to those detected in patients with schizophrenia.

Brief reactive psychosis and brief psychotic disorder

In DSM-III, the essential feature of brief reactive psychosis is the sudden onset of psychotic symptoms shortly after a recognizable psychosocial stressor, persisting for no more than 2 weeks, and with a full return to the premorbid level of functioning. In DSM-IIIR, the maximum duration of the disorder has been increased from 2 to 4 weeks, and there is acknowledgement that the stressors may be cumulative.

In DSM-IV, brief reactive disorder is listed as a subtype of a new category labelled brief psychotic disorder. The disorder is subdivided into three subtypes: with marked stressor(s), corresponding to the definition of brief reactive psychosis; without marked stressor(s); and with postpartum onset.

Schizophreniform disorder

The essential features of this disorder are identical to those of schizophrenia, with the exception that the duration is less than 6 months (but at least 1 month). Two subtypes may be specified, according to the presence or absence of 'good prognostic features' such as rapid onset, confusion or perplexity, good premorbid functioning and absence of blunted or flat affect.

There is little support for 'schizophreniform disorder' as a distinct diagnostic entity and a subtype of schizophrenia or affective illness. The clinical utility of the diagnosis is limited because it identifies a heterogeneous group of patients with new-onset schizophrenia, schizoaffective disorder and atypical affective disorder and only a small subgroup with a remitting non-affective psychosis, and a substantial number of patients are being rediagnosed during follow-up as schizophrenic. A review suggests that patients meeting criteria for schizophreniform disorder should instead be diagnosed as having 'psychotic disorder not otherwise specified' until additional clinical information (e.g. course of illness) becomes available (Strakowski 1994). Furthermore, the recent demonstration of impaired antioxidant defence and higher plasma lipid peroxides in unmedicated schizophreniform disorder than in normal controls was similar to the findings in unmedicated patients with first-episode schizophrenia (Mahadik et al. 1998). In addition, significantly higher soluble interleukin 2 receptor (sIL-2R) levels than normal controls were found in the sera of patients with both schizophrenia and schizophreniform disorder, thus implicating similar immunological mechanisms in both (Gaughran et al. 1998).

Schizoaffective disorder

The definition of schizoaffective disorder has been modified from DSM-III to DSM-IIIR, and again from DSM-IIIR to DSM-IV. In DSM-IV, the diagnosis is given to individuals who have had an uninterrupted period of illness during which, at some time, there was a major depressive episode or manic episode concurrent with symptoms of schizophrenia. During the same period of illness, there must have been delusions and hallucinations for at least 2 weeks in the absence of prominent mood symptoms. In addition, symptoms meeting criteria for a mood episode must be present for a substantial portion of the total duration of the illness.

Shared psychotic disorder

The DSM-IV definition of shared delusional disorder corresponds to the original description of folie à deux given by Lasègue and Falret (1877). A critical review of 61 case reports from 1942 to 1943 reveals that:
1 males and females were affected with equal frequency;
2 prevalence was equal in younger and older patients;
3 the majority of shared psychoses (90.2%) were equally distributed among married couples, siblings and parent–child dyads;
4 comorbid dementia, depression and mental retardation were common;
5 hallucinations were common; and
6 the majority of dyads (67.3%) were socially isolated.
The article concludes that shared psychotic disorder probably occurs in premorbidly disposed individuals in the context of social isolation that is shared with a psychotic person (Silveira & Seeman 1995).

Schizotypal personality disorder

In DSM-III, DSM-IIIR and DSM-IV, schizotypal disorder is listed among the personality disorders.

Atypical psychotic disorders in ICD-10

In ICD-10 (WHO 1992; Sartorius et al. 1993), atypical psychotic disorders (as defined here) are subdivided into five groups:
1 persistent delusional disorders;
2 acute and transient psychotic disorders;
3 induced delusional disorder;
4 schizoaffective disorder;
5 schizotypal disorder.
The ICD-10 classification of atypical psychotic disorders is presented in Table 5.4.

Persistent delusional disorder

The group of persistent delusional disorders includes a variety of disorders in which long-standing delusions constitute the only, or the most conspicuous, clinical characteristic, and which can-

Table 5.4 ICD-10 classification of non-organic atypical psychotic disorders.

F21	Schizotypal disorder	
F22	Persistent delusional disorders	
	F22.0	Delusional disorder (the following types may be specified if desired: persecutory, litigious, self-referential, grandiose, hypochondriacal, jealous, erotomanic
	F22.8	Other persistent delusional disorders
	F22.9	Persistent delusional disorder, unspecified
F23	Acute and transient psychotic disorders	
	F23.0	Acute polymorphic psychotic disorder without symptoms of schizophrenia
	F23.1	Acute polymorphic psychotic disorder with symptoms of schizophrenia
	F23.2	Acute schizophrenia-like psychotic disorder
	F23.3	Other acute predominantly delusional psychotic disorder
	F23.8	Other acute and transient psychotic disorders
	F23.9	Acute and transient psychotic disorders, unspecified

A fifth character may be used to identify the presence or absence of associated acute stress:
F23.x0 Without associated acute stress
F23.x1 With associated acute stress

F24	Induced delusional disorder	
F25	Schizoaffective disorders	
	F25.0	Schizoaffective disorder, manic type
	F25.1	Schizoaffective disorder, depressed type
	F25.2	Schizoaffective disorder, mixed type
	F25.8	Other schizoaffective disorders
	F25.9	Schizoaffective disorder, unspecified
F28	Other non-organic psychotic disorders	
F29	Unspecified non-organic psychosis	

not be classified as organic, schizophrenic or affective. They are probably heterogeneous and have uncertain relationships to schizophrenia. The relative importance of genetic factors, personality characteristics and life circumstances in their genesis is uncertain and probably variable.

The category is subdivided into delusional disorder, other persistent delusional disorder and unspecified persistent delusional disorder.

Delusional disorder is characterized by the development of either a single delusion or a set of related delusions other than those listed as typically schizophrenic. The delusions are highly variable in content, the most common examples being persecutory, grandiose, hypochondriacal, jealous or erotic. They must be present for at least 3 months; they are usually persistent and sometimes lifelong. Persistent hallucinations in any modality must not be present and the general criteria of schizophrenia must not be fulfilled. Depressive symptoms may be present intermittently, provided that the delusions persist at times when there is no disturbance of mood. The following subtypes may be specified: persecutory, litigious, self-referential, grandiose, hypochondriacal or somatic, jealous and erotomanic.

The diagnostic criteria for research that are posed in ICD-10 for delusional disorder are presented in Table 5.5.

The category 'other persistent delusional disorders' should be used to classify disorders in which delusions are accompanied by persistent hallucinatory voices or by schizophrenic symptoms that are insufficient to meet the criteria for schizophrenia.

Acute and transient psychotic disorders

ICD-10 explicitly recognizes that systematic clinical information that should provide definite guidance on the classification of acute and transient psychotic disorders is not yet available, and the limited data and clinical tradition that must therefore be used instead do not give rise to concepts that can be clearly defined and separated from each other.

The general diagnostic criteria for research that are proposed in ICD-10 for the group of acute and transient psychotic disorders are presented in Table 5.6.

To classify the disorders in this group, ICD-10 uses a diagnostic sequence that reflects the order of priority given to selected key features. Acute and transient psychotic disorders are subdivided according to whether the onset is acute (within a period of 2 weeks or less) or abrupt (within 48 h or less), whether the typical syndrome is polymorphic or typical of schizophrenia, and whether or not it is associated with acute stress. None of the disorders in the group meets the criteria for manic or depressive episodes, although emotional changes may be prominent from time to time. The disorders are also defined by the absence of

Table 5.5 Delusional disorder: ICD-10 diagnostic criteria for research.

A   A delusion or set of related delusions, other than those listed as typically schizophrenic (i.e. other than completely impossible or culturally inappropriate), must be present. The most common examples are persecutory, grandiose, hypochondriacal, jealous or erotic delusions

B   The delusion(s) in the first criterion must be present for at least 3 months

C   The general criteria for schizophrenia are not fulfilled

D   There must be no persistent hallucinations in any modality (but there may be transitory or occasional auditory hallucinations that are not in the third person or giving a running commentary)

E   Depressive symptoms (or even a depressive episode) may be present intermittently, provided that the delusions persist at times when there is no disturbance of mood

F   Most commonly used exclusion criteria. There must be no evidence of primary or secondary organic mental disorder, or of a psychotic disorder as a result of psychoactive substance use

Specification for possible subtypes. The following types may be specified if desired: persecutory, litiginous, self-referential, grandiose, hypochondriacal (somatic), jealous, erotomanic

Table 5.6 Acute and transient psychotic disorders: ICD-10 diagnostic criteria for research.

G1   There is acute onset of delusions, hallucinations, incomprehensible or incoherent speech, or any combination of these. The interval between the first appearance of any psychotic symptoms and the presentation of the fully developed disorder should not exceed 2 weeks

G2   If transient states of perplexity, misidentification or impairment of attention and concentration are present, they do not fulfil the criteria for organically caused clouding of consciousness

G3   The disorder does not meet the symptomatic criteria for manic episode, depressive episode or recurrent depressive disorder

G4   There is insufficient evidence of recent psychoactive substance use to fulfil the criteria for intoxication, harmful use, dependence or withdrawal states. The continued moderate and largely unchanged use of alcohol or drugs in amounts or with the frequency to which the individual is accustomed does not necessarily rule out the use of this category; this must be decided by clinical judgement and the requirements of the research project in question

G5   Most commonly used exclusion clause. There must be no organic mental disorder or serious metabolic disturbances affecting the central nervous system (this does not include childbirth)

A fifth character should be used to specify whether the acute onset of the disorder is associated with acute stress (occurring 2 weeks or less before evidence of first psychotic symptoms)

For research purposes it is recommended that change of the disorder from a non-psychotic to a clearly psychotic state is further specified as either abrupt (onset within 48 h) or acute (onset in more than 48 h but less than 2 weeks)

organic causation and should not be diagnosed in the presence of obvious intoxication by a psychoactive substance.

The syndrome called 'polymorphic' is defined as a rapidly changing and variable state in which hallucinations, delusions, perceptual disturbances and emotional turmoil with intense feelings of happiness and ecstasy or anxiety and irritability are obvious but markedly variable, changing from day to day or even from hour to hour.

The most appropriate duration of acute and transient psychotic disorders is specified with regard to the duration of symptoms required for a diagnosis of schizophrenia and persistent delusional disorders. In ICD-10, the diagnosis of schizophrenia depends upon the presence of typical schizophrenic symptoms that persist for at least 1 month. When schizophrenic symptoms are consistently present during an acute psychotic disorder, the diagnosis should be changed to schizophrenia if the schizophrenic symptoms persist for more than 1 month. For patients with psychotic, but non-schizophrenic, symptoms that persist beyond 1 month, there is no need to change the diagnosis until the duration requirement of delusional disorder is reached (3 months).

Fifty-one patients with ICD-10 acute and transient psychotic disorder were followed up by a Danish team (Jorgensen *et al.* 1996). According to DSM-IV criteria these patients were classified into three diagnostic categories: schizophreniform disorder (41%), brief psychotic disorder (33%) and psychotic disorder not otherwise classified (25%). After a 1-year follow-up, the authors found that 52% of the patients had diagnostic stability. The rest had their diagnosis changed to either affective disorder (28%) or schizophrenia (15%). Demographic, social and clinical data could not differentiate between patients who changed their diagnosis and those who did not. Patients with an unchanged diagnosis continued to functioned fairly well throughout the year psychosocially, but brief psychotic episodes with an acute onset may also be an early manifestation of severe mental disorder (Jorgensen *et al.* 1997).

Induced delusional disorder

The ICD-10 definition of induced delusional disorder corresponds to the original description by Lasègue and Falret (1877).

Schizoaffective disorders

According to ICD-10, schizoaffective disorders are episodic disorders in which both affective and schizophrenic symptoms are prominent within the same episode of illness, and concurrently for at least part of the episode. The diagnosis rests upon an approximate equilibrium between the number, severity and duration of schizophrenic and affective symptoms. The disorder is subdivided into manic, depressive and mixed types. Two further subtypes may be specified according to the longitudinal development of the disorder, i.e. to whether or not schizophrenic symptoms persist beyond the duration of affective symptoms.

Table 5.7 Schizotypal disorder: ICD-10 diagnostic criteria for research.

A   The subject must have manifested at least four of the following over a period of at least 2 years, either continuously or repeatedly:
  1   Inappropriate or constricted affect, with the individual appearing cold and aloof
  2   Behaviour or appearance that is odd, eccentric or peculiar
  3   Poor rapport with others and a tendency to social withdrawal
  4   Odd beliefs or magical thinking, influencing behaviour and inconsistent with subcultural norms
  5   Suspiciousness or paranoid ideas
  6   Ruminations without inner resistance, often with dysmorphophobic, sexual or aggressive contents
  7   Unusual perceptual experiences, including somatosensory (bodily) or other illusions, depersonalization or derealization
  8   Vague, circumstantial, metaphoric, overelaborate or often stereotyped thinking, manifested by odd speech or in other ways, without gross incoherence
  9   Occasional transient quasipsychotic episodes with intense illusions, auditory or other hallucinations and delusion-like ideas, usually occurring without external provocation

B   The subject must never have met the criteria for schizophrenia

Schizotypal disorder

In ICD-10, schizotypal disorder is listed together with schizophrenia and delusional disorders. The diagnostic criteria for research that are proposed in ICD-10 for schizotypal disorder are presented in Table 5.7.

Conclusions

Atypical psychotic disorders represent a heterogeneous and poorly understood group of disorders. The nomenclature of these disorders is as uncertain as their nosological status. Little empirical evidence has been available up to now, and the limited data and clinical tradition used instead to define these disorders have generated concepts that remain controversial. However, there seems to be considerable international consensus as to which of these disorders should be classified, at least provisionally, apart from schizophrenia and the mood disorders. It is hoped that the specified atypical psychotic disorders that have been included in recent classification systems will lead to widespread critical appraisal of their usefulness and to increasingly rigorous empirical investigations into their true clinical value.

References

Almeida, O.P., Howard, R.J., Levy, R., *et al.* (1995) Clinical and cognitive diversity of psychotic states arising in late life (late paraphrenia). *Psychological Medicine* 25, 699–714.

American Psychiatric Association (1981) *Diagnostic and Statistical Manual of Mental Disorder (DSM-III)*, 3rd edn. American Psychiatric Association, Washington, DC.

American Psychiatric Association (1987) *Diagnostic and Statistical Manuel of Mental Disorder (DSM-IIIR)*, revised 3rd edn. American Psychiatric Association, Washington, DC.

American Psychiatric Association (1994) *Diagnostic and Statistical Manuel of Mental Disorder (DSM-IV)*, 4th edn. American Psychiatric Association, Washington, DC.

Anderson, D.N. & Williams, E. (1994) The delusion of inanimate doubles. *Psychopathology* **27**, 220–225.

Ballet, G. (1911) La psychose hallucinatoire chronique. *Encéphale* **11**, 401–411.

Bergem, A.M., Dahl, A.A., Guldberg, C.A. & Hansen, H. (1990) Langfeldt's schizophreniform psychoses fifty years later. *British Journal of Psychiatry* **157**, 351–354.

Berrios, G.E. & Luque, R. (1995a) Cotard's delusion or syndrome? A conceptual history. *Comprehensive Psychiatry* **36**, 218–223.

Berrios, G.E. & Luque, R. (1995b) Cotard's syndrome: analysis of 100 cases. *Acta Psychiatrica Scandinavica* **91**, 185–188.

Berson, R.J. (1983) Capgras' syndrome. *American Journal of Psychiatry* **140**, 969–978.

Breitner, B.C.C. & Anderson, D.N. (1994) The organic and psychological antecedents of delusional jealousy in old age. *International Journal of Geriatric Psychiatry* **9**, 703–707.

Brockington, I.F., Kendell, R.E. & Leff, J.P. (1978) Definitions of schizophrenia: concordance and prediction of outcome. *Psychological Medicine* **8**, 387–398.

Brockington, I.F., Perris, C., Kendell, R.E., Hillier, V.E. & Wainwright, S. (1982) The course and outcome of cycloid psychosis. *Psychological Medicine* **12**, 97–105.

Campana, A., Gambini, O. & Scarone, S. (1998) Delusional disorder and eye tracking dysfunction: preliminary evidence of biological and clinical heterogeneity. *Schizophrenia Research* **30**, 51–58.

Capgras, J. & Reboul-Lachaux, J. (1923) L'illusion des 'sosies' dans un délire systématisé chronique. *Annales Médico-Psychologiques* **81**, 186–193.

de Clérambault, G. (1942) *Oeuvre Psychiatrique*. Presses Universitaires de France, Paris.

Cotard, J. (1880) Du délire hypochondriaque dans une forme grave de la mélancolie anxieuse. *Annales Médico-Psychologiques* **38**, 168–174.

Cotard, J. (1882) Du délire des négations. *Archives de Neurologie* **11**, 152–170; and **12**, 282–296.

Cutting, J.C., Clarke, A.W. & Mann, A.H. (1978) Cycloid psychosis: an investigation of the diagnostic concept. *Psychological Medicine* **8**, 637–648.

Debruille, J.B. & Stip, E. (1996) Capgras syndrome: evolution of hypotheses. *Canadian Journal of Psychiatry* **41**, 181–187.

Dupré, E. & Logre, L. (1911) Les délires d'imagination: mythomanie délirante. *Encéphale* **10**, 209–232.

Edelstyn, N.M. & Oyebode, F. (1999) A review of the phenomenology and cognitive neuropsychological origins of the Capgras' syndrome. *International Journal of Geriatric Psychiatry* **14**, 48–59.

Ellis, H.D. (1994) The role of the right hemisphere in the Capgras delusion. *Psychopathology* **27**, 177–185.

Ellis, H.D., Quayle, A.H., de Pauw, K.W., *et al.* (1996) Delusional misidentification of inanimate objects: a literature review and neuropsychological analysis of cognitive deficits in two cases. *Cognitive Neuropsychiatry* **1**, 27–40.

Ellis, P. & Mellsop, G. (1985) De Clérambault's syndrome: a nosological entity? *British Journal of Psychiatry* **146**, 90–95.

Faergeman, P.M. (1963) *Psychogenic Psychoses: A Description and Follow-Up of Psychoses Following Psychological Stress*. Butterworths, London.

Ferrey, G. & Zebdi, S. (1999) Evolution et pronostic des troubles psychotiques aigus (bouffée délirante polymorphe). *Encéphale* **25**, 26–32.

Forsell, Y. & Henderson, A.S. (1998) Epidemiology of paranoid symptoms in an elderly population. *British Journal of Psychiatry* **172**, 429–432.

Franzek, E., Becker, T., Hofmann, E. *et al.* (1996) Is computerized tomography ventricular abnormality related to cycloid psychosis? *Biological Psychiatry* **40**, 1255–1266.

Garmezy, N. (1968) Process and reactive schizophrenia: some conceptions and issues. In: *The Role and Methodology of Classification in Psychiatry and Psychopathology* (eds M.M. Katz, J.O. Cole & W.E. Barton), pp. 419–430. Government Printing Office, Washington, DC.

Gaughran, F., O'Neil, E., Cole, M., *et al.* (1998) Increased soluble interleukin 2 receptor levels in schizophrenia. *Schizophrenia Research* **29**, 263–267.

Gelder, M., Gath, D. & Mayou, R. (1989) Paranoid symptoms and paranoid syndromes. *Oxford Textbook of Psychiatry*, 2nd edn, pp. 324–344. Oxford University Press, Oxford.

Gerrans, P. (2000) Refining the explanation of Cotard's delusion. *Mind and Language* **15**, 111–122.

Gottesman, I. & Bertelsen, A. (1989) Dual mating studies in psychiatry: offspring of inpatients with examples from reactive (psychogenic) psychoses. *International Review of Psychiatry* **1**, 287–295.

Grahame, P.S. (1984) Schizophrenia in old age (late paraphrenia). *British Journal of Psychiatry* **145**, 493–495.

Guldberg, C.A., Dahl, A.A., Hansen, H. & Bergem, A.M. (1991) Were Langfeldt's schizophreniform psychoses really affective? *Psychopathology* **24**, 270–276.

Hatta, S.M. (1996) A Malay crosscultural worldview and forensic review of amok. *Australian and New Zealand Journal of Psychiatry* **30**, 505–510.

Hoffler, J., Braunig, P., Kruger, S. & Ludvik, M. (1997) Morphology according to cranial computed tomography of first episode cycloid psychosis and its long-term course differences compared to schizophrenia. *Acta Psychiatrica Scandinavica* **96**, 184–187.

Holden, N.L. (1987) Late paraphrenia or the paraphrenias? A descriptive study with a 10-year follow-up. *British Journal of Psychiatry* **150**, 635–639.

Howard, R., Casde, D., Wessely, S. & Murray, R. (1993) A comparative study of 470 cases of early-onset and late-onset schizophrenia. *British Journal of Psychiatry* **163**, 352–357.

Howard, R., Almeida, O. & Levy, R. (1994) Phenomenology, demography and diagnosis in late paraphrenia. *Psychological Medicine* **24**, 397–410.

Jordan, H.W. & Howe, G. (1980) De Clérambault syndrome (erotomania): a review and case presentation. *Journal of the National Medical Association* **72**, 979–985.

Jorgensen, P., Bennedsen, B., Christensen, J. & Hyllested, A. (1996) Acute and transient psychotic disorder: comorbidity with personality disorder. *Acta Psychiatrica Scandinavica* **94**, 460–464.

Jorgensen, P., Bennedsen, B., Christensen, J. & Hyllested, A. (1997) Acute and transient psychotic disorder: a 1-year follow-up study. *Acta Psychiatrica Scandinavica* **96**, 150–154.

Kendell, R.E. (1993) Paranoid disorders. In: *Companion to Psychiatric Studies* (eds R.E. Kendell & A.K. Zealley), pp. 459–471. Churchill Livingstone, Edinburgh.

Kendler, K.S., McGuire, M., Gruenberg, A.M., *et al.* (1993) The Roseommon Family Study. II. The risk of non-schizophrenic non-affective psychoses in relatives. *Archives of General Psychiatry* 50, 645–652.

Kendler, S.K. (1980) The nosologic validity of paranoia (simple delusional disorder): a review. *Archives of General Psychiatry* 37, 699–706.

Kendler, S.K., Gruenberg, A.M. & Strauss, J.S. (1981) An independent analysis of the Copenhagen sample of the Danish Adoption Study of schizophrenia. *Archives of General Psychiatry* 38, 985–987.

Kendler, S.K., Masterson, C.C. & Davis, K.L. (1985) Psychiatric illness in first-degree relatives of patients with paranoid psychosis, schizophrenia and medical illness. *British Journal of Psychiatry* 147, 524–531.

Kendler, S.K., Spitzer, R.L. & Williams, J.B.W. (1989) Psychotic disorders in DSM-IIIR. *American Journal of Psychiatry* 146, 953–962.

Kety, S.S., Rosenthal, D., Wender, P.H., Schulsinger, F. & Jacobson, B. (1978) The biologic and adoptive families of adopted individuals who became schizophrenic: prevalence of mental illness and other characteristics. In: *The Nature of Schizophrenia* (ed. L.D. Wynne). John Wiley & Sons, New York.

Kirrane, R.M. & Siever, L.J. (2000) New perspectives on schizotypal personality disorder. *Current Psychiatry Reports* 2, 62–66.

Kon, Y. (1994) Amok. *British Journal of Psychiatry* 165, 685–689.

Kraepelin, E. (1899) *Psychiatrie: Ein Lehrbuch Fur Studierende und Aerzte*, 6th edn. Barth, Leipzig.

Kraepelin, E. (1909–15) *Psychiatrie. Ein Lehrbuch Fur Studierende und Aerzte*, 8th edn. Barth, Leipzig.

Kretschmer, E. (1918) *Der Sensitive Beziehungswahn*. Springer-Verlag, Berlin.

Lanczik, M., Fritze, J. & Beckmann, H. (1990) Puerperal and cycloid psychoses: results of a retrospective study. *Psychopathology* 23, 220–227.

Langfeldt, G. (1939) *The Schizophreniform States*. Munsksgaard, Copenhagen/Oxford University Press, Oxford.

Langfeldt, G. (1961) The erotic jealousy syndrome: a clinical study. *Acta Psychiatrica Scandinavica Supplement* 151.

Lasègue, C. & Falret, J. (1877) La folie à deux ou folie communiquée. *Annales Médico-Psychologiques* 18, 321.

Legrain, M. (1886) *Du Délire Chez les Dégénérés*. Deshaye et Lecrosoier, Paris.

Leong, G.B., Silva, J.A., Garza-Trevino, E.S. *et al.* (1994) The dangerousness of persons with the Othello syndrome. *Journal of Forensic Sciences* 39, 1445–1454.

Leonhard, K. (1957) *Aufteilung der Endogenen Psychosen*. Akademie Verlag, Berlin.

Lindvall, M., Hagnell, O. & Ohman, R. (1990) Epidemiology of cycloid psychosis. *Psychopathology* 23, 228–232.

Magnan, V. & Legrain, M. (1895) *Les Dégénérés (Etat Mental et Syndromes Episodiques)*. Rueff et Cie, Paris.

Mahadik, S.P., Mukherjee, S., Scheffer, R., Correnti, E.F. & Mahadik, J.S. (1998) Elevated plasma lipid peroxes at the onset of non-affective psychosis. *Biological Psychiatry* 43, 674–679.

Maj, M. (1990) Cycloid psychotic disorder: validation of the concept by means of a follow-up and a family study. *Psychopathology* 23, 196–204.

Manschreck, T.C. (1996) Delusional disorder: the recognition and management of paranoia. *Journal of Clinical Psychiatry* 57 (Suppl. 3), 32–38.

Mowat, R.R. (1966) *Morbid Jealousy and Murder*. Tavistock, London.

Mullen, P.E. & Maack, L.H. (1985) Jealousy, pathological jealousy and aggression. In: *Aggression and Dangerousness* (eds D.P. Farington & J. Gunn), pp. 103–126. Wiley, Chicester.

Mullen, P.E., Pathé, M. & Purcell, R. (2000) *Stalkers and Their Victims*. Cambridge University Press, Cambridge.

Munro, A. & Mok, H. (1995) An overview of treatment in paranoia/delusional disorder. *Canadian Journal of Psychiatry* 40, 616–622.

Odom-White, A., de Leon, J., Stanilla, J. *et al.* (1995) Misidentification syndromes in schizophrenia: case reviews with implications for classification and prevalence. *Australian and New Zealand Journal of Psychiatry* 29, 63–68.

Opjordsmoen, S. & Retterstol, N. (1987) Hypochondriacal delusions in paranoid psychoses: course and outcome compared with other types of delusions. *Psychopathology* 20, 272–284.

de Pauw, K.W. (1994a) Delusional misidentification: a plea for an agreed terminology and classification. *Psychopathology* 27, 123–129.

de Pauw, K.W. (1994b) Psychodynamic approaches to the Capgras delusion: a critical historical review. *Psychopathology* 27, 154–160.

Perris, C. (1974) A study of cycloid psychoses. *Acta Psychiatrica Scandinavica Supplement* 253.

Pfuhlmann, B., Stöber, G., Franzek, E. & Beckmann, H. (1998) Cycloid psychoses predominate in severe postpartum psychiatric disorders. *Journal of Affective Disorders* 50, 125–134.

Pichot, P. (1983) *A Century of Psychiatry*. Roger Dacosta, Paris.

Pichot, P. (1990) The diagnosis and classification of mental disorders in the French-speaking countries: background, current values and comparison with other classifications. In: *Sources and Traditions of Classification in Psychiatry* (eds N. Sartorius, A. Jablensky, D.A. Regier *et al.*), pp. 7–58. Hofgrete & Huber, Toronto.

Pichot, P. & Debray, H. (1971) *Hospitalisation Psychiatrique: Statistique Descriptive*. Sandoz Editions, Paris.

Pitta, J.C.N. & Blay, S.L. (1997) Psychogenic (reactive) and hysterical psychoses: a cross-system reliability study. *Acta Psychiatrica Scandinavica* 95, 112–118.

Pull, C.B., Pull, M.C. & Pichot, P. (1987) Des critères empiriques francais pour les psychoses. III. Algorithmes et arbre de décision. *Encéphale* 13, 59–66.

Raskin, D.E. & Sullivan, K.E. (1974) Erotomania. *American Journal of Psychiatry* 131, 1033–1035.

Ravindran, A.V., Yatham, L.N. & Munro, A. (1999) Paraphrenia redefined. *Canadian Journal of Psychiatry* 44, 133–137.

Remington, G. & Book, H. (1984) Case report of de Clérambault syndrome, bipolar affective disorder, and response to lithium. *American Journal of Psychiatry* 141, 1285–1287.

Roth, M. (1955) The natural history of mental disorder in old age. *Journal of Mental Science* 101, 281–301.

Sartorius, N., Jablenski, A., Korten, A. *et al.* (1986) Early manifestations and first contact incidence of schizophrenia in different cultures: a preliminary report on the initial evaluation phase of the WHO Collaborative Study on Determinants of Outcome of Severe Mental Disorders. *Psychological Medicine* 16, 909–928.

Sartorius, N., Kaelber, C.T. Cooper, J.E. *et al.* (1993) Progress toward achieving a common language in psychiatry: results from the field trial of the Clinical Guidelines accompanying the WHO Classification of Mental and Behavioural Disorders in ICD-10. *Archives of General Psychiatry* 50, 115–124.

Schanda, H. (2000) Paranoia and dysphoria: historical developments, current concepts. *Psychopathology* 33, 204–208.

Schanda, H. & Gabriel, E. (1988) Position of affective symptomatology in the course of delusional psychoses. *Psychopathology* 21, 1–11.

Schmidt-Degenhard, M. (1998) The history and psychopathology of paranoia. *Fortschritte der Neurologie-Psychiatrie* 66, 313–325.

Sérieux, P. & Capgras, J. (1909) *Les Folies Raisonnantes: le Délire d'Interprétation*. Felix Arcan, Paris.

Shepherd, M. (1961) Morbid jealousy: some clinical and social aspects of a psychiatric symptom. *Journal of Mental Science* **107**, 687–753.

Sigmund, D. & Mundt, C. (1999) The cycloid type and its differentiation from core schizophrenia: a phenomenological approach. *Comprehensive Psychiatry* **40**, 4–18.

Signer, S.F. (1991a) 'Les psychoses passionnelles' reconsidered: a review of de Clérambault's cases and syndrome with respect to mood disorders. *Journal of Psychiatry and Neuroscience* **16**, 81–90.

Signer, S.F. (1991b) Erotomania. *American Journal of Psychiatry* **148**, 1276.

Signer, S.F. (1994) Localization and lateralization in the delusion of substitution. *Psychopathology* **27**, 168–176.

Signer, S.F. & Cummings, J.L. (1987) De Clérambault's syndrome in organic affective disorder: two cases. *British Journal of Psychiatry* **151**, 404–407.

Signer, S.F. & Swinson, R.P. (1987) Two cases of erotomania (de Clérambault's syndrome) in bipolar affective disorder. *British Journal of Psychiatry* **151**, 853–855.

Silva, J.A., Ferrari, M.M., Leong, G.B. & Penny, G. (1998) The dangerousness of persons with delusional jealousy. *Journal of the American Academy of Psychiatry and the Law* **26**, 607–623.

Silveira, J.M. & Seeman, M.V. (1995) Shared psychotic disorder: a critical review of the literature. *Canadian Journal of Psychiatry* **40**, 389–395.

Sims, A. & Reddie, M. (1976) The de Clérambault and Capgras history. *British Journal of Psychiatry* **129**, 95–96.

Sims, A. & White, A. (1973) Coexistence of Capgras and de Clérambault's syndromes: a case history. *British Journal of Psychiatry* **123**, 635–637.

Staner, L. (1991) Sleep, dexamethasone suppression test, and response to somatic therapies in an atypical affective state presenting as erotomania: a case report. *European Psychiatry* **6**, 269–271.

Stöber, G., Kocher, I., Franzek, E. & Beckmann, H. (1997) First trimester maternal gestation infection and cycloid psychosis. *Acta Psychiatrica Scandinavica* **96**, 319–324.

Strakowski, S.M. (1994) Diagnostic validity of schizophreniform disorder. *American Journal of Psychiatry* **151**, 815–824.

Strik, W.K., Fallgatter, A.J., Stöber, G., Franzek, E. & Beckmann, H. (1997) Specific P300 features in cycloid psychosis. *Acta Psychiatrica Scandinavica* **95**, 67–72.

Strömgren, E. (1974) Psychogenic psychoses. In: *Themes and Variations in European Psychiatry* (eds S.R. Hirsch & M. Shepherd), pp. 97–117. Wright & Sons, Bristol.

Strömgren, E. (1989) The development of the concept of reactive psychoses. *British Journal of Psychiatry* **154**, 47–50.

Tsai, S.-J., Hwang, J.-P., Yang, C.-H. & Liu, K.-M. (1997) Delusional jealousy in dementia. *Journal of Clinical Psychiatry* **58**, 492–494.

Vauhkonen, K. (1968) On the pathogenesis of morbid jealousy. *Acta Psychiatrica Scandinavica Supplement* **202**, 1–261.

Weinstein, E.A. (1994) The classification of delusional misidentification syndromes. *Psychopathology* **27**, 130–135.

Wimmer, A. (1916) Psykogene Sindssygdomsformer. *Sct. Hans Mental Hospital 1816–1916*, Jubilee Publication, pp. 85–216. Gad, Copenhagen.

World Health Organization (1992) *The ICD-10 Classification of Mental and Behavioural Disorders: Clinical Descriptions and Diagnostic Guidelines*. World Health Organization, Geneva.

World Health Organization (1993) *The ICD-10 Classification of Mental and Behavioural Disorders: Diagnostic Criteria for Research*. World Health Organization, Geneva.

Yamada, N., Nakajima, S. & Noguchi, T. (1998) Age at onset of delusional disorder is dependent on the delusional theme. *Acta Psychiatrica Scandinavica* **97**, 122–124.

Young, A.W., Leafhead, K.M. & Szulecka, T.K. (1994) The Capgras and Cotard delusions. *Psychopathology* **27**, 226–231.

6

Late-onset schizophrenia

R. Howard and D. V. Jeste

This chapter considers what has historically been a contentious area. Schizophrenia is generally regarded as an illness with onset in early adult life, yet cases of an illness that shows only minor phenotypical differences can arise for the first time in middle age and late life. Psychiatrists initially squabbled over whether or not such cases really existed. Once it was established that they did, researchers then disagreed about how they might relate to more 'typical' schizophrenia and what to call them. It may be difficult to understand the current view of these psychoses without some consideration of the historical development of the concepts and diagnoses involved.

Historical development

Both Kraepelin (1913) and Bleuler (1911) observed that there was a relatively small group of patients with schizophrenia who had an illness onset in late middle or old age and who, on clinical grounds, closely resembled those who had an onset in early adult life. Utilizing a very narrow conception of dementia praecox and specifically excluding cases of paraphrenia, Kraepelin (1913) reported that only 5.6% of 1054 patients had an onset after the age of 40 years. If the age of onset was set at 60 years or greater, only 0.2% of patients could be included.

Manfred Bleuler (1943) carried out the first specific and systematic examination of late-onset patients and defined late schizophrenia as follows:
1 onset after the age of 40;
2 symptomatology that does not differ from that of schizophrenia occurring early in life (or, if it does differ, it should not do so in a clear or radical way); and
3 it should not be possible to attribute the illness to a neuropathological disorder because of the presence of an amnestic syndrome or associated signs of organic brain disease.
Bleuler found that between 15% and 17% of two large series of schizophrenia patients had an onset after the age of 40. Of such late-onset cases, only 4% had become ill for the first time after the age of 60. Later authors confirmed that while onset of

schizophrenia after the age of 40 was unusual, onset after 60 should be considered even more rare. From 264 elderly schizophrenia patients admitted in Edinburgh in 1957, only seven had an illness that had begun after the age of 60 (Fish 1958). Using very broad criteria for the diagnosis of schizophrenia (including schizoaffective, paraphrenic and other non-organic non-affective psychoses) and studying 470 first contacts with the Camberwell Register, Howard *et al.* (1993) found 29% of cases to have been over 44 years at onset. Based on a literature review, Harris and Jeste (1988) noted that 23% of all schizophrenia inpatients reportedly had onset of their illness after age 40. There seemed to be a progressive decline in the number of patients with onset in later years.

Kraepelin and E. Bleuler both considered late-onset cases to have much in common with more typically early-onset schizophrenia and this view was supported by M. Bleuler's report (1943) of only very mild phenomenological variance from early-onset cases. However, his 126 late-onset cases were symptomatically milder, had less affective flattening and were less likely to have formal thought disorder than patients with a younger onset. Fish (1960) reported that the clinical picture presented by 23 patients with onset after 40 years did not differ importantly from patients who were younger at onset, but he believed that with increasing age at onset schizophrenia took on a more 'paraphrenic' form.

The European use of late paraphrenia

The notion of paraphrenia as a distinct diagnostic entity had been discredited by Mayer's follow-up of Kraepelin's 78 original cases. At least 40% of these patients had developed clear signs of dementia praecox within a few years and only 36% could still be classified as paraphrenic. Many of the paraphrenic patients had positive family histories of schizophrenia and the presenting clinical picture of those patients who remained 'true' paraphrenics did not differ from those who were later to develop signs of schizophrenia. Roth and Morrisey (1952) resurrected both the terminology and the controversy with their choice of the term 'late paraphrenia' to describe patients who they believed had schizophrenia, but with an onset delayed until after the age of 55 or 60 years. The term was intended to be descriptive: to distinguish the illness from the chronic schizophrenia patients seen in psychiatric institutions at the time and to emphasize the clinical similarities with the illness described by Kraepelin. Choice of the term was perhaps unfortunate because two particular points of misconception often seem to arise in relation to it and it is vital to set these straight. Late paraphrenia was never intended to mean the same thing as paraphrenia and Kraepelin certainly did not emphasize late age of onset as a feature of the illness. Kay and Roth (1961) studied a group of 39 female and three male patients diagnosed with late paraphrenia in Graylingwell Hospital between 1951 and 1955. All but six of these cases were followed up for 5 years. The case records of 48 female and nine male late paraphrenia patients admitted to a hospital in Stockholm between 1931 and 1940 were also collected and these cases were followed up till death or until 1956. Over 40% of the Graylingwell late paraphrenia patients were living alone, compared with 12% of affective disorder patients and 16% of those with organic psychoses who were of comparable ages. Late paraphrenia patients were also socially isolated. Although the frequency of visual impairment at presentation (15%) was no higher than that in comparison groups with other diagnoses, some impairment of hearing was present in 40% of late paraphrenic patients and this was considered severe in 15%. Deafness was only present in 7% of affective disorder patients. Focal cerebral disease was identified in only 8% of late paraphrenic patients at presentation. Primary delusions, feelings of mental or physical influence and hallucinations were all prominent and the prognosis for recovery was judged to be poor. From a detailed analysis of 1250 first admissions to a hospital in Gothenburg, Sjoegren (1964) identified 202 elderly individuals who conformed to the French concept of paraphrenia (Magnan 1893): well-organized and persistent paranoid delusions with hallucinations occurring in clear consciousness. Sjoegren argued cogently that, together with constitutional factors, ageing itself produced effects (feelings of isolation and loneliness, social and economic insecurity and heightened vulnerability) which contributed to the development of paranoid reactions.

Post (1966) collected a sample of 93 patients to whom he gave the non-controversial and self-explanatory label 'persistent persecutory states' and made a point of including cases regardless of coexisting organic brain change. Within this broad category he recognized three clinical subtypes: a schizophrenic syndrome (34 of 93 patients), a schizophreniform syndrome (37 patients) and a paranoid hallucinosis group (22 patients). Post regarded those patients with the schizophrenic syndrome as having a delayed form of the illness with only partial expression. Post's patients were treated with phenothiazines and he was able to demonstrate that the condition was responsive to antipsychotic medication. Success or failure of treatment was related to the adequacy of phenothiazine treatment and its long-term maintenance.

From a series of 45 female and two male late paraphrenic patients (identified using the same criteria as Kay & Roth's) admitted to St Francis' Hospital in Hayward's Heath between 1958 and 1964, Herbert and Jacobson (1967) confirmed many of Kay and Roth's (1961) observations. In addition, these investigators found an unexpectedly high prevalence of schizophrenia among the mothers (4.4%) and siblings (13.3%) of their patients.

Current diagnosis of patients within ICD-10 and DSM-IV

Diagnostic guidelines published by authoritative organizations such as the World Health Organization (WHO) or the American Psychiatric Association (APA) reflect the views of many contemporary clinicians who were consulted at the draft and field trial stages. Inclusion or exclusion of a particular diagnosis in published diagnostic schemes thus reflects the current credence given to the nosological validity of that diagnosis plus an indication of its general usefulness in clinical practice.

Late paraphrenia, included within ICD-9, has not survived as a separate codeable diagnosis into ICD-10. There are three possible diagnostic categories available for the accommodation of patients previously diagnosed as late paraphrenic: schizophrenia, delusional disorder and other persistent delusional disorders. It seems likely that most cases will be coded under schizophrenia (F20.0) (Quintal et al. 1991; Howard et al. 1994a), although the category of delusional disorder (F22.0) is suggested as a replacement for 'paraphrenia (late)' in the diagnostic guidelines. Distinction between cases of schizophrenia and delusional disorder within ICD-10 is very much dependent on the quality of auditory hallucinations experienced by patients and is subject to some unhelpful ageism. The guidelines for delusional disorder (F22.0) in ICD-10 state that: 'clear and persistent auditory hallucinations (voices) . . . are incompatible with this diagnosis'. Rather confusingly, the guidelines for a diagnosis of delusional disorder suggest that: 'occasional or transitory auditory hallucinations, particularly in elderly patients, do not rule out this diagnosis, provided that they are not typically schizophrenic and form only a small part of the overall clinical picture'. To add further to diagnostic dilemma, the guidelines also include the suggestion that: 'disorders in which delusions are accompanied by persistent hallucinatory voices or by schizophrenic symptoms that are insufficient to meet criteria for schizophrenia' should be coded under the category of other persistent delusional disorders (F22.8). Because the majority of late paraphrenic patients who hear distinct hallucinatory voices also have a rich variety of schizophrenic core symptoms, very few will be diagnosed as having other persistent delusional disorders.

The inclusion within DSM-IIIR (American Psychiatric Association 1987) of a separate category of late-onset schizophrenia for cases with an illness onset after the age of 44 years seems largely to have been a reaction to the unsatisfactory and arbitrary upper age limit for onset that had been included for DSM-III (American Psychiatric Association 1980) for a diagnosis of schizophrenia. DSM-IV (American Psychiatric Association 1994) contains no separate category for late-onset schizophrenia and this presumably reflects the current general North American view that there is a direct continuity between cases of schizophrenia whatever their age at onset.

Terminology and classification for the future

The important questions now are: have ICD-10 and DSM-IV been fair to abandon any facility for coding late-onset within schizophrenia, and do we need diagnostic categories that distinguish the functional psychoses with onset in later life from schizophrenia? These questions provided the spur to establish an international consensus on diagnosis and terminology (Howard *et al.* 2000), which may form the basis for consideration of these patients within future revisions of DSM and ICD. When the late-onset schizophrenia international consensus group met in 1998, it agreed that the available evidence from the areas of epidemiology, phenomenology and pathophysiology supported heterogeneity within schizophrenia with increasing age at onset up to the age of 60 years. Schizophrenia-like psychosis with onset after the age of 60 years (i.e. what some psychiatrists used to call late paraphrenia) was considered to be distinct from schizophrenia. The consensus group recommended that schizophrenia with onset between 40 and 59 years be termed late-onset schizophrenia and that chronic psychosis with onset after 60 years should be called very-late-onset schizophrenia-like psychosis (VLOSLP). The latter term is long-winded and unmemorable but at least is unambiguous and had the unprecedented support of both European and North American geriatric psychiatrists. There was no consensus regarding the exact age cut-offs of 40 and 60 years for defining late-onset schizophrenia and VLOSLP, and these were considered provisional until further research established evidence-based cut-points. From this point in this chapter the term late paraphrenia will be used only for patients already described as such in the literature.

Clinical features

Schizophrenic symptoms

Although Bleuler (1943) believed that it was not possible to separate early- and late-onset patients on clinical grounds, he acknowledged that a later onset was accompanied by less affective flattening and a more benign course. Formal thought disorder is seen in only about 5% of cases of DSM-IIIR late-onset schizophrenia (Pearlson *et al.* 1989) and could not be elicited from any of 101 late paraphrenic patients (Howard *et al.* 1994a). The first-rank symptoms of Schneider are seen, but may be somewhat less prevalent in later onset cases. Thought-insertion, block and withdrawal seem to be particularly uncommon (Grahame 1984; Pearlson *et al.* 1989; Howard *et al.* 1994b) and negative symptoms are less severe (Almeida *et al.* 1995a). In a multicentre study of late-onset schizophrenia, Jeste

et al. (1988) found that delusions, particularly of persecution, and auditory hallucinations were prominent in these patients. Late-onset schizophrenia typically resembled the paranoid subtype of early-onset schizophrenia. Other subtypes of schizophrenia, including catatonic and disorganized types, were very rare in old age. In studies at San Diego, Jeste *et al.* (1997) and Palmer *et al.* (2001) compared similarly aged patients with middle-age- and early-onset schizophrenia. The clinical symptoms were rated on the various scales used: Brief Psychiatric Rating Scale (BPRS), Scale for the Assessment of Positive Symptoms (SAPS), and Scale for the Assessment of Negative Symptoms (SANS) (Overall & Gorham 1962). The severity of positive symptoms was similar in the two groups, and both groups had significantly more positive symptoms, including thought disorder, than did normal subjects. Early-onset schizophrenia patients had more severe negative symptoms, including affective blunting, alogia, avolition and inattention, than did middle-age-onset schizophrenia patients. However, although middle-age-onset schizophrenia patients had less severe negative symptoms than early-onset schizophrenia patients, they still had consistently worse negative symptoms than normal subjects. These results suggest that middle-age-onset schizophrenia patients do have thought disorder and negative symptoms. It is worth noting that, by definition, patients with paranoid subtype lack a prominence of negative symptoms, and most patients with middle-age-onset schizophrenia have a paranoid type of schizophrenia (Andreasen 1982; Andreasen & Olsen 1982).

Delusions

Persecutory delusions usually dominate the presentation although, in a series of 101 late paraphrenic patients, delusions of reference (76%), control (25%), grandiose ability (12%) and of a hypochondriacal nature (11%) were also present (Howard *et al.* 1994a). Partition delusions are found in about two-thirds of cases and refer to the belief that people, animals, materials or radiation can pass through a structure that would normally constitute a barrier to such passage. This barrier is generally the door, ceiling, walls or floor of a patient's home and the source of intrusion is frequently a neighbouring residence (Herbert & Jacobson 1967; Pearlson *et al.* 1989; Howard & Levy 1992).

Affective symptoms

The coexistence of affective features in late-onset schizophrenia is well recognized clinically but there have been no controlled studies comparing such features in early- and late-onset cases. Atypical, schizoaffective and cycloid psychoses are all characterized by affective features, tend to arise later in life and affect women more than men (Cutting *et al.* 1978; Levitt & Tsuang 1988). Among late paraphrenic patients, Post (1966) reported depressive admixtures in 60% of cases, while Holden (1987) considered that 10 of his 24 'functional' late paraphrenic patients had affective or schizoaffective disorders. These patients also had a better outcome in terms both of institutionalization and 10-year survival compared with paranoid patients. Such observations have led to the suggestion that some later onset schizophrenic or late paraphrenic patients may have variants of primary affective disorder (Murray *et al.* 1992).

Cognitive deficits

Attempts to identify and characterize the patterns of cognitive impairment associated with these conditions began with Hopkins and Roth (1953), who administered the vocabulary subtest from the Wechsler–Bellevue Scale, a shortened form of Raven's Progressive Matrices, and a general test of orientation and information, to patients with a variety of diagnoses. Twelve late paraphrenic patients performed as well as a group of elderly depressive patients and better than patients with dementia on all three tests.

Naguib and Levy (1987) evaluated 43 late paraphrenic patients (having already excluded subjects with a diagnosable dementia) with the Mental Test Score (MTS), Digit Copying Test (DCT) and the Digit Symbol Substitution Test. Patients performed less well than age-matched controls on both the MTS and DCT.

Miller *et al.* (1991) have published neuropsychological data on patients with what they term 'late life psychosis'. These patients performed less well than age-matched controls on the Mini-Mental State Examination (MMSE), the Wechsler Adult Intelligence Scale–Revised, the Wisconsin Card Sorting Test, Logical Memory and Visual Reproduction subtests from the Wechsler Memory Scale, a test of verbal fluency and the Warrington Recognition Memory Test. However, patients were not well matched with controls for educational attainment and premorbid intelligence and some of the patients clearly had affective psychoses and dementia syndromes (Miller *et al.* 1992), so it is probably not fair to equate them with late paraphrenia or late-onset schizophrenia patients.

Almeida *et al.* (1995a) carried out a detailed neuropsychological examination of 40 patients with late paraphrenia in south London. Using cluster analysis of the results he identified two groups of patients. The first was a 'functional' group characterized by impairment restricted to executive functions, in particular a computerized test assessing extra- and intradimensional attention set shift ability and a test of planning. Such patients had a high prevalence and severity of positive psychotic symptoms and lower scores on a scale of neurological abnormalities. A second 'organic' group of late paraphrenic patients showed widespread impairment of cognitive functions together with a lower frequency of positive psychotic symptoms and a high prevalence of abnormalities on neurological examination (Almeida *et al.* 1995b).

Heaton *et al.* (1994, 2001) assessed cognitive performance with an expanded version of the Halstead–Reitan test battery in over 200 subjects. Overall, late-onset schizophrenia was similar to early-onset schizophrenia in terms of the pattern of neuropsychological impairment (Heaton *et al.* 1994). The neuropsychological deficit scores (corrected for age, gender and education) were similar among the schizophrenia groups and different from (intermediate between) those in the normal subjects and Alzheimer's disease patients. There was a dissociation in terms of learning and retaining information. The schizophrenia patients had mild to moderate impairment on learning but normal retention of information, whereas the patients with Alzheimer's disease were markedly impaired on both. Although the overall pattern of normal neuropsychological functioning for late- and early-onset schizophrenia groups was similar, there were some differences between late- and early-onset schizophrenia; these were in terms of learning and abstraction/flexibility of thinking, with the late-onset schizophrenia group being less impaired on these measures. Schizophrenia patients classified as having a normal learning and memory pattern had an older age of onset than patients with abnormal learning and memory profiles (Paulsen *et al.* 1995). Also, age of onset of schizophrenia was positively associated with total recall across learning trials and negatively associated with evidence of retrieval problems.

Paulsen *et al.* (1996) characterized the integrity of semantic memory in both late- and early-onset schizophrenia patients and found that the organization of semantic memory was almost normal in the late-onset schizophrenia patients, whereas it was significantly impaired in the early-onset schizophrenia patients.

Aetiology

Genetic factors

Reviewing the literature of family history in schizophrenia, Gottesman and Shields (1982) reported that the overall risk of schizophrenia in the relatives of an affected proband was about 10%, compared with a risk of around 1% for the general population. Kendler *et al.* (1987) concluded that there was no consistent relationship between age at onset and familial risk for schizophrenia, but data from patients with an onset in old age were not included in this analysis. The literature on familiality in late-onset schizophrenia and related psychoses of late life is sparse and inconclusive, partly because of variations in illness definition and age at onset, but principally because of the difficulties inherent in conducting family studies in patients who often have only a small number of surviving first-degree relatives. The results of the few studies specifically of late-onset psychoses, reviewed by Castle and Howard (1992), suggest a trend for increasing age at onset of psychosis to be associated with reduced risk of schizophrenia in first-degree relatives. Thus, studies involving subjects with illness onset after the age of 40 or 45 years have reported rates of schizophrenia in relatives of between 4.4% and 19.4% (Bleuler 1943; Huber *et al.* 1975; Pearlson *et al.* 1989), while those with onsets delayed to 50 or 60 years have yielded rates of between 1.0% and 7.3% (Funding 1961; Post 1966; Herbert & Jacobson 1967). More recently, studies of patients with psychosis onset after the age of 50 (Brodaty *et al.* 1999) and 60 years (Howard *et al.* 1997) reported no increase in the prevalence of schizophrenia among relatives of patients and those of healthy comparison subjects. In a controlled family study involving data from 269 first-degree relatives of patients with onset after 60 years and 272 relatives of healthy elderly subjects, the estimated lifetime risk for schizophrenia with an onset range of 15–90 years was 2.3% for the relatives of patients and 2.2% for the relatives of controls (Howard *et al.* 1997). In another study comparing patients with middle-age- with early-onset schizophrenia, there was no significant group difference in the proportion of first-degree relatives with schizophrenia (Jeste *et al.* 1997). Both the groups of schizophrenia patients had a significantly greater likelihood of having a first-degree relative with schizophrenia than normal subjects.

Brain abnormalities seen with imaging

Exclusion from computerized tomography (CT) studies of patients with obvious neurological signs or a history of stroke, alcohol abuse or dementia has shown that structural abnormalities other than large ventricles in patients with late paraphrenia are probably no more common than in healthy elderly controls. Despite adhering to such exclusions, Flint *et al.* (1991) found unsuspected cerebral infarction on the scans of five out of 16 of their late paraphrenic patients. Most of these infarcts were subcortical or frontal and they were more likely to occur in patients who had delusions but no hallucinations. The results of this study need to be interpreted with some caution, because only 16 of a collected sample of patients had actually undergone CT scanning and it is possible that these represented the more 'organic' cases, or at least those that were thought most likely to have some underlying structural abnormality.

The superiority of magnetic resonance imaging (MRI) over CT, both in terms of grey/white matter resolution and visualization of deep white matter, is established. The results of MRI studies of changes in periventricular and deep white matter in patients with paranoid psychosis, however, must be viewed with some caution because few have assessed abnormalities in white matter in any kind of standardized manner and appropriate control populations, matched for cerebrovascular risk factors, are rarely used. Miller *et al.* (1989, 1991, 1992) have reported the results of structural MRI investigations in patients with what they termed 'late life psychosis'. They have reported that 42% of non-demented patients with an onset of psychosis after the age of 45 (mean age at scanning 60.1 years) had white matter abnormalities on MRI, compared with only 8% of a healthy age-matched control group. The appearance of large patchy white matter lesions (WMLs) was six times more likely in the temporal lobe and four times more common in the frontal lobes of patients than controls (Miller *et al.* 1991). These authors hypothesized that, although insufficient to give rise to focal neurological signs, WMLs might produce dysfunction in the overlying frontal and temporal cortex and that this could contribute to psychotic symptomatology. They acknowledged that because WMLs in the occipital lobes could also be implicated, it might not be pos-

sible to pinpoint an isolated anatomical white matter lesion that predisposed to psychosis. When comparisons were made between the patients who had structural brain abnormalities on MRI (10) with those who did not (7), there were no significant differences in age, educational level, IQ or performance on a wide battery of neuropsychological tests. Measurements of ventricle–brain ratio (VBR) indicated a non-significant increase in patients (10.6%) compared with controls (8.8%). The DSM-IIIR (American Psychiatric Association 1987) diagnoses of the 24 patients at entry to this study were schizophrenic disorder (late-onset type) (10), delusional disorder (7), schizophreniform psychosis (2) and psychosis not otherwise specified (5), but at least 12 were shown to have organic cerebral conditions. Studies by Howard *et al.* (1995) of white matter signal hyperintensities among patients with late paraphrenia, from whom the authors have tried to exclude organic cases, have suggested that they may be no more common in such patients than in healthy community-living elderly controls.

Pearlson *et al.* (1993) have reported the results of a volumetric MRI study of late-onset schizophrenia patients based on a sample of 11 individuals with an illness onset after the age of 55 years. Third ventricle volume was significantly greater in late-onset schizophrenia patients than in an age-matched control group. VBR estimations were greater among the late-onset schizophrenia patients (mean 9.0) than controls (mean 7.1), but this difference did not reach statistical significance.

Howard *et al.* (1994b) have reported the results of volumetric MRI studies, based on the scans of 47 patients with late paraphrenia, 31 of whom satisfied ICD-10 criteria for a diagnosis of schizophrenia and 16 for delusional disorder. While total brain volume was not reduced in the patients compared with 35 elderly community-living controls, lateral and third ventricle volumes were increased. Measurements of the frontal lobes, hippocampus, parahippocampus, thalamus and basal ganglia structures failed to demonstrate further differences between patient and control subjects.

Symonds *et al.* (1997) found no significant differences among age-comparable late-onset schizophrenia, early-onset schizophrenia and normal control groups in terms of clinically relevant structural brain abnormalities such as strokes, tumours, cysts or other lesions that are obvious to a clinical neuroradiologist reporting on the MRI (Breitner *et al.* 1990). We believe that if there is a patient with a relevantly located stroke or brain tumour who develops new-onset psychosis, the diagnosis should be psychosis not otherwise specified or psychosis secondary to a general medical condition, rather than labelling it late-onset schizophrenia with stroke or tumour.

Corey-Bloom *et al.* (1995) performed a computerized quantitative analysis of grey matter, white matter and fluid volumes in different regions of the brain in a subset of the subjects (Jernigan *et al.* 1990, 1991). Comparing the three groups, late-onset schizophrenia, early-onset schizophrenia and normal controls (*n* = 16, 14 and 28, respectively), similar in age (all over 45), gender and education, the only significant differences in MRI measures were in ventricular and thalamic volumes. There were no significant differences between late- and early-onset schizophrenia groups in terms of non-specific structural brain abnormalities: ventricular enlargement and white matter hyperintensities. The ventricles were significantly larger in late-onset schizophrenia patients than in normal subjects, with early-onset schizophrenia being intermediate. The late-onset schizophrenia patients had a significantly larger thalamus than early-onset schizophrenia patients, with normal subjects being intermediate. (The difference in ventricular volume between early-onset schizophrenia and normal subjects, or in thalamic volume between either schizophrenia group and normal subjects was not significant, probably because of small sample sizes.) The functions of the thalamus include filtering stimuli, sensory gating and focusing attention (Sherman & Koch 1990), all of which are impaired in schizophrenia. Several studies have found a reduced neuronal number or density in the dorsomedial nucleus of thalamus in early-onset schizophrenia (Treff & Hempel 1958; Pakkenberg 1990, 1992). Andreasen et al. (1990, 1994) found a reduced thalamic volume on MRI, primarily on the right, and Buchsbaum et al. (1996) reported a reduced metabolic rate on positron emission tomography (PET), primarily in the right posterior and left anterior portions of the thalamus in neuroleptic-naive patients with schizophrenia. All of these investigations were restricted to early-onset schizophrenia patients. Hence, the preliminary finding of a larger thalamus in late-onset schizophrenia, if replicated, may have relevance to the differential age of onset of schizophrenia.

Gender

The female preponderance of individuals who have an onset of schizophrenia or a schizophrenia-like psychosis in middle or old age is a consistent finding. Among late-onset schizophrenia patients (onset after 40–50 years) females have been reported to constitute 66% (Bleuler 1943), 72% (Klages 1961), 82% (Gabriel 1978), 85% (Marneros & Deister 1984) and 87% (Pearlson et al. 1989) of patients. In studies of patients with an illness onset at 60 years or greater, the female preponderance is even greater: 75% (Sternberg 1972), 86% (Howard et al. 1994a), 88% (Kay & Roth 1961) and 91% (Herbert & Jacobson 1967).

Two recent reports have indicated the presence of a subgroup of female schizophrenia patients with later illness onset who typically do not have a positive family history of schizophrenia (Shimizu & Kurachi 1989; Gorwood et al. 1995). Typically, later illness onset, particularly in females, is associated with a milder symptom profile and better outcome, better premorbid social adjustment and a lower prevalence of structural brain abnormalities than in (mostly male) patients with early illness onset. This has led to the suggestion that sex differences in schizophrenia may reflect different psychiatric disorders. Lewine (1981) proposed two competing theories to account for age of onset and gender differences – the timing model and the subtype model. According to the timing model, men and women have the same form of schizophrenia but the age at onset of illness is different. There may be an earlier onset for men or a delayed onset for women because of biological and/or psychosocial gender differences. In this model, the age of onset would account for most of the gender differences. According to the subtype model, there are two distinct forms of schizophrenia: 'male' schizophrenia and 'female' schizophrenia. Castle and Murray (1991) have suggested that early-onset, typically male schizophrenia is essentially a heritable neurodevelopmental disorder, while late-onset schizophrenia in females may have aetiologically more in common with affective psychosis than with the illness seen in males.

In contrast, Lindamer et al. (2002) believe that the gender differences are better explained by Lewine's timing model. The less severe symptoms and more favourable course of schizophrenia seen in women might be related to the delayed onset of illness (for most disorders, the later the onset, the longer the period for normal premorbid functioning and the better the prognosis.) Because the evidence to support gender differences in heritability, neuropsychological impairment, structural brain abnormalities and treatment response is inconclusive, the hypothesis that there are two subtypes of schizophrenia based on gender is weakened. Given the lack of consistent evidence for important psychosocial factors in the age at onset differential, biological factors gain more credence as possible mediators of the timing effect. As a potential way of explaining gender differences in the distribution of age at onset in this 'timing' model, several lines of evidence suggest that oestrogen could act as one important neuroendocrine mediator to delay and/or protect against the illness.

Seeman has long proposed an important role for sex hormones, especially oestrogen, in the development of schizophrenia (Seeman 1981, 1999; Seeman & Lang 1990). It is hypothesized that those women with a genetic predisposition to schizophrenia are afforded protection between puberty and menopause from oestrogen, therefore delaying the onset of the illness (Riecher-Rossler et al. 1994; Lindamer et al. 2000). Direct evidence to support this hypothesis is so far lacking.

Sensory deficits

Deafness has been experimentally and clinically associated with the development of paranoid symptoms. Deficits of moderate to severe degree affect 40% of patients with late paraphrenia (Kay & Roth 1961; Herbert & Jacobson 1967) and are more prevalent than in elderly depressed patients or normal controls (Post 1966; Naguib & Levy 1987). Deafness associated with late-life psychosis is more usually conductive than degenerative (Cooper et al. 1974) and is generally of early onset, long duration, bilateral and profound (Cooper 1976; Cooper & Curry 1976). Corbin and Eastwood (1986) suggested that deafness may reinforce a pre-existing tendency to social isolation, withdrawal and suspiciousness. Further, auditory hallucinations are the psychopathological phenomena most consistently associated with deafness (Keshavan et al. 1992). There are several reports of improvement in psychotic symptoms after the fitting of a hearing aid (Eastwood et al. 1981; Khan et al. 1988; Almeida et al.

1993), although it has to be said that clinical practice suggests that this is not usually the case. Visual impairment, most commonly a consequence of cataract or macular degeneration, is also more common in elderly paranoid psychosis patients than those with affective disorder and there is a higher coincidence of visual and hearing impairment in paranoid than affective patients (Cooper & Curry 1976). An association between visual impairment and the presence of visual hallucinations (Howard *et al.* 1994a) echoes Keshavan's findings with deafness.

Somewhat different results were observed in a study by Prager and Jeste (1993). The authors conducted a case–control study involving a comparison of schizophrenic patients (early- and late-onset schizophrenia) with mood disorder patients and normal control subjects in terms of visual and auditory impairment. The results showed that all the psychiatric groups were similar to normal controls on uncorrected vision or hearing, but were significantly more impaired on corrected sensory function (i.e. with eyeglasses or hearing aids). These results suggest that the association between sensory impairment and late-life psychosis may be, at least in part, a result of insufficient correction of sensory deficits in older schizophrenia patients compared with normal controls. This could reflect a difficulty for these patients to access optimal health care, especially for the treatment of sensory impairment. In other words, the sensory deficits *per se* do not seem to predispose to late-onset schizophrenia but, rather, the sensory deficits remain largely uncorrected in older patients with schizophrenia. Alternatively, the causes for sensory deficits might be such that in this group the deficits are not correctable.

Premorbid personality and other factors

Premorbid personality in patients with late and mid-life paranoid psychoses and the quality of premorbid relationships within families and with friends were assessed retrospectively by Kay *et al.* (1976). This study is an important one because, through use of structured patient and informant interviews, it represented a first effort to overcome some of the problems inherent in any retrospective attempt at defining premorbid personality. From a consecutive series of first admissions to a psychiatric hospital, the authors selected 54 cases of paranoid and 57 of affective psychosis over the age of 50. Patients and close relatives or friends were independently given a semistructured clinical interview, designed to cover a wide range of paranoid traits. The paranoid patients were rated more highly, both by themselves and informants, on items that suggested that they had greater difficulty in establishing and maintaining satisfactory relationships premorbidly. They had also been significantly more shy, reserved, touchy and suspicious and less able to display sympathy or emotion. Through principal component analysis of the results, the authors derived a 'prepsychotic schizoid personality factor' consisting of unsociability, reticence, suspiciousness and hostility.

Retterstol (1966) has argued that because personality deviations in paranoid patients are recognizable at a very early age, factors in the childhood and adolescence of patients are important in determining a predisposition to paranoid psychosis later in life. Key experiences in the later development of paranoid psychoses are proposed to be those that provoke feelings of insecurity or that damage the self-image of an individual whose personality is already overtly sensitive. Gurian *et al.* (1992) have also provided evidence for the importance of childhood experiences in the development of paranoid psychosis in late life. Among nine Israeli patients with delusional disorder, these authors found a high prevalence of 'war refugees'. These were individuals who had survived the Armenian or Nazi holocausts or been forced to leave their native country. The authors proposed an association between the presence of extremely life-threatening experiences in childhood, a failure to produce progeny and the development of paranoid delusional symptoms in late life in response to a stressful situation such as widowhood. Just how early the threatening experience needs to be is not clear. Cervantes *et al.* (1989) found the risk of developing a paranoid psychosis to be doubled in immigrants from Mexico and Central America who were escaping war or political unrest, compared with those who had moved for economic reasons. Thus, the period during which a personality may be rendered sensitive to the later development of paranoid psychosis by exposure to trauma is presumably not limited to early childhood.

Exactly how important abnormalities in personality functioning are in the aetiology and onset of late-life paranoid psychoses is unclear. While there is evidence linking social trauma in childhood or early adult life to the later development of psychosis, it is perhaps more plausible to view the abnormal premorbid personality as an early marker of impending psychosis rather than to regard the psychosis as an indication of earlier personality dysfunction.

In a small study, Lohr *et al.* (1997) found that middle-age-onset schizophrenia patients, similar to early-onset schizophrenia patients, had a greater number of minor physical anomalies than normal subjects and patients with Alzheimer's disease. This is an interesting finding because, as is generally accepted for early-onset schizophrenia patients, it suggests aberrations in the neurodevelopment of middle-age-onset schizophrenia patients.

According to the neurodevelopmental model (Weinberger 1987), the brain lesions putatively related to the pathogenesis of schizophrenia are of developmental origin and are not progressive or degenerative in nature. Studies by Jeste *et al.* (1997) suggest that the neurodevelopmental model also applies to late-onset schizophrenia. Differences in severity and specific locations or nature of these 'lesions' may account for a delay in the onset of schizophrenia. Wong *et al.* (1984) suggest that the later age of onset and a better prognosis for schizophrenia in women may relate to a later peak and a delayed regression of dopaminergic activity.

Management/treatment

There is limited published research addressing the treatment of late-onset schizophrenia. The available studies are generally characterized by small sample sizes and are often case reports or case series rather than well-controlled double-blind studies. Because the number of reports in late-onset schizophrenia is limited, we also include studies related to other psychotic disorders (e.g. early-onset schizophrenia, delusional disorder) in late life. Studies related to these other disorders may be applicable to patients with late-onset schizophrenia.

Establishing a therapeutic relationship

Although these patients are often described as hostile and their relationships with neighbours, primary care physicians and the local police may be affected by their psychotic symptoms by the time psychiatric referral is considered, the authors' experience is that they are often extremely lonely. Without entering into any kind of collusion, it is always possible to at least take the time to listen to the patient's account of his or her persecution and not difficult to express sympathy for the distress he or she is experiencing. Sometimes a brief admission to hospital or the establishment of regular community psychiatric nurse (CPN) visits can be rendered acceptable as an attempt to 'get to the bottom' of whatever is going on. Once a relationship of trust and support has been established, patients will often accept medication and visits from members of the psychiatric team. Use of compulsory admission powers should be reserved until all else has failed. Relatives and friends should be advised to encourage the patient to reserve discussion of such complaints to the time when the CPN visits if this is possible. However, there is no single strategy which is best for all patients. For most patients, interventions delivered to their own homes (CPN or volunteer visits, home helps and meals-on-wheels) seem to be most acceptable; although some will respond well to the activities and company provided by a day hospital or centre, some may decline to attend. The potential role of psychological treatments in the management of psychotic symptoms in younger patients is becoming clearer, but older psychotic patients are not routinely considered for these, which is unfortunate and unfair (Aguera-Ortiz & Reneses-Prieto 1999).

Rehousing

Because these patients may have highly restricted and encapsulated delusional systems, their complaints about neighbours or the home environment are sometimes taken at face value by social services staff. Hence, by the time of first psychiatric referral, a patient might have been rehoused at least once in the preceding months. As a general rule, even if it results in a brief reduction of complaints from the patient, provision of new accommodation is followed within a few weeks by a re-emergence of symptoms. The obvious distress this causes is sufficient reason always to advise patients and social workers against such moves unless they are being considered for non-delusional reasons or following successful treatment of psychosis.

Cognitive and behavioural interventions

Cognitive–behaviour therapy and social skills training have been found to be useful in younger adults with schizophrenia. Preliminary studies with older patients, including some with late-onset illness, suggest that age-appropriate combined cognitive behavioural–social skills training interventions may help to improve psychopathology and everyday functioning in older patients too (McQuaid et al. 2001; Granholm et al. 2002).

Antipsychotic medication

In general, neuroleptic or antipsychotic medications are the most effective symptomatic treatment for early- and late-onset chronic schizophrenia as these drugs improve both the acute symptoms and prevent relapses (Jeste et al. 1993). However, alterations in pharmacokinetics and pharmacodynamics complicate pharmacotherapy in older patients. In comparison to younger patients, geriatric patients show an increased variability of response and an increased sensitivity to medications (Salzman 1990).

Rabins et al. (1984) found no, or only a partial, response to neuroleptics in 43% of schizophrenic patients with an onset after 44 years, while Pearlson et al. (1989) reported that 54% of their patients fell into this category. In reports of patients with late paraphrenia, the comparable rates range from 49% (Post 1966) to 75% (Kay & Roth 1961). The general conclusion from such studies is that while drugs relieve some target symptoms, the overall treatment response to medication is modest.

It would be useful to know which illness parameters are associated with poor response to medication. Pearlson et al. (1989) found a poor response to neuroleptics to be associated with the presence of thought disorder and with schizoid premorbid personality traits. The presence of first-rank symptoms, family history of schizophrenia and gender had no effect on treatment response. In a late paraphrenic patient group, Holden (1987) found auditory hallucinations and affective features to predict a favourable response. However, this may simply reflect a better natural history in such patients.

Among a group of 64 late paraphrenic patients prescribed neuroleptic medication for at least 3 months, 42.2% showed no response, 31.3% a partial response and 26.6% a full response to treatment (Howard & Levy 1992). Compliance with medication, receiving depot rather than oral medication, and use of a community psychiatric nurse if the patient was an outpatient all had a positive effect on treatment response. Patients prescribed depot medication received on average a lower daily dose in chlorpromazine equivalents than those prescribed oral medication.

Rockwell et al. (1994) studied middle-aged and elderly patients with late-onset psychosis with somatic delusions (e.g. a delusional belief that the person has some physical defect, disorder or disease) with a mean age of 63. The delusional patients showed poor compliance with psychiatric treatment recommendations and rarely benefited from short-term psychopharmacological (mainly neuroleptic) intervention.

Dosage

In four North American clinical centres, the mean daily dosage prescribed to late-onset schizophrenia patients was several times lower than that in a group of young patients with schizophrenia (Jeste & Zisook 1988). Moreover, Jeste *et al.* (1997) found that the mean daily dosage of antipsychotics used in patients with late-onset schizophrenia was significantly smaller than that prescribed to age-comparable patients with early-onset schizophrenia.

Tardive dyskinesia

There is a serious risk associated with long-term use of typical neuroleptics. Patients may develop tardive dyskinesia (TD), a movement disorder characterized by involuntary, irregular or repetitive abnormal movements. In one study (Saltz *et al.* 1991) of elderly patients, ranging in age from 55 to 99 years, the incidence of TD was 31% after 43 weeks of cumulative neuroleptic treatment. Jeste *et al.* (1999b) reported the cumulative incidence of dyskinetic movements in elderly patients to be 29% following 12 months of typical neuroleptic use. This cumulative annual incidence of TD in older adults is five to six times that reported in younger adults. Higher dosage and longer duration of neuroleptic treatment, as well as other factors including alcohol dependence and subtle movement disorder at baseline, were found to increase the risk of TD in the older patient population (Jeste *et al.* 1995).

Novel antipsychotic medications

Because of its relatively weak blockade of striatal dopamine D_2-receptors, low-dose clozapine seemed a promising drug for the treatment of elderly psychotic patients who have individual sensitivity to extrapyramidal symptoms caused by typical neuroleptics. However, clozapine has anticholinergic, hypotensive and sedating effects and has been shown to impair memory function and, despite a few early positive case reports, has not found favour with those who regularly prescribe for older patients. Risperidone is a benzisoxazole derivative with strong binding affinity for serotonin $5-HT_2$-receptors, dopamine D_2-receptors and α_1- and α_2-adrenergic and histamine H_1-receptors. Of all the atypical antipsychotics, clinical experience with risperidone in the older patient group has so far been most extensive. Early reports with this drug suggested that activity at $5-HT_2$-receptors appeared to be important in the treatment of complex visual hallucinations, which had been traditionally regarded as treatment-resistant. Risperidone has efficacy in the treatment of hallucinations and delusions in elderly patients at low doses (typically, 0.5–2 mg/day). Jeste *et al.* (1999a) compared the 9-month cumulative incidence of TD with risperidone to that with haloperidol in older patients. Sixty-one patients on risperidone

were matched with 61 patients from a larger sample of patients who received haloperidol in terms of age, diagnosis and length of pre-enrolment neuroleptic intake. The median daily dose of each medication was 1 mg. Results suggested that, over this 9-month period, risperidone was associated with a fivefold lower cumulative incidence of TD than haloperidol in a high-risk group of older patients. Risperidone should be prescribed to patients with late-onset schizophrenia at considerably lower dosage than those recommended for younger adults. The initial doses of risperidone should be between 0.25 and 0.5 mg/day, with increases not to exceed 0.5 mg/day. Maximum dosage in patients with schizophrenia should remain at 3 mg/day or less. The risk of extrapyramidal symptoms, postural hypotension and somnolence increases with higher dosage.

Olanzapine has a similar receptor-binding profile to clozapine but does not appear to cause the anticholinergic problems seen with the earlier agent. A starting dosage of 2.5–5 mg/day is generally well tolerated and can be increased to 10 or even 15 mg/day if no adverse events appear. Although data on the incidence of TD in elderly patients treated with olanzapine have not yet been reported, preliminary evidence indicates a low risk for extrapyramidal symptoms in this population and the risk of TD in young olanzapine-treated adults appears to be low (Tollefson *et al.* 1997). Anecdotal evidence suggests that olanzapine is less likely to cause extrapyramidal symptoms but more likely to produce sedation and weight gain.

Quetiapine, a newer atypical antipsychotic, also has a low risk of extrapyramidal symptoms, and probably of TD. It may cause sedation and postural hypotension at higher dosage. The recommended starting dosage is 25–50 mg/day, and the maintenance dosage range in older patients is 100–200 mg/day.

At this time, there is very little published information on ziprasidone in elderly patients with schizophrenia.

Comparative trials of different atypical antipsychotics are needed in older schizophrenia patients.

Guidelines for prescribing

There is no real evidence that any particular drug is more effective in this group of patients. The choice of drug for each individual patient should thus be based on considerations of concomitant physical illness and other treatments received, together with the specific side-effect profile of the drug (Tran-Johnson *et al.* 1994). Treatment should usually be commenced at a low dosage of an oral preparation and it is easy to argue that this should be one of the atypical agents because of the reduced risk of early and delayed emergent motor side-effects. Patients who do not respond to oral treatment (whether because of poor compliance or genuine treatment resistance) can be treated with depot. Successful treatment of patients with depot can often be at very modest dosage. For example, the mean dosage of prescribed depot in Howard and Levy's (1992) study was 14.4 mg flupenthixol decanoate or 9 mg fluphenazine decanoate every fortnight. Over the next few years we can expect to see the development of depot preparations of the atypical anti-psychotics. Indeed, trials of depot risperidone are in progress at the time of writing. If these trials prove successful, we have little doubt that this will represent the optimal way of delivering antipsychotic treatment to at least some of these patients.

Conclusions

The history of schizophrenia and schizophrenia-like psychoses that have onset in later life is a long one, but it is only in the last three decades that any real attempts have been made to study patients with these conditions and understand how they might relate to psychoses which arise earlier in the life cycle. The aetiological roles of premorbid personality functioning, degenerative and genetic factors are still not fully elucidated, although most recent brain imaging studies indicate that gross degenerative changes are not present. If compliance with neuroleptic medication can be established and maintained, and supplemented by psychosocial therapy, the prognosis for symptomatic and functional improvement can be favourable.

Acknowledgements

This work was supported, in part, by the National Institute of Mental Health grants MH43695, MH49671 and MH19934 and by the Department of Veterans Affairs.

References

Aguera-Ortiz, L. & Reneses-Prieto, B. (1999) *The Place of Non-Biological Treatments*. In: *Late-Onset Schizophrenia* (eds R. Howard, P.V. Rabins & D.J. Castle), pp. 233–261. Wrightson Biomedical, Petersfield.

Almeida, O., Forstl, H., Howard, R. & David, A.S. (1993) Unilateral auditory hallucinations. *British Journal of Psychiatry* 162, 262–264.

Almeida, O.P., Howard, R.J., Levy, R. & David, A.S. (1995a) Psychotic states arising in late life (late paraphrenia): psychopathology and nosolgy. *British Journal of Psychiatry* 165, 205–214.

Almeida, O.P., Howard, R.J., Levy, R. et al. (1995b) Clinical and cognitive diversity of psychotic states arising in late life (late paraphrenia). *Psychological Medicine* 25, 699–714.

American Psychiatric Association (1980) *Diagnostic and Statistical Manual of Mental Disorders*, 3rd edn. American Psychiatric Press, Washington, DC.

American Psychiatric Association (1987) *Diagnostic and Statistical Manual of Mental Disorders–Revised*, 3rd edn. American Psychiatric Press, Washington, DC.

American Psychiatric Association (1994) *Diagnostic and Statistical Manual of Mental Disorders*, 4th edn. American Psychiatric Press, Washington, DC.

Andreasen, N.C. (1982) Negative symptoms in schizophrenia: definition and reliability. *Archives of General Psychiatry* 39, 784–788.

Andreasen, N.C. & Olsen, S. (1982) Negative vs. positive schizophrenia: definition and validation. *Archives of General Psychiatry* 39, 789–794.

Andreasen, N.C., Ehrhardt, J.C., Swayze, V.W. et al. (1990) Magnetic resonance imaging of the brain in schizophrenia. *Archives of General Psychiatry* 47, 35–44.

Andreasen, N.C., Arndt, S., Swayze, V.W. et al. (1994) Thalamic abnormalities in schizophrenia visualized through magnetic resonance image averaging. *Science* 266, 294–298.

Bleuler, E.P. (1911) *Dementia Praecox or the Group of Schizophrenias*. Deuticke, Leipzig.

Bleuler, M. (1943) Die spatschizophrenen krankheitsbilder. *Fortschritte der Neurologie Psychiatrie* 15, 259–290.

Breitner, J., Husain, M., Figiel, G., Krishnan, K. & Boyko, O. (1990) Cerebral white matter disease in late-onset psychosis. *Biological Psychiatry* 28, 266–274.

Brodaty, H., Sachdev, P., Rose, N., Rylands, K. & Prenter, L. (1999) Schizophrenia with onset after age 50 years. 1. Phenomenology and risk factors. *British Journal of Psychiatry* 175, 410–415.

Buchsbaum, M.S., Someya, T., Teng, C.Y. et al. (1996) PET and MRI of the thalamus in never-medicated patients with schizophrenia. *American Journal of Psychiatry* 153, 191–199.

Castle, D.J. & Howard, R. (1992) What do we know about the aetiology of late-onset schizophrenia. *European Psychiatry* 7, 99–108.

Castle, D.J. & Murray, R.M. (1991) The neurodevelopmental basis of sex differences in schizophrenia. *Psychological Medicine* 21, 565–575.

Cervantes, R.C., Salgado-Snyder, V.N. & Padilla, A.M. (1989) Post-traumatic stress in immigrants from Central American and Mexico. *Hospital Community Psychiatry* 40, 615–619.

Cooper, A.F. (1976) Deafness and psychiatric illness. *British Journal of Psychiatry* 129, 216–226.

Cooper, A.F. & Curry, A.R. (1976) The pathology of deafness in the paranoid and affective psychoses of later life. *Journal of Psychosomatic Research* 20, 97–105.

Cooper, A.F., Curry, A.R., Kay, D.W.K., Garside, R.F. & Roth, M. (1974) Hearing loss in paranoid and affective psychoses of the elderly. *Lancet* 2, 851–854.

Corbin, S.L. & Eastwood, M.R. (1986) Sensory deficits and mental disorders of old age: causal or coincidental associations? *Psychological Medicine* 16, 251–256.

Corey-Bloom, J., Jernigan, T., Archibald, S., Harris, M.J. & Jeste, D.V. (1995) Quantitative magnetic resonance imaging of the brain in late-life schizophrenia. *American Journal of Psychiatry* 152, 447–449.

Cutting, J.C., Clare, A.W. & Mann, A.H. (1978) Cycloid psychosi: investigation of the diagnostic concept. *Psychological Medicine* 8, 637–648.

Eastwood, R., Corbin, S. & Reed, M. (1981) Hearing impairment and paraphrenia. *Journal of Otolaryngology* 10, 306–308.

Fish, F. (1958) A clinical investigation of chronic schizophrenia. *British Journal of Psychiatry* 104, 34–54.

Fish, F. (1960) Senile schizophrenia. *Journal of Mental Science* 106, 938–946.

Flint, A.J., Rifat, S.I. & Eastwood, M.R. (1991) Late-onset paranoia: distinct from paraphrenia? *International Journal of Geriatric Psychiatry* 6, 103–109.

Funding, T. (1961) Genetics of paranoid psychosis of later life. *Acta Psychiatrica Scandinavica* 37, 267–282.

Gabriel, E. (1978) *Die Langfristige Entwicklung der Spatschizophrenien*. Karger, Basel.

Gorwood, P., Leboyer, M., Jay, M., Payan, C. & Feingold, J. (1995) Gender and age at onset in schizophrenia: impact of family history. *American Journal of Psychiatry* 152, 208–212.

Gottesman, I.I. & Shields, J. (1982) *Schizophrenia: the Epigenetic Puzzle.* Cambridge University Press, Cambridge.

Grahame, P.S. (1984) Schizophrenia in old age (late paraphrenia). *British Journal of Psychiatry* **145**, 493–495.

Granholm, E., McQuaid, J.R., McClure, F.S., Pedrelli, P. & Jeste, D.V. (2002) A randomized controlled pilot study of cognitive behavioral social skills training for older patients with schizophrenia. *Schizophrenia Research* **53**, 167–169.

Gurian, B.S., Wexler, D. & Baker, E.H. (1992) Late-life paranoia: possible association with early trauma and infertility. *International Journal of Geriatric Psychiatry* **7**, 277–284.

Harris, M.J. & Jeste, D.V. (1988) Late-onset schizophrenia: an overview. *Schizophrenia Bulletin* **14**, 39–55.

Heaton, R., Paulsen, J., McAdams, L.A. *et al.* (1994) Neuropsychological deficits in schizophrenia: relationship to age, chronicity and dementia. *Archives of General Psychiatry* **51**, 469–476.

Heaton, R.K., Gladsjo, J.A., Palmer, B. *et al.* (2001) The stability and course of neuropsychological deficits in schizophrenia. *Archives of General Psychiatry* **58**, 24–32.

Herbert, M.E. & Jacobson, S. (1967) Late paraphrenia. *British Journal of Psychiatry* **113**, 461–469.

Holden, N.L. (1987) Late paraphrenia or the paraphrenias: a descriptive study with a 10-year follow-up. *British Journal of Psychiatry* **150**, 635–639.

Hopkins, B. & Roth, M. (1953) Psychological test performance in patients over sixty. II. Paraphrenia, arteriosclerotic psychosis and acute confusion. *Journal of Mental Science* **99**, 451–463.

Howard, R. & Levy, R. (1992) Which factors affect treatment response in late paraphrenia? *International Journal of Geriatric Psychiatry* **7**, 667–672.

Howard, R., Castle, D., Wessely, S. & Murray, R.M. (1993) A comparative study of 470 cases of early and late-onset schizophrenia. *British Journal of Psychiatry* **163**, 352–357.

Howard, R., Almeida, O. & Levy, R. (1994a) Phenomenology, demography and diagnosis in late paraphrenia. *Psychological Medicine* **24**, 397–410.

Howard, R.J., Almeida, O., Levy, R., Graves, P. & Graves, M. (1994b) Quantitative magnetic resonance imaging volume try distinguishes delusional disorder from late-onset schizophrenia. *British Journal of Psychiatry* **165**, 474–480.

Howard, R., Cox, T., Almeida, O. *et al.* (1995) White matter signal hyperintensities in the brains of patients with late paraphrenia and the normal community-living elderly. *Biological Psychiatry* **38**, 86–91.

Howard, R., Graham, C., Sham, P. *et al.* (1997) A controlled family study of late-onset non-affective psychosis (late paraphrenia). *British Journal of Psychiatry* **170**, 511–514.

Howard, R., Rabins, P.V., Seeman, M.V. & Jeste, D.V. and the International Late-Onset Schizophrenia Group (2000) Late-onset schizophrenia and very-late-onset schizophrenia-like psychosis: an international consensus. *American Journal of Psychiatry* **157**, 172–178.

Huber, G., Gross, G. & Schuttler, R. (1975) Spat schizophrenie. *Archiv Fur Psychiatrie und Nervenkrankheiten* **22**, 53–66.

Jernigan, T.L., Press, G.A. & Hesselink, J.R. (1990) Methods for measuring brain morphologic features on magnetic resonance images: validation and normal aging. *Archives of Neurology* **47**, 27–32.

Jernigan, T.L., Zisook, S., Heaton, R.K. *et al.* (1991) Magnetic resonance imaging abnormalities in lenticular nuclei and cerebral cortex in schizophrenia. *Archives of General Psychiatry* **48**, 881–890.

Jeste, D.V. & Zisook, S. (1988) Preface to psychosis and depression in the elderly. *Psychiatric Clinics of North America* **11**, xiii–xv.

Jeste, D.V., Harris, M.J., Pearlson, G.D. *et al.* (1988) Late-onset schizophrenia: studying clinical validity. *Psychiatric Clinics of North America* **11**, 1–14.

Jeste, D.V., Lacro, J.P., Gilbert, P.L., Kline, J. & Kline, N. (1993) Treatment of late-life schizophrenia with neuroleptics. *Schizophrenia Bulletin* **19** (4), 817–830.

Jeste, D.V., Caligiuri, M.P., Paulsen, J.S. *et al.* (1995) Risk of tardive dyskinesia in older patients: a prospective longitudinal study of 266 patients. *Archives of General Psychiatry* **52**, 756–765.

Jeste, D.V., Symonds, L.L., Harris, M.J. *et al.* (1997) Non-dementia non-praecox dementia praecox? Late-onset schizophrenia. *American Journal of Geriatric Psychiatry* **5**, 302–317.

Jeste, D.V., Lacro, J.P., Palmer, B. *et al.* (1999a) Incidence of tardive dyskinesia in early stages of neuroleptic treatment for older patients. *American Journal of Psychiatry* **156**, 309–311.

Jeste, D.V., Lacro, J.P., Palmer, B.W. *et al.* (1999b) Incidence of tardive dyskinesia in early stages of low-dose treatment with typical neuroleptics in older patients. *American Journal of Psychiatry* **156**, 309–311.

Kay, D.W.K. & Roth, M. (1961) Environmental and hereditary factors in the schizophrenias of old age ('late paraphrenia') and their bearing on the general problem of causation in schizophrenia. *Journal of Mental Science* **107**, 649–686.

Kay, D.W.K., Cooper, A.F., Garside, R.F. & Roth, M. (1976) The differentiation of paranoid from affective psychoses by patients' premorbid characteristics. *British Journal of Psychiatry* **129**, 207–215.

Kendler, K.S., Tsuang, M.T. & Hays, P. (1987) Age at onset in schizophrenia: a familial perspective. *Archives of General Psychiatry* **44**, 881–890.

Keshavan, M.S., David, A.S., Steingard, S. & Lishman, W.A. (1992) Musical hallucinations: a review and synthesis. *Neuropsychiatry, Neuropsychology and Behavioural Neurology* **5**, 211–223.

Khan, A.M., Clark, T. & Oyebode, F. (1988) Unilateral auditory hallucinations. *British Journal of Psychiatry* **152**, 297–298.

Klages, W. (1961) *Die Spatschizophrenie.* Enke, Stuttgart.

Kraepelin, E. (1913) *Psychiatrie, Ein Lehrbuch Fur Studierende und Artze.* Barth, Leipzig.

Levitt, J.J. & Tsuang, M.T. (1988) The heterogeneity of schizoaffective disorder: implications for treatment. *American Journal of Psychiatry* **145**, 926–936.

Lewine, R. (1981) Sex differences in schizophrenia: timing or subtype? *Psychological Bulletin* **90**, 432–444.

Lindamer, L.A., Harris, M.J., Gladsjo, J.A. *et al.* (2000) Gender and schizophrenia. In: *Sex Hormones, Aging, and Mental Disorders* (ed. M. Morrison), pp. 223–239. National Institute of Mental Health, Washington, DC.

Lindamer, L.A., Dunn, L.B. & Jeste, D.V. (2002) Gender and age of onset in schizophrenia: Lewine's hypothesis revisited. In: *Women's Health and Psychiatry* (eds K. Pearson & S.S. Rosenbaum). Lippincott Williams & Wilkins, New York.

Lohr, J.B., Alder, M., Flynn, K., Harris, M.J. & McAdams, L.A. (1997) Minor physical anomalies in older patients with late-onset schizophrenia, early-onset schizophrenia, depression, and Alzheimer's disease. *American Journal of Geriatric Psychiatry* **5**, 318–323.

McQuaid, J.R., Granholm, E., Roepke, S. *et al.* (2000) Development of an integrated cognitive–behavioral, social skills training intervention for older patients with schizophrenia. *Journal of Psychotherapy Research and Practice* **9**, 149–156.

Magnan, V. (1893) *Lecons Cliniques Sur les Maladies Mentales.* Bureaux de Progres Medical, Paris.

Marneros, A. & Deister, A. (1984) The psychopathology of 'late schizophrenia'. *Psychopathology* **17**, 264–174.

Miller, B.L., Lesser, I.M., Boone, K. *et al.* (1989) Brain white-matter lesions and psychosis. *British Journal of Psychiatry* **155**, 73–78.

Miller, B.L., Lesser, I.M., Boone, K.B. *et al.* (1991) Brain lesions and cognitive function in late-life psychosis. *British Journal of Psychiatry* **158**, 76–82.

Miller, B.L., Lesser, I.M., Mena, I. *et al.* (1992) Regional cerebral blood flow in late-life-onset psychosis. *Neuropsychiatry, Neuropsychology and Behavioural Neurology* **5**, 132–137.

Murray, R.M., O'Callaghan, E., Castle, D.J. & Lewis, S.W. (1992) A neurodevelopmental approach to the classification of schizophrenia. *Schizophrenia Bulletin* **18**, 319–332.

Naguib, M. & Levy, R. (1987) Late paraphrenia. neuropsychological impairment and structural brain abnormalities on computed tomography. *International Journal of Geriatric Psychiatry* **2**, 83–90.

Overall, J.E. & Gorham, D.R. (1962) The Brief Psychiatric Rating Scale. *Psychological Reports* **10**, 799–812.

Pakkenberg, B. (1990) Pronounced reduction of total neuron number in mediodorsal thalamic nucleus and nucleus accumbens in schizophrenia. *Archives of General Psychiatry* **47**, 1023–1028.

Pakkenberg, B. (1992) The volume of the mediodorsal thalamic nucleus in treated and untreated schizophrenics. *Schizophrenia Research* **7**, 95–100.

Palmer, B.W., McClure, F. & Jeste, D.V. (2001) Schizophrenia in late-life: findings challenge traditional concepts. *Harvard Review of Psychiatry* **9**, 51–58.

Paulsen, J.S., Heaton, R.K., Sadek, J.R. *et al.* (1995) The nature of learning and memory impairments in schizophrenia. *Journal of the International Neuropsychological Society* **1**, 88–99.

Paulsen, J.S., Romero, R., Chan, A. *et al.* (1996) Impairment of the semantic network in schizophrenia. *Psychiatry Research* **63**, 109–121.

Pearlson, G.D., Kreger, L., Rabins, R.V. *et al.* (1989) A chart review study of late-onset and early-onset schizophrenia. *American Journal of Psychiatry* **146**, 1568–1574.

Pearlson, G.D., Tune, L.E., Wong, D.F. *et al.* (1993) Quantitative D_2 dopamine receptor PET and structural MRI changes in late onset schizophrenia. *Schizophrenia Bulletin* **19**, 783–795.

Post, F. (1966) *Persistent Persecutory States of the Elderly.* Pergamon Press, London.

Prager, S. & Jeste, D.V. (1993) Sensory impairment in late-life schizophrenia. *Schizophrenia Bulletin* **19**, 755–772.

Quintal, M., Day-Cody, D. & Levy, R. (1991) Late paraphrenia and ICD-10. *International Journal of Geriatric Psychiatry* **6**, 111–116.

Rabins, P., Pauker, S. & Thomas, J. (1984) Can schizophrenia begin after age 44? *Comprehensive Psychiatry* **25**, 290–293.

Retterstol, N. (1966) *Paranoid and Paranoiac Psychoses: A Personal Follow-Up Investigation with Special Reference to Aetiological, Clinical and Prognostic Aspects.* Thomas Springfield. Oslo Universitetsforlaget.

Riecher-Rossler, A., Hafner, H., Stumbalum, M., Maurer, K. & Schmidt, R. (1994) Can estradiol modulate schizophrenic symptomatology? *Schizophrenia Bulletin* **20**, 203–213.

Rockwell, E., Krull, A.J., Dimsdale, J. & Jeste, D.V. (1994) Late-onset psychosis with somatic delusions. *Psychosomatics* **35**, 66–72.

Roth, M. & Morrisey, J.D. (1952) Problems in the diagnosis and classification of mental disorders in old age. *Journal of Mental Science* **98**, 68–80.

Saltz, B.L., Woerner, M.G., Kane, J.M. *et al.* (1991) Prospective study of tardive dyskinesia incidence in the elderly. *Journal of the American Medical Association* **266**, 2402–2406.

Salzman, C. (1990) Principles of psychopharmacology. In: *Verwoerdt's Clinical Geropsychiatry* (ed. D. Bienenfeld), pp. 235–249. Williams & Wilkins, Baltimore, MD.

Seeman, M.V. (1981) Gender and the onset of schizophrenia: neurohumoral influences. *Psychiatric Journal of the University of Ottawa* **6**, 136–138.

Seeman, M.V. (1999) Oestrogens and psychosis. In: *Late Onset Schizophrenia* (eds. R. Howard, P.V. Rabins & D.J. Castle), pp. 165–180. Biomedical Publishing, Wrightson, Philadelphia.

Seeman, M.V. & Lang, M. (1990) The role of estrogens in schizophrenia gender differences. *Schizophrenia Bulletin* **16**, 185–194.

Sherman, S.M. & Koch, C. (1990) Thalamus. In: *The Synaptic Organization of the Brain*, 3rd end (eds. G.M. Shepherd), pp. 246–278. Oxford University Press, New York.

Shimizu, A. & Kurachi, M. (1989) Do women without a family history of schizophrenia have a later onset of schizophrenia? *Japanese Journal of Psychiatry and Neurology* **43**, 133–136.

Sjoegren, H. (1964) Paraphrenic, melancholic and psychoneurotic states in the pre-senile and senile periods of life. *Acta Psychiatrica Scandinavica Supplement* **176**.

Sternberg, E. (1972) Neuere forschungsergebnisse bei spatschizophrenen psychosen. *Fortschritte der Neurologie Psychiatrie* **40**, 631–646.

Symonds, L.L., Olichney, J.M., Jernigan, T.L. *et al.* (1997) Lack of clinically significant structural abnormalities in MRIs of older patients with schizophrenia and related psychoses. *Journal of Neuropsychiatry and Clinical Neuroscience* **9**, 251–258.

Tollefson, G.D., Beasley, C.M., Tamura, R.N., Tran, P.V. & Potvin, J.H. (1997) Blind, controlled, long-term study of the comparative incidence of treatment-emerged tardive diskinesia with olanzapine or haloperidol. *American Journal of Psychiatry* **154**, 1248–1254.

Tran-Johnson, T.K., Harris, M.J. & Jeste, D.V. (1994) Pharmacological treatment of schizophrenia and delusional disorders of late life. In: *Principles and Practices of Geriatric Psychiatry* (eds J.R.M. Copeland, M.T. Abou-Saleh & D.G. Blazer), pp. 685–692. John Wiley, New York.

Treff, W.M. & Hempel, K.J. (1958) Die Zelldichte bei Schizophrenen und klinisch Gesunden. *Journal für Hirnforschung* **4**, 314–369.

Weinberger, D.R. (1987) Implications of normal brain development for the pathogenesis of schizophrenia. *Archives of General Psychiatry* **44**, 660–669.

Wong, D.F., Wagner, H.N. Jr, Dannals, R.F. *et al.* (1984) Effects of age on dopamine and serotonin receptors measured by positron emission tomography in the living human brain. *Science* **226**, 1393–1396.

7 The schizophrenia spectrum personality disorders

K. O'Flynn, J. Gruzelier, A. Bergman and L.J. Siever

European phenomenologically orientated psychiatrists such as Kraeplin and Bleuler were among the first to observe that there may be gradations of schizophrenia-related disorders, with relatives of schizophrenic patients displaying mild psychotic-like symptoms and asociality similar but less severe than the signs and symptoms observed in chronic schizophrenia (Kraeplin 1919/1971; Bleuler 1950). More recently, the adoption studies of Kety *et al.* (1975) described the clinical profiles of probands and relatives with diagnoses of 'borderline schizophrenia' or 'latent schizophrenia'. These case histories were reviewed and the features identified provided the basis for the diagnosis 'schizotypal personality disorder' (SPD) which was included for the first time in DSM-III (Table 7.1; American Psychiatric Association 1980).

SPD is part of the 'odd' cluster of the personality disorders. Analogous to symptoms of chronic schizophrenia, the features of SPD may be viewed as psychotic-like (ideas of reference, magical thinking, suspiciousness) and deficit-related symptoms (social isolation, inadequate rapport). SPD represents the first personality disorder defined in part by its genetic relationship to schizophrenia and is the prototype of the schizophrenia-related personality disorders in the schizophrenia spectrum.

Studies of the phenomenology, genetics, biology, cognition, outcome and treatment response of SPD have consistently supported a close relationship of SPD to schizophrenia. Schizotypal patients do not, by definition, suffer from chronic psychosis, they have not been exposed to long-term medication, are usually not on current medication and are generally free from the effects of multiple hospital admissions or long-term institutionalization. These patients are therefore spared the multiple artefacts that potentially confound research in schizophrenia. Study of SPD patients may afford an opportunity to disentangle the factors which interact to determine the schizophrenic process. In this chapter, we present an up to date perspective on research in this relatively novel and expanding area.

Phenomenology

Diagnostic criteria for schizotypal personality disorder or schizotypal disorder consist of attenuated psychotic-like symptoms such as ideas of reference and cognitive–perceptual distortions, as well as deficit-like symptoms of constricted affect, social isolation and related criteria reflecting eccentric appearance and speech. The ideas of reference of schizotypal personality disorder, while not held with the conviction characteristic of the chronic schizophrenic, are often persistent and disturbing to the patient. Schizotypal individuals may feel that others are staring at them or talking about them when they enter a bus or attend a social occasion. They often entertain unusual beliefs that are outside the social norms of their culture, sometimes in a superstitious or religious context and other times in an idiosyncratic fashion. For example, they may manifest 'magical thinking' such as the belief that one's thoughts anticipate tragic events such as accidental deaths. Illusions and other perceptual experiences are common, particularly in situations where information is ambiguous, such as in a darkened room, or in an altered state, such as drowsiness or fatigue. Schizotypal individuals may be socially isolated and have few friends in whom they confide and to whom they feel close in an enduring way. Their affect may be constricted, and they may be difficult to engage interpersonally. Rapport with others may be severely lacking. At other times, they may smile inappropriately and react emotionally in a way that appears incongruent with the content of

Table 7.1 DSM-IV diagnostic criteria for schizotypal personality disorder (American Psychiatric Association 1994).

A   A pervasive pattern of social and interpersonal deficits marked by acute discomfort with, and reduced capacity for, close relationships as well as by cognitive or perceptual distortions and eccentricities of behaviour, beginning by early adulthood and present in a variety of contexts, as indicated by five (or more) of the following:

  1   Ideas of reference (excluding delusions of reference)
  2   Odd beliefs or magical thinking that influences behaviour and is inconsistent with subcultural norms (e.g. superstitiousness, belief in clairvoyance, telepathy or 'sixth sense'; in children or adolescents, bizarre fantasies or preoccupations)
  3   Unusual perceptual experiences, including bodily illusions
  4   Odd thinking and speech (e.g. vague, circumstantial, metaphorical, overelaborate, or stereotyped)
  5   Suspiciousness or paranoid ideation
  6   Inappropriate or constricted affect
  7   Behaviour or appearance that is odd, eccentric or peculiar
  8   Lack of close fiends or confidants other than first-degree relatives
  9   Excessive social anxiety that does not diminish with familiarity and tends to he associated with paranoid fears rather than negative judgements about self

B   Does not occur exclusively during the course of Schizophrenia, a Mood Disorder With Psychotic Features, another Psychotic Disorder, or a Pervasive Developmental Disorder

---

Note: If criteria are met prior to the onset of schizophrenia, add 'premorbid', e.g. 'schizotypal personality disorder (premorbid)'.

their speech context. They tend to be suspicious and guarded, attributing negative or persecutory intents to others. Their behaviour and appearance may also appear odd with idiosyncratic movements, expressions, mannerisms and style of dress. Their speech may also be unusual and may be concrete and impoverished or extraordinarily elaborate with frequent non-sequiturs.

The diagnostic criteria for paranoid personality disorder emphasize suspicious and mistrustful traits; distortions in cognition and perception may not be present. Thus, persons with this disorder have an expectancy of malevolent intent and behaviour on the part of others. They constantly question the loyalty of friends and close colleagues and see hidden threatening meanings that tend to justify their preconceptions. Because of their fear of the ill-will of others, they are reluctant to confide in them and are often volatile in response to perceived slights.

In contrast, schizoid personality disorder is grounded in the core traits of asociality and lack of enjoyment of interpersonal engagement. The schizoid person, like the schizotypal individual, may have no close friends or confidants, although people with schizoid personality disorder do not necessarily have the cognitive–perceptual distortions that are criteria for schizotypal personality disorder. The schizoid individual appears to prefer being alone and does not evidence desire for, or pleasure from, close relationships, whether friendly or intimate. Such individu-

als often appear indifferent to criticism and praise, and share with the schizotypal individual an aloof detached constricted appearance.

Schizotypal, schizoid and paranoid disorders are highly overlapping in clinical samples (Kalus *et al.* 1996). Schizoid personality is least common in the clinical setting, perhaps because these individuals are stably isolated and thus do not experience the dysphoria, disruption of relationships and work function, along with the more eccentric appearance associated with the cognitive peculiarities of schizotypal and paranoid personality disorders. Paranoid and schizotypal personality disorders are highly overlapping in most clinical studies (Kalus *et al.* 1996), which is not surprising given the overlap between the criteria. However, it is not clear whether there is perhaps a group of individuals with paranoid personality disorder distinct from individuals meeting criteria for schizotypal personality disorder, who may be more closely related to delusional disorder or, in some cases, to the histrionic and dramatic spectrum of personality disorders. Further uncertainty involves the role of affect; in one study up to 40% of SPD patients had experienced episodes of major depression, a comorbidity also found in paranoid personality disorder (Bernstein *et al.* 1996; Siever *et al.* 1996).

The generally high comorbidity of these disorders and close relationship of their criteria raise the question of whether they are defining distinct disorders or are actually gradations of severity along the schizophrenia spectrum. According to the latter conception, schizoid personality disorder would represent one end of the continuum, at the other end of which is schizophrenia, with schizotypal personality disorder located between the two. Obviously, as one moves towards the more schizoid end of the spectrum, the relationship to schizophrenia is less strong and specific. However, from an aetiological point of view, heterogeneity might be found throughout the spectrum, because a variety of pathophysiological processes may lead to a final outcome of chronic schizophrenia.

There is also an overlap between schizophrenia spectrum personality disorders and borderline and avoidant personality disorders. However, the overlap with borderline personality disorder has been diminished as the criteria for each have become refined (Kavoussi & Siever 1992). The psychotic-like symptoms of borderline personality disorder are viewed as transient and often dissociative, in contrast to those of schizotypal personality disorder, which are more persistent and pervasive, and are accompanied by affective instability. Conceptually, avoidant personality disordered individuals yearn for social relationships but require an unusually strong degree of acceptance before engaging in them because of their anxiety, while schizoid and schizotypal individuals do not actively want or seek these relationships. However, in practice these distinctions are difficult to make. Schizotypal and schizotoid individuals may acknowledge a wistfulness for relationships and experience the limitations of their isolation. Furthermore, avoidant individuals may at times appear aloof and distant, and on neuropsychological testing show cognitive impairment (Cohen *et al.* 1996) that may not be clearly distinct in character from the neuropsy-

While findings of premorbid schizoid and schizotypal personality traits in schizophrenic patients lend support to the notion of a schizophrenia spectrum, it must also be noted that not all schizophrenic patients evidence abnormal personality traits before the onset of schizophrenia. In fact, one study found that a normal personality was the most frequent premorbid characterization of the schizophrenic sample (44%; Peralta *et al.* 1991). Another report indicated that 42% of the sample had no premorbid diagnosis based on the schedule for interviewing DSM-III personality disorders (SIDP), although when the Million Multiaxial Clinical Inventory (MMCI-I) was used, 70% of the same sample had at least one personality disorder diagnosis (Hogg *et al.* 1990). Once again, the heterogeneous nature of schizophrenia seems apparent.

In conclusion, it seems likely that a subgroup of schizophrenic patients can be characterized by premorbid personality disorders that are clearly related to schizophrenia. However, the relationship between abnormal personality traits and later schizophrenia is not clear. It may be that the presence of schizophrenia spectrum personality disorders is indicative of a higher morbidity for the development of schizophrenia, or that these personality disorders are part of the extended phenotype of schizophrenia. Furthermore, it is not clear whether a schizophrenia spectrum personality disorder is a necessary transitional stage occurring before the development of schizophrenia, which would indicate that all schizophrenic patients have a premorbid personality disturbance. Research investigating schizophrenia spectrum personality disorders in a variety of populations, including the premorbid personalities of schizophrenic patients, non-affected relatives of schizophrenic patients and clinically referred personality disordered patients, may help to answer some of the questions regarding the role of early personality disturbances in the development of schizophrenia.

Genetics

Adoption and family studies have provided strong evidence for a genetic relationship between schizophrenia and SPD (Kendler *et al.* 1981, 1993a, 1994; Frangos *et al.* 1985; Kendler 1985, 1988; Gershon *et al.* 1988; Maier *et al.* 1993). There is an increased incidence of SPD among the relatives of schizophrenic probands compared with the relatives of control subjects (Kendler *et al.* 1981, 1993b; Baron *et al.* 1982; Gunderson *et al.* 1983). An increased incidence of SPD has been reported in relatives of schizotypal probands, supporting a genetic basis for this personality disorder. An increase of schizophrenia-related disorders (Siever *et al.* 1990b) and of schizophrenia itself (Schulz *et al.* 1986; Battaglia *et al.* 1995) has been reported in the families of patients with SPD. The likelihood of having a schizophrenic relative is comparable for probands diagnosed with either SPD or schizophrenia (6.9% vs. 6.5%), further supporting common genetic substrates for the two disorders (Kendler *et al.* 1993a).

A further subject of investigation is the heritability of the factor structure of schizotypy. Certain SPD features suggest a closer genetic relationship to schizophrenia than others (Webb & Levinson 1993; Ingraham & Kety 2000). For example, an analysis of the Provincial sample of the Danish Adoption Study found suspiciousness, flat or spotty affectivity and reclusive withdrawn behaviour most frequent among the non-schizophrenic biological relatives of schizophrenic adoptees and each feature was significantly more common than among the biological relatives of controls. Psychotic-like symptoms, on the other hand, were not more prevalent among the biological relatives of schizophrenic adoptees than controls (Ingraham & Kety 2000). Several family studies have observed that, in contrast to positive psychotic-like SPD symptoms, the deficit-like SPD traits, primarily reflecting social and cognitive deficits, better characterized the relatives of schizophrenic probands compared with those of normal controls or other comparison groups (Gunderson *et al.* 1983; Kendler 1985; Torgersen *et al.* 1993; Webb & Levinson 1993; Maier *et al.* 1994). A study of twins from a non-clinical population (Kendler *et al.* 1991) found that positive and negative symptoms associated with SPD represent two relatively independent strongly heritable dimensions. However, only negative symptoms were related to other characteristics also associated with schizophrenia (Grove *et al.* 1991). These symptoms appear to underlie the core pathology across the spectrum, possibly reflecting a common neurodevelopmental abnormality.

It has been questioned whether there is a phenomenological difference between SPD patients who are relatives of schizophrenics and those who are identified clinically (Raine & Lencz 1995). For example, clinical patients may have more prominent psychotic-like symptoms. This may lead to an overlap in diagnosis between patients with borderline personality disorder and SPD patients where positive symptomatology is the prominent feature. This overlap was found to be considerable when DSM-III diagnostic criteria were used. An attempt to differentiate the psychotic-like symptoms of borderline personality disorder as transient, often dissociative and associated with periods of affective symptoms, as opposed to those of SPD which are more persistent and independent of affective symptoms, has been incorporated into DSM-IV (American Psychiatric Association 1994). As diagnostic criteria are refined, we are moving towards a more homogeneous SPD group, which will render interpretation of studies more meaningful. Studies involving populations from family, clinical and community sources may further clarify the underlying dimensions of schizotypy.

Psychophysiology (see also Chapter 16, which
pertains to adults and patients with schizophrenia *per se*)

Prepulse inhibition

Dysfunctions at very early stages of sensory gating and information processing have been putatively associated with clinical features such as perceptual aberrations, hallucinations and distraction, which have been considered as potential precursors of sensory overload, cognitive fragmentation and disorganization. Among psychophysiological measures one approach has involved the startle reflex with the prepulse inhibition (PPI) paradigm. PPI refers to the inhibitory effect of a weak auditory prestimulus on the acoustic startle blink reflex to a loud noise. At short lead intervals this has the effect of markedly attenuating or 'gating' the amplitude of the startle response and facilitating its latency (Braff et al. 1991). Disruption of PPI occurs with agonists of dopamine and serotonin and with glutamate/N-methyl-D-aspartate (NMDA) antagonists (Swerdlow & Geyer 1998). Neurodevelopmental studies have shown that PPI is reduced by rearing rats in isolation, an effect which may be reversed by typical and atypical antipsychotic drugs. Furthermore, in rats with neonatal neurotoxic lesions of the hippocampus PPI is impaired after puberty, suggesting that early developmental lesions of the hippocampus create a vulnerability to hormonal influences on neuronal circuits that accompany puberty (Lipska et al. 1995).

Applications to the schizophrenia spectrum have shown that PPI is diminished in schizophrenia (Braff et al. 1991; Grillon et al. 1992; Bolino et al. 1994) and in schizotypal patients with positive and negative symptoms (Cadenhead et al. 1993). At the same time there have been disconfirmatory reports in both schizophrenia (Dawson et al. 1993) and in both positive and negative dimensions of schizotypy measured with the Chapman scales of perceptual aberration/magical ideation and anhedonia (Cadenhead et al. 1996). More subtle individual differences than simple positive–negative syndromes may assist with syndrome correlates. Swerdlow et al. (1995) reported an association with low Minnesota Multiphasic Personality Inventory (MMPI) hysteria scores, i.e. low scores on somatic anxiety, lassitude, social naivety and inhibited aggression, features in keeping with an activated syndrome (Gruzelier 1999a, 2002; Gruzelier et al. 2002).

The acoustic startle reflex is thought to involve inhibitory influences from descending frontolimbic circuitry elucidated in animals with pharmacological studies showing modulation by the hippocampal and medial prefrontal cortices and the basolateral amygdala. Accordingly, top-down modulatory influences may be important to control experimentally, as shown in recent-onset relatively asymptomatic schizophrenic patients (Dawson et al. 1993). Whereas PPI was normal in the conventional passive attention paradigm, there was a deficit in conditions where attention was required to the prepulse. Indeed, in schizophrenia higher level cognitive deficits have been associated with PPI attenuation and these include thought disorder, Wisconsin Card Sorting Test (WCST) performance, distractability on the Continuous Performance Test (CPT) and lateralized inattention on the Posner task (Karper et al. 1996). At the same time, Swerdlow et al. (1995) found no association in schizotypal individuals with cognitive tasks measuring disinhibition while Cadenhead et al. (1996) found no association with lower level processes including habituation of startle, visual backward masking and reaction time.

P50 suppression

Another measure of sensory gating involves a two-stimulus (S1, S2) evoked potential paradigm where normally the positive-going potential at 50 ms (P50) to the second stimulus (S2) is attenuated. A gating deficit at short interstimulus intervals is measured by a reduced ratio or difference between the two positive-going response amplitudes (P50s) at around 50 ms. This is typically interpreted as a failure to inhibit the response to the second stimulus, referred to as the P50 suppression anomaly. Neural underpinning is thought to involve desensitization of the alpha-7 nicotinic receptor (Griffith et al. 1998), which is modulated at the CA3 hippocampal level (Flach et al. 1996) and is linked with the same gene locus as schizophrenia (Freedman et al. 1997).

P50 suppression has been found deficient in many schizophrenic patients, their first-degree relatives and in SPD patients, as defined in Table 7.1 (Siegel et al. 1984; Waldo et al. 1991; Clementz et al. 1998; Cadenhead et al. 2000). Whereas symptom relations and the putative link with perceptual abnormalities have proved elusive in schizophrenia, a psychometric study in the normal population has found the unreality dimension to characterize those with abnormal P50 suppression (Croft et al. 2001). This relation was found not with P50 suppression per se but was caused by an attenuated amplitude to the first stimulus (S1), as well as to a failure of habituation of S2 amplitude, indicating the need for a closer look at the nature of the S1–S2 effect.

From a study of parents who carry the genetic inheritance, Freedman et al. concluded that the gating deficit may predispose to schizophrenia but that additional hippocampal pathology was necessary for the psychosis to develop (Harris et al. 1996). They found that while parents shared attentional deficits with patients, verbal learning deficits were only found in patients. Furthermore, in a sibling study, while schizophrenic and non-schizophrenic siblings shared the P50 gating deficit, hippocampal volumes, which correlated with IQ, were reduced only in those siblings with schizophrenia (Waldo et al. 1994). However, as will be shown below, short-term verbal learning deficits are not uncommon in schizotypes.

Habituation

Abnormalities in the response to novel stimuli and in the habituation of the response with stimulus repetition have also contributed to evidence of early stage anomalies of processing in schizophrenia and schizotypy. Habituation is a prerequisite for flexibility in selective attention and the redistribution of processing resources while the orienting response indexes the focusing of attention and a call for processing resources.

The more extensive examination of habituation in the schizophrenia spectrum has concerned electrophysiological approaches involving autonomic recording, electrodermal orienting activity in particular. A variety of abnormalities has been demonstrated, varying from over- to under-responsivity. In schizotypy, while a similar range of anomalies has been represented, irregular patterns of orienting and habituation are the most common and may coincide with cognitive disorganization (Gruzelier & Raine 1994; Raine *et al.* 1997). Interest in habituation deficits has extended to the P50 (Croft *et al.* 2001) and to habituation of the startle reflex (Bolino *et al.* 1992; Braff *et al.* 1992). In both cases, delayed habituation has been found to correlate with P50 and PPI deficits, as outlined in previous sections, suggesting shared central mechanisms (Schwarzkopf *et al.* 1993; Croft *et al.* 2001).

N100 and P300 evoked potentials

The N100 wave has provided a useful index of attentional allocation, often measured with simple paradigms requiring the detection of target stimuli among trains of standard stimuli: paradigms most commonly used to assess the P300 to the target or oddball stimuli. Attenuation of the N100 has been found in various schizophrenic subgroups, more so than attenuation of later P200 and P300 components (Boutros *et al.* 1997). These reductions have been found in obligate carriers (Frangou *et al.* 1997) although not in children at genetic risk (Freedman *et al.* 1988), while patients with SDP have shown results intermediate between schizophrenic patients and controls (Trestman *et al.* 1996). Waldo *et al.* (1988) have reported the coexistence of P50 suppression failure and N100 diminution in schizophrenic patients, whereas in those relatives with P50 suppression impairment the N100 amplitudes were larger than normal, interpreted as a compensatory mechanism.

Amplitude reduction of the P300 is often found in schizophrenia (McCarley *et al.* 1993), in patients with schizotypal personality disorder (Blackwood *et al.* 1986; Trestman *et al.* 1996) as well as in borderline personality disorder (Blackwood *et al.* 1986). While P300 reduction has been assumed to accompany negative or deficit symptoms, there is as yet no clear symptom relation in schizophrenia (Gruzelier 1999a) or schizotypal personality disorder (Siever 1991), although in the New York High-Risk Project a negative social–interpersonal dimension was associated with P300 and verbal working memory deficits (Squires-Wheeler *et al.* 1997). A cognitive measure of allusive thinking has also been found to correlate with P300 amplitude reduction in students (Kutcher *et al.* 1989).

Lateral asymmetry in the P300 may more readily yield syndrome relations in the schizophrenia spectrum (Strik *et al.* 1994; Gruzelier *et al.* 1999b). In the latter study activated–withdrawn syndrome relations were associated with P300 asymmetry and they were also found to hold for the earlier N100 and P200 components, suggestive of a generalized thalamocortical activation imbalance rather than a circumscribed memory deficit often theoretically associated with the P300 deficit.

Eye movements

Of theoretical relevance to disorders of visual perception and attention, eye movement recording has disclosed a range of abnormalities in schizophrenia and family members. One takes the form of deviant smooth pursuit eye tracking through intrusive and anticipatory saccadic eye movements (Grove *et al.* 1991; Clementz *et al.* 1994; Ross *et al.* 1996, 1998), another a failure to inhibit reflexive saccades following instruction (Clementz *et al.* 1994; Katsanis *et al.* 1997; McDowell & Clementz 1997). In support of a genetic vulnerability factor disinhibition along with a failure to suppress anticipatory saccades in smooth pursuit has been found to characterize those parents with a history of chronic schizophrenia in comparison to their spouses without a family history (Ross *et al.* 1998).

Tracking abnormalities have been found in patients with SPD and not in other personality disorders, and have been associated with schizotypy in college students (Siever *et al.* 1984, 1989, 1990a). Evidence of a functional basis to the deficit follows demonstration in recent-onset schizophrenia of improvement by attentional manipulations, suggesting an association with diminished voluntary attention in keeping with frontal involvement in smooth pursuit (White & Yee 1997).

Syndromal considerations have linked poor tracking with negative symptoms through association with the Chapman scales of physical anhedonia (Simons & Katkin 1985) and social anhedonia (Clementz *et al.* 1992), and in clinical samples with deficit-like rather than psychotic-like symptoms (Siever 1991; Siever *et al.* 1993). Perceptual aberration has been implicated along with physical anhedonia as a correlate of poor eye tracking in students (Simons & Katkin 1985; O'Driscoll *et al.* 1998), while O'Driscoll *et al.* (1998) found perceptual aberrations to accompany both antisaccade and smooth pursuit deficits.

Information processing and cognitive function

Visual processing

Clinical evidence, such as Klosterkotter *et al.*'s (1992) report that visual symptoms far outnumbered auditory symptoms in predicting the development of first-rank symptoms in first-episode schizophrenia when combined with experimental results on visual processing, is stimulating new research on the schizophrenia spectrum. Visual processing involves complementary and reciprocally related dorsal magnocellular (fast/transient cell) and the ventral parvocellular (slow/sustained cell) systems (Breitmeyer & Ganz 1976). The magnocellular transient-processing channel (retinal gangion, lateral geniculate nucleus, striate, prestriate, superior temporal sulcus, posterior parietal cortex) exhibits selectivity for low spatial frequencies by virtue of its high temporal resolution and primarily responds to the movement of stimuli and their appearance/disappearance. The magnocellular system is specialized for the precise timing of visual events, playing a major part in motion perception, spatial location and eye movement control including smooth pursuit eye movements. This system is not specific to vision but is also involved in the very rapid temporal coding required for the coherence of visual, auditory and olfactory perception, for cross-modal integration and for motor control. The parvocellular pathway (retinal ganglion, striate, prestriate, inferior temporal cortex) is a sustained-processing channel favouring high spatial frequencies having a low spatial resolution and is involved in pattern analysis. It is concerned with object recognition, colour perception and high-resolution form perception.

Magnocellular function deficits in motion sensitivity have been found in both schizophrenic patients with positive or mixed positive/negative symptoms and in dyslexic subjects, who have often been characterized by positive symptom schizotypy (Richardson *et al.* 1994). Motion sensitivity together with visual direction sense was also found to be impaired in students with positive features of schizotypy but not in those with negative features (Richardson & Gruzelier 1994). A comparison of magnocellular tasks of motion perception and location with parvocellular tasks of spatial frequency and pattern finding deficits implicated the magno and not the parvo system (O'Donnell *et al.* 1996). In the same study, more severe than the perceptual impairment in motion detection was a recognition deficit involving working memory which was attributed to prefrontal involvement.

Both magno and parvo systems are dynamically involved in backward masking. This is the phenomenon where the presentation of a stimulus following a target at short interstimulus intervals has the effect of hampering or masking target detection, the interference seemingly working backwards in time. The transient system first locates the target and responds to its offset, having meanwhile given over identifying the target to the sustained system. More than one abnormality has been disclosed in schizophrenia (Braff *et al.* 1991; Green *et al.* 1994; Slaghuis & Bakker 1995). In keeping with a parvocellular abnormality, some patients have abnormal threshold durations for identifying the target stimulus without the mask (critical stimulus duration) which suggests longer iconic persistence, also demonstrated with two-pulse temporal resolution measures. This deficit appears to be associated with negative rather than positive symptoms (Gruzelier 1999b).

Magnocellular deficits have been more commonly invoked as an explanation for the masking deficits. The nature of such an aberrant transient system deficit is unclear, but its disruptive consequences suggest overactivity of some kind: easily triggered transients, abnormally potent transients, prolonged transient channel activity or additive transient susceptibility, i.e. susceptibility to multiple transient bursts in a short period of time (Merritt & Balogh 1989). Masking deficits have coexisted with both positive and negative symptoms in schizophrenic patients and in association with the unreality dimension of schizotypy (Saccuzzo *et al.* 1981; Merritt & Balogh 1989; Schuck & Lee 1989), yet there is a clear preference in the reports towards an association with positive symptoms and positive features of schizotypy.

Green *et al.* (1997) went on to delineate early sensory–perceptual components from the later attentional disengagement components in backward masking, comparing siblings with schizophrenia and unaffected siblings. Masking deficits relating to both magnocellular and parvocellular systems were disclosed, with the earlier sensory–perceptual components providing the vulnerability marker in the unaffected siblings.

Frontal and executive functions

An implication from more than one investigation of early stages of information processing where higher cognitive functions were also examined was that predisposition to schizophrenia resided with lower level processes while higher cognitive deficits were necessary for the manifestation of psychosis (Harris *et al.* 1996; Green *et al.* 1997). This attractive hypothesis has not been confirmed. Cognitive deficits have been well documented in schizotypy, although severity of deficit does appear frequently to be greater in schizophrenia than in schizotypy, at least when the conclusion is based on group comparisons.

Deficits include executive functions involving the frontal lobe such as set changing and perseveration measured with the WCST, which have characterized many schizophrenic patients, patients with SPD and schizotypes in the normal population (Lyons *et al.* 1991; Raine *et al.* 1992; Battaglia *et al.* 1994; Trestman *et al.* 1995; Voglmaier *et al.* 1997). In studies of patients and their relatives, a range of higher level cognitive deficiencies have been reported including set alternation frequency, verbal fluency, abstraction, verbal memory and Trail Making (Franke *et al.* 1993; Keefe *et al.* 1994).

Addressing the question of specificity, Tien *et al.* (1992) found by assessing the type of error made on the WCST that perseveration was associated with schizotypal traits as distinct from paranoid and schizoid traits. Similarly, Keefe *et al.* (1994) found relatives of patients with schizophrenia to have more perseverative errors than other personality disorders, to sort fewer categories and to take more time to complete Trail Making B, although they were no different in verbal fluency or in general intelligence. These results were similar to those found in schizotypal patients by Trestman *et al.* (1995). A failure in maintaining response set on the WCST has been found to characterize high-scoring students on the perceptual aberration scale (Park *et al.* 1995).

Continuous performance test

Executive functions include the control and maintenance of attention. A widely used behavioural measure of sustained attention is the CPT. This involves the random brief rapid visual presentation of letters or digits with the instruction to press a key to target stimuli. The task may be made more difficult by degrading stimuli that place a load on perceptual processing or by increasing the load on working memory. Deficits have been demonstrated in schizophrenia, including patients in remission, in children with a schizophrenic parent and other first-degree relatives and in SPD patients (Cornblatt & Keilp 1994; Roitman *et al.* 1997). The deficits tend not to increase within the session, implying that the disability is not one of sustaining attention *per se*.

In support of perceptual involvement, an association between CPT deficit and schizotypy in the form of perceptual aberration (PAS) as well as the negative Schizotypal Personality Questionnaive (SPQ) (Raine 1991) interpersonal factor was shown in a Taiwanese study (Chen *et al.* 1997). Furthermore, when combined with poor CPT performance the similar schizotypy features of perceptual distortion and social anhedonia have characterized subjects performing poorly on frontal lobe tests including the WCST, Trail Making and verbal fluency (Obiols *et al.* 1999). This is in keeping with frontal lobe involvement in components of the task involving working memory and the control of attention.

Thought disorder and disinhibition

Another type of attentional deficit is distractability which is thought to underpin cognitive disorganization including thought disorder. These features form a major component of positive schizophrenic symptomatology and have been considered one fundamental aspect of schizotypy exemplified by Meehl's (1962) concept of cognitive slippage. At the same time this is one of the least well-defined aspects of schizotypy. The syndrome constellation may include distractability, odd speech, disorganization, cognitive activation and disinhibition, together with odd behaviour and non-conformity.

A diversity of measures has been applied to schizotypy. Using a Thought Disorder Index (TDI) derived from the Rorschach test which reflects a loosening of associations, abnormalities have been found in both clinical SPD and schizophrenia, as well as in siblings of schizophrenic patients and non-clinical samples with high perceptual aberration scores (Edell 1987; Hain *et al.* 1995; Coleman *et al.* 1996). Communication deviance has been examined in the parents of schizophrenic patients where it was found to be associated with both schizotypy and distractability (Docherty *et al.* 1998). Another approach has been to explore mentalizing or the ability to maintain representations of mental states of oneself and others. Using a false-belief picture sequencing task, normal subjects were categorized according to mentalizing ability and examined for differences in SPQ factors (Langdon & Coltheart 1999). In different experiments, the interpersonal factor and the cognitive–perceptual/disorganized factors were implicated. The pattern of deficits supported an impairment in inferring and representing mental states as distinct from executive planning or a failure of disengagement.

A number of cognitive disinhibitory deficits have been examined and, on the whole, they have been associated with positive symptoms. One such phenomenon is latent inhibition. By virtue of repeated pre-exposure to a stimulus without reinforcement consequences, the learning of subsequent associations with the stimulus is retarded. This has been studied as an animal model for schizophrenia because the dopamine agonist amphetamine disrupts latent inhibition and is reversed by typical neuroleptics. However, evidence of a disruption of latent inhibition in schizophrenia is controversial with both affirmative (Baruch *et al.* 1988a; Gray *et al.* 1995) and negative reports (Lubow *et al.* 1987; Swerdlow *et al.* 1995). Consideration of the conflicting evidence has led to the attribution of latent inhibition disruption to a highly circumscribed aspect of the early schizophrenic process, one without, as yet, any clearly demarcated symptom or process correlates. Latent inhibition has also been associated with the predominantly positive symptom Claridge Schizotypal Personality (STA) scale (Baruch *et al.* 1988b; Lipp & Vaitl 1992) and with Eysenck's Psychoticism measure (Baruch *et al.* 1988b).

Cognitive disinhibition manifested by reduced negative priming has also been associated with positive symptoms in schizophrenia (Beech *et al.* 1989; Williams 1995), in schizotypy in the normal population (Peters *et al.* 1994; Moritz & Mass 1997) as well as in the relatives of schizophrenic and neurotic patients (Claridge & Beech 1996). Disinhibition has also been implicated in an analysis of the content of verbal fluency tests (Duchene *et al.* 1998), which disclosed that high-scoring subjects on the magical ideation scale produced more low-frequency words, interpreted as a disinhibition of semantic networks that may underpin thought disorder and creativity.

Memory

Consistent with the view that explicit declarative memory is one of the cardinal neuropsychological deficits in schizophrenia (Gruzelier *et al.* 1988; Saykin *et al.* 1994), declarative memory has been found deficient in relatives (Keefe *et al.* 1994) and in siblings with a schizotypal personality (Cannon *et al.* 1994). In contrast to this, implicit memory may not be affected (Ferraro & Okerlund 1995). Furthermore, reduced performance on the California Verbal Learning Test has been demonstrated in SPD patients compared with other personality disorders. This deficit has been found accompanied by WCST deficits but not by a range of other deficits interpreted as a profile in support of a left temporofrontal deficit (Voglmaier *et al.* 1997).

Working memory which involves frontal functions has been found deficient in schizophrenia (Park & Holzman 1992; Keefe *et al.* 1997) and in first-degree relatives (Park *et al.* 1995). In relation to schizotypy with a battery of cognitive tasks verbal working memory was found in SPD patients to be mid-way between that of normal subjects and schizophrenic patients, as was general intellectual performance together with recognition memory, abstract reasoning, cognitive inhibition and measures of attention (Cadenhead *et al.* 1999). Visuospatial working memory impairment has also been identified in SPD patients and the extent found to be greater than in other personality disorders (Roitman *et al.* 2000). Working memory was identified as the source of the visuospatial deficit rather than perceptual abilities *per se* (Farmer *et al.* 2000).

At the same time, perceptual symptoms have been associated with working memory deficits. Working memory deficits have been shown to be related to both positive unreality (PAS, magical ideation or MIS) and social anhedonia features of schizotypy, as well as correlating with WCST performance in support of frontal involvement (Gooding *et al.* 1999). In normal schizotypes identified by PAS, working memory deficits were disclosed on a delayed spatial response task (Park *et al.* 1995). The working memory deficit was accompanied by set maintenance deficits on the WCST, whereas in a subsequent report the same subjects failed to show verbal working memory deficits (Lenzenweger & Gold 2000). Conflicts as to the verbal or non-verbal nature of the working memory deficit may arise from differences between studies in the composition of various dimensions of schizotypy.

Lateralization

Left hemisphere dysfunction has been a widely researched hypothesis in schizophrenia and while there is a good deal of support for left temporolimbic deficits, functional deficits in the right hemisphere have also been disclosed, and there is some structural evidence of a loss of normal asymmetry in the planum temporale (Gruzelier 1999a). As in schizophrenia, reports in schizotypy on the nature and direction of functional asymmetries have diverged. Claridge and co-workers, with predominantly positive schizotypy scales (STA), have reported evidence with a range of techniques for an imbalance in excitation–inhibition: the right hemisphere excitatory and the left inhibitory. A deficiency in left hemisphere-mediated smooth pursuit has characterized schizotypy measured with the MMPI (Kelly & Bakan 1999). Males with MIS have disclosed olfactory detection deficits implicating the left temporal lobe (Mohr *et al.* 2001), while in females MIS has been associated with excess left hemisphere inhibition indexed by right hemi-space neglect with a modified Corsi block task (Nalcaci *et al.* 2000). In contrast, Raine and Manders (1988) reported neuropsychological evidence for the opposite state of imbalance, as has Jutai (1989), while Goodarzi *et al.* (2000) found a global perceptual processing deficit implicating the right hemisphere in association with unusual experiences and the STA scale.

Consideration of syndrome relations may unravel some of the complexity in the laterality of functional deficits in the schizophrenia spectrum (Gruzelier 1999a). Characterizing schizophrenic patients on the basis of cognitive or electrophysiological asymmetry delineated a positive activated syndrome which was accompanied by left > right functional preference, and a negative withdrawn syndrome accompanied by right > left functional preference activity (Gruzelier *et al.* 1988, 1999a, c; Gruzelier 1999a). Hallucinations and delusions of first-rank were independent of these two syndromes, and constituted a third syndrome which showed inconsistent associations with functional asymmetry.

A similar three-factor solution of activated, withdrawn and unreality factors was demonstrated in schizotypy in the normal population measured with the Raine SPQ accompanied by Thayer activation scales (Gruzelier 1996). Furthermore, tests of verbal and non-verbal recognition memory in schizotypy disclosed the same activated–withdrawn syndrome asymmetry relations as in schizophrenia, with unreality showing inconsistent relations with asymmetry (Gruzelier *et al.* 1995; Gruzelier &

Doig 1996). Congruent relations with a test of lateral visual direction sense, a putative magnocellular measure, were also disclosed with the Oxford–Liverpool Inventory psychosis-proneness scales (OLIFE; Gruzelier & Richardson 1994; Mason *et al.* 1997), as were relations with electrodermal asymmetries in relation both to self-reported social anhedonia in unmedicated schizophrenic patients (Gruzelier & Davis 1995) and to positive schizotypal features in the normal population (Mason *et al.* 1997). Prospective evidence arose serendipitously from a student whose outlying face > word asymmetry predicted a withdrawn/unreality syndrome profile in subsequent first and second schizophrenic episodes (Gruzelier *et al.* 1995).

There is a range of evidence in support of an association between inconsistent functional lateralization and the unreality dimension. High-scoring subjects on MIS were equipotential for either visual field in a lexical decision task on which low-scoring subjects showed a right visual field advantage (Leonhard & Brugger 1998). Inconsistent handedness (as distinct from strong left-handedness) has been associated with unreality and unusual experiences (Richardson 1994; Gruzelier & Doig 1996; Shaw *et al.* 2001). In fact, the incidence and impact of non-righthandedness assessed by handedness questionnaires has been one of the more replicable neurocognitive findings in schizotypy (Chapman & Chapman 1985; Kelly & Coursey 1992; Kim *et al.* 1992; Richardson 1994; Gruzelier & Doig 1996; Shaw *et al.* 2001). This supports the role of developmental influences, as does the ontology of functional asymmetry.

Animal and human evidence shows that functional asymmetries are subject to the influence of genes, hormones and early experiences, and remain vulnerable to stressors throughout the life span (Gruzelier 1999a). Of importance to the nature of the activated and withdrawn syndrome asymmetry findings, it has been shown that after birth and prior to the development of both language and visuoconstructive skills in children, spontaneous asymmetries in gesture and emotion have been documented, described as influencing the approach–withdrawal balance in social encounters (Trevarthen 1996). Also relevant to schizotypy and Meehl's concept of schizotaxia may be the developmental processes that determine variations in neuronal connectivity such as synaptogenesis influenced by pubertal timing. Replicable associations with early and late pubertal timing when compared with normal maturation have been shown with the unreality dimension of schizotypy (Gruzelier & Kaiser 1996; Kaiser & Gruzelier 1999a), while some implications for brain connectivity were supported through measurement of evoked potential latencies and EEG connectivity through coherence in response to photic driving (Kaiser & Gruzelier 1996, 1999b).

Neurochemistry

The dopamine (DA) hypothesis that the schizophrenic process is secondary to an excess of dopamine has long been the cornerstone of research into the pathophysiology of schizophrenia. Although supported, at least in part, by the efficacy of neuroleptic

covered by umbrella concepts of psychotic-like or unreality experiences.

The problems of heterogeneity and the allied issue of diagnostic specificity are among the most pressing in research on the schizophrenia spectrum. Their study promotes the teasing apart of multiple domains of pathophysiological dysfunction. The study of schizotypal individuals offers the methodological advantage of providing an opportunity to obtain a more homogeneous behavioural sample ascertained through questionnaire assessment of a large number of normal individuals or clinical assessment of community volunteers. In addition, this advantage may be combined with the relative freedom in schizotypal individuals from the confounds of hospitalization, medication, chronic psychosis and other consequences of a long-term psychiatric diagnosis. By combining this strategy with the study of SPD patients, who also suffer fewer of the confounds encountered with schizophrenic patients, valuable insights may be provided into the pathophysiology of schizophrenia.

References

Abi-Dhargam, A., Gil, R., Krystal, J. *et al.* (1998) Increased striatal dopamine transmission in schizophrenia: confirmation in a second cohort. *American Journal of Psychiatry* **155**, 761–767.

American Psychiatric Association (1980) *Diagnostic and Statistical Manual of Mental Disorders*, 3rd edn. American Psychiatric Association, Washington DC.

American Psychiatric Association (1994) *Diagnostic and Statistical Manual of Mental Disorders*, 4th edn. American Psychiatric Association, Washington DC.

Amin, F., Siever, L.J., Silverman, J.M. *et al.* (1997) *Plasma HVA in Schizotypal Personality Disorder Plasma Homovanillic Studies in Schizophrenia, Implications for Presynaptic Dopamine Dysfunction* (eds A.J. Fruedhoff & F. Amin), pp. 133–149. Progress in Psychiatry Series, American Psychiatric Press, Washington, DC.

Andreasen, N.C., Paradiso, S. & O'Leary, D.S. (1998) 'Cognitive dysmetria' as an integrative theory of schizophrenia: a dysfunction in cortical-subcortical-cerebullar circuitry? *Schizophrenia Bulletin* **24**, 203–218.

Baron, M., Gruen, R., Rainer, J.D. *et al.* (1982) Schizoaffective illness, schizophrenia, and affective disorders: morbidity risk and genetic transmission. *Acta Psychiatrica Scandinavica* **65**, 253–262.

Barthell, C. & Holmes, D. (1968) High school yearbooks: a nonreactive measure of social isolation in graduates who later became schizophrenic. *Journal of Abnormal Psychology* **78**, 313–316.

Baruch, I., Hemsley, D.R. & Gray, A. (1988a) Differential performance of acute and chronic schizophrenics in a latent inhibition task. *Journal of Nervous and Mental Disease* **176**, 598–606.

Baruch, I., Hemsley, D.R. & Gray, A. (1988b) Latent inhibition and 'psychotic proneness' in normal subjects. *Personality and Individual Differences* **1988**, 777–783.

Battaglia, M., Abbruzzese, M., Ferri, S. *et al.* (1994) An assessment of the Wisconsin Card Sorting Test as an indicator of liability to schizophrenia. *Schizophrenia Research* **14**, 39–45.

Battaglia, M., Bernardeschi, L. Franchini, L. *et al.* (1995) A family study of schizotypal disorder. *Schizophrenia Bulletin* **21**, 33–46.

Battaglia, M., Cavallini, M.C., Macciardi, F. & Bellodi, L. (1997) The structure of DSM-IIIR schizotypal personality disorder diagnosed by direct interview. *Schizophrenia Bulletin* **23**, 83–92.

Beech, A., Powell, T., McWilliam, J. & Claridge, G. (1989) Evidence of reduced 'cognitive inhibition' in schizophrenia. *British Journal of Clinical Psychology* **28**, 109–116.

Bentall, R.P., Claridge, G.S. & Slade, P.D. (1989) The multidimensional nature of schizotypal traits: a factor analytic study with normal subjects. *British Journal of Clinical Psychology* **28**, 363–375.

Bernstein, D.P., Useda, D. & Siever, L.J. (1996) Paranoid personality disorder. In: *DSM-IV Sourcebook*, Vol. 2 (eds T.A. Widiger, A.J. Frances, H.A. Pincus, R. Ross, M.B. First & W.W. Davis), pp. 665–674. American Psychiatric Association, Washington, DC.

Blackwood, D.H.R., St Clair, D.M. & Kutcher, S.P. (1986) P300 event-related potential abnormalities in borderline personality disorder. *Biological Psychiatry* **21**, 557–560.

Bleuler, E. (1950) *Dementia Praecox or the Group of Schizophrenias*. International Universities Press, New York.

Bolino, F., Manna, V. DiCicco, L. *et al.* (1992) Startle reflex habituation in functional psychoses: a controlled study. *Neuroscience Letters* **145**, 126–128.

Bolino, F., Di Michele, V., DiCicco, L. *et al.* (1994) Sensorimotor gating and habituation evoked by electro-cutaneous stimulation in schizophrenia. *Biological Psychiatry* **36**, 670–679.

Boutros, N.N., Nasrallah, H., Leighty, R. *et al.* (1997) Auditory evoked potentials: clinical versus research applications. *Psychiatry Research* **24**, 183–195.

Bower, E.M., Schellhammer, T.A. & Daily, J.A. (1960) School characteristics of male adolescents who later become schizophrenic. *American Journal of Orthopsychiatry* **30**, 712–729.

Braff, D.L., Saccucco, D.P., Geyer & M.A. (1991) Information processing dysfunctions in schizophrenia: studies of visual backward masking, sensorimotor gating, and habituation. In: *Handbook of Schizophrenia*, Vol. 5 *Neuropsychology, Psychophysiology and Information Processing* (eds S.R. Steinhauser, J.H. Gruzelier & J. Zubin), pp. 303–334. Elsevier, Amsterdam.

Braff, D.L., Grillon, C. & Geyer, M.A. (1992) Gating and habituation of the startle reflex in schizophrenic patients. *Archives of General Psychiatry* **49**, 206–215.

Breitmeyer, B. & Ganz, L. (1976) Implications of sustained and transient channels for theories of visual pattern masking. *Psychological Review* **83**, 1–36.

Buchsbaum, M.S., Someya, T. & Tang, C.Y. (1996) PET and MRI of the thalamus of never-medicated patients with schizophrenia. *American Journal of Psychiatry* **153**, 191–199.

Buchsbaum, M.S., Yang, S., Hazlett, E. *et al.* (1997a) Ventricular volume and asymmetry in schizotypal personality disorder and schizophrenia assessed with magnetic resonance imaging. *Schizophrenia Research* **27**, 45–53.

Buchsbaum, M.S., Trestman, R.J., Hazlett, E. *et al.* (1997b) Regional cerebral blood flow during the Wisconsin Card Sort test in schizotypal personality disorder. *Schizophrenia Research* **27**, 21–28.

Buchsbaum, M.S., Nenadic, I., Hazlett, E. *et al.* (2002) Differential metabolic rates in prefrontal and temporal Brodman areas in schizophrenia and schizotypal personality disorder. *Schizophrenia Research* **54**, 141–150.

Byne, W., Buchsbaum, M.S., Kemether, E. *et al.* (2001) MRI assessment of medial and dorsal pulvinar nuclei of the thalamus in schizophrenia and schizotypal personality disorder. *Archives of General Psychiatry* **58**, 133–140.

Cadenhead, K.S., Geyer, M.A. & Braff, D.L. (1993) Impaired startle prepulse inhibition and habituation in patients with schizotypal personality disorder. *American Journal of Psychiatry* **150**, 1862–1867.

Cadenhead, K.S., Perry, W. & Braff, D.L. (1996) The relationship of information-processing deficits and clinical symptoms in schizotypal personality disorder. *Biological Psychiatry* **40**, 853–858.

Cadenhead, K.S., Perry, W., Shafer, K. & Braff, D.L. (1999) Cognitive functions in schizotypal personality disorder. *Schizophrenia Research* **37**, 123–132.

Cadenhead, K.S., Light, G.A., Geyer, M.A. & Braff, D.L. (2000) Sensory gating deficits assessed by the P50 event-related potential in subjects with schizotypal personality disorder. *American Journal of Psychiatry* **157**, 55–59.

Cannon, T.D., Mednick, S.A. & Parnas, J. (1990) Antecedents of predominantly negative- and predominantly positive-symptom schizophrenia in a high risk population. *Archives of General Psychiatry* **47**, 622–632.

Cannon, T.D., Zorrilla, L.E., Shtasel, D. *et al.* (1994) Neuropsychological functioning in siblings discordant for schizophrenia and healthy volunteers. *Archives of General Psychiatry* **51**, 651–661.

Cazzulo, V.A., Giobbio, G.M. *et al.* (1991) Cerebral structural abnormalities in schizophreniform disorder and in schizophrenia spectrum disorders. In: *Advances in Neuropsychiatry and Psychopharmacology* (eds C.A. Tamminga & S.C. Schulz).

Chapman, L.J. & Chapman, J.P. (1985) Psychosis proneness. In: *Controversies in Schizophrenia: Changes and Constancies* (ed. M. Alpert), pp. 157–174. Guilford Press, New York.

Chapman, L.J., Chapman, J.P. & Raulin, M.L. (1976) Scales for physical and social anhedonia. *Journal of Abnormal Psychology* **85**, 374–382.

Chapman, L.J., Chapman, J.P. & Raulin, M.L. (1978) Body-image aberration in schizophrenia. *Journal of Abnormal Psychology* **87**, 399–407.

Chen, W.J., Hsiao, C.K. & Lin, C.C. (1997) Schizotypy in community samples: the three-factor structure and correlation with sustained attention. *Journal of Abnormal Psychology* **106**, 649–654.

Claridge, G. & Beech, A. (1996) Schizotypy and lateralised negative priming in schizophrenics' and neurotics' relatives. *Personality and Individual Differences* **20**, 193–199.

Claridge, G. & Broks, P. (1984) Schizotypy and hemisphere function I. Theoretical considerations and the measurement of schizotypy. *Personality and Individual Differences* **5**, 633–648.

Clementz, B.A., Grove, W.M., Iacono, W.G. & Sweeney, J. (1992) Smooth pursuit eye movement dysfunction and liability for schizophrenia: implications for genetic modelling. *Journal of Abnormal Psychology* **101**, 117–129.

Clementz, B.A., McDowell, J.E. & Zisook, S. (1994) Saccadic system functioning among schizophrenia patients and their first-degree biological relatives. *Journal of Abnormal Psychology* **103**, 277–287.

Clementz, B.A., Geyer, M.A. & Braff, D.L. (1998) Poor P50 suppression among schizophrenia patients and their first-degree biological relatives. *American Journal of Psychiatry* **155**, 1691–1694.

Cohen, L.J., Hollander, E., DeCaria, C.M. *et al.* (1996) Specificity of neuropsychological impairment in obsessive–compulsive disorder: a comparison with social phobic and normal control subjects. *Journal of Neuropsychiatry and Clinical Neurosciences* **8**, 82–85.

Coleman, M.J., Levy, D.L., Lenzenweger, M.F. & Holzman, P.S. (1996) Thought disorder, perceptual aberrations, and schizotypy. *Journal of Abnormal Psychology* **105**, 469–473.

Cornblatt, B.A. & Keilp, J.G. (1994) Impaired attention, genetics and the pathophysiology of schizophrenia. *Schizophrenia Bulletin* **20**, 31–46.

Croft, R.J., Lee, A., Bertolot, J. & Gruzelier, J.H. (2001) Associations of P50 suppression and habituation with perceptual and cognitive features of 'unreality' in schizotypy. *Biological Psychiatry* **50**, 441–446.

Crow, T.J., Done, D.J. & Sacker, A. (1995) Birth cohort study of the antecedents of psychosis: ontogeny as witness to phylogenetic origins. In: *Search for the Causes of Schizophrenia*, Vol. 3 (eds H. Haefner & W.F. Gattaz), pp. 3–20. Springer, Berlin.

Csernansky, J., Murphy, G. & Faustman, W. (1991) Limbic/mesolimbic connections and the pathogenesis of schizophrenia. *Biological Psychiatry* **30**, 383–400.

Davidson, M. & Davis, K.L. (1988) A comparison of plasma homovanillic concentrations in schizophrenics and normal controls. *Archives of General Psychiatry* **45**, 561–563.

Davis, K.L., Davidson, M., Mohs, R.C. *et al.* (1985) Plasma homovanillic acid concentration and the severity of schizophrenic illness. *Science* **227**, 1601–1602.

Davis, K.L., Kahn, R.S., Ko. G. & Davidson, M. (1991) Dopamine and schizophrenia: a reconceptualisation. *American Journal of Psychiatry* **148**, 1474–1486.

Dawson, M.E., Hazlett, A.E., Filion, D.L. *et al.* (1993) Attention and schizophrenia: impaired modulation of the startle reflex. *Journal of Abnormal Psychology* **102**, 633–641.

Dickey, C.C., McCarley, R.W., Volgmaier, M., *et al.* (1999) Schizotypal personality disorder and MRI abnormalities of temporal lobe grey matter. *Biological Psychiatry* **45**, 1393–1402.

Docherty, N.M., Rhinewine, J.P., Labhart, R.P. & Gordinier, S.W. (1998) Communication disturbances and family psychiatric history in parents of schizophrenic patients. *Journal of Nervous and Mental Disease* **186**, 761–768.

Downhill, J.E., Buchsbaum, M.S., Wei, T.S. *et al.* (2000) Temporal lobe volume determined by magnetic resonance imaging in schizotypal personality disorder and schizophrenia. *Schizophrenia Research* **42**, 193–208.

Duchene, A., Graves, R.E. & Brugger, P. (1998) Schizotypal thinking and associative processing: a response commonality analysis of verbal fluency. *Journal of Psychiatry and Neuroscience* **23**, 56–60.

Eckblad, M. & Chapman, L.J. (1983) Magical ideation as an indicator of schizotypy. *Journal of Consulting and Clinical Psychology* **51**, 215–225.

Edell, W.S. (1987) Role of structure in disordered thinking in borderline and schizophrenic disorders. *Journal of Personality Assessment* **51**, 23–41.

El-Guebaly, N., Offord, D.R., Sullivan, K.T. & Lynch, G.W. (1978) Psychosocial adjustment of the offspring of psychiatric inpatients: the effect of alcoholic, depressive, and schizophrenic parentage. *Canadian Psychiatric Association Journal* **23**, 281–289.

Farmer, C.M., O'Donnell, B.F., Niznikiewicz, M.A. *et al.* (2000) Visual perception and working memory in schizotypal personality disorder. *American Journal of Psychiatry* **157**, 781–788.

Fenton, T.S. & McGlashan, T.H. (1989) Risk of schizophrenia in character disordered patients. *American Journal of Psychiatry* **146**, 1280–1284.

Ferraro, R.R. & Okerlund, M. (1995) Implicit memory of nonclinical schizotypal individuals. *Perceptual and Motor Skills* **80**, 371–376.

Fish, B. (1986) Antecedents of an acute schizophrenic break. *Journal of the American Academy of Child Psychiatry* **25**, 595–600.

Flach, K.A., Adler, L.E., Gerhardt, G.A. *et al.* (1996) Sensory gating in a computer model of the CA3 neural network of the hippocampus. *Biological Psychiatry* **40**, 1230–1245.

Foerster, A., Lewis, S., Owen, M. & Murray, R. (1991a) Premorbid adjustment and personality in psychosis: effects of sex and diagnosis. *British Journal of Psychiatry* **158**, 171–176.

Foerster, A., Lewis, S., Owen, M. & Murray, R. (1991b) Low birth weight and a family history of schizophrenia predict poor premorbid functioning in psychosis. *Schizophrenia Research* **5**, 13–20.

Frangos, E., Athenassanas, G., Tsitouorides, S., Katsanou, N. &

Alexandrakou, P. (1985) Prevalence of DSM-III schizophrenia among first-degree relatives of schizophrenic probands. *Acta Psychiatrica Scandinavica* **72**, 382–386.

Frangou, S., Sharma, T., Alarcon, G. *et al.* (1997) The Maudsley Family Study. II. Endogenous event-related potentials in familial schizophrenia. *Schizophrenia Research* **23**, 45–53.

Franke, P., Maier, W., Hardt, J. & Hain, C. (1993) Cognitive functioning and anhedonia in subjects at risk for schizophrenia. *Schizophrenia Research* **10**, 77–84.

Freedman, R., Coon, H., Myles-Worsley, M. *et al.* (1997) Linkages of a neurophysiological deficit in schizophrenia to chromosome 15 locus. *Proceedings of the National Academy of Sciences, USA* **94**, 587–592.

Freedman, L.R., Rock, D., Roberts, S.A., Cornblatt, B.A. & Erlenmeyer-Limling, L. (1998) The New York High-Risk Project: attention, anhedonia and social outcome. *Schizophrenia Research* **30**, 1–9.

Gershon, E.S., DeLisi, L.E., Hamovit, J. *et al.* (1988) A controlled family study of chronic psychoses. *Archives of General Psychiatry* **45**, 328–336.

Glish, M.A., Erlenmeyer-Kimling, L. & Watt, N.F. (1982) Parental assessment of the social and emotional adaptation of children at high risk for schizophrenia. In: *Advances in Child Clinical Psychology* (eds B. Lahey & A. Kazdin). Wiley, New York.

Goldberg, S.C., Schulz, C., Schulz, M. *et al.* (1986) Borderline and schizotypal personality disorders treated with low dose thioxene vs. placebo. *Archives of General Psychiatry* **43**, 680–686.

Goodarzi, M.A., Wykes, T. & Hemsley, D.R. (2000) Cerebral lateralization of global–local processing in people with schizotypy. *Schizophrenia Research* **45**, 115–121.

Gooding, D.C., Kwapil, T.R. & Tallent, K.A. (1999) Wisconsin Card Sorting Test deficits in schizotypic individuals. *Schizophrenia Research* **40**, 201–209.

Goodman, M., Mitropoulou, V., New, A.S., Koeningsberg, H. & Siever, L.J. (2000) Frontal cortex dysfunction and dopaminergic activity in schizophrenia spectrum. *Biological Psychiatry* **47**, 34S.

Gray, N.S., Pilowsky, L.S., Gray, J.A. & Kerwin, R.W. (1995) Latent inhibition in drug naïve schizophrenics: relationship to duration of illness and dopamine D_2 binding using SPET. *Schizophrenia Research* **17**, 95–107.

Green, M.F., Nuechterlein, K.H. & Mintz, J. (1994) Backward masking in schizophrenia and mania. II. Specifying the visual channels. *Archives of General Psychiatry* **51**, 945–951.

Green, M.F., Nuechterlein, K.H. & Breitmeyer, B. (1997) Backward masking performance in unaffected siblings of schizophrenic patients: evidence for a vulnerability indicator. *Archives of General Psychiatry* **54**, 465–472.

Griffith, J.M., O'Neill, J.E., Petty, F. *et al.* (1998) Nicotinic receptor desensitization and sensory gating deficits in schizophrenia. *Biological Psychiatry* **44**, 98–106.

Grillon, C., Ameli, R., Charney, D.S., Krystal, J. & Braff, D. (1992) Startle gating deficits occur across prepulse intensities in schizophrenic patients. *Biological Psychiatry* **32**, 939–943.

Grove, W.M., Lebow, B.S., Clementz, B.A. *et al.* (1991) Familial prevalence and coaggregation of schizotypy indicators: a multitrait family study. *Journal of Abnormal Psychology* **100**, 115–121.

Gruzelier, J.H. (1996) The factorial structure of schizotypy. I. Affinities and contrasts with syndromes of schizophrenia. *Schizophrenia Bulletin* **22**, 611–620.

Gruzelier, J. (1999a) Functional neuro-psychophysiological asymmetry in schizophrenia: a review and reorientation. *Schizophrenia Bulletin* **25**, 91–120. (Special issue on Lateralization.)

Gruzelier, J. (1999b) A review of the implications of early sensory processing and subcortical involvement for cognitive dysfunction in schizophrenia. In: *Review of Psychiatry* (ed. J. Oldham), pp. 29–76. American Psychiatric Association, Washington, DC.

Gruzelier, J.H. (2002) A Janusian perspective on the nature, development and structure of schizophrenia and schizotypy. *Schizophrenia Research* **54**, 95–103.

Gruzelier, J. & Davis, S. (1995) Social and physical anhedonia in relation to cerebral laterality and electrodermal habituation in unmedicated psychotic patients. *Psychiatry Research* **56**, 163–172.

Gruzelier, J. & Doig, A. (1996) The factorial structure of schizotypy. II. Patterns of cognitive asymmetry, arousal, handedness and gender. *Schizophrenia Bulletin* **22**, 621–634.

Gruzelier, J.H. & Kaiser, J. (1996) Syndromes of schizotypy and timing of puberty. *Schizophrenia Research* **21**, 183–194.

Gruzelier, J. & Raine, A. (1994) Schizophrenia, schizotypal personality, syndromes, cerebral lateralisation and electrodermal activity. *International Journal of Psychophysiology* **16**, 1–16.

Gruzelier, J. & Richardson, A. (1994) Patterns of cognitive asymmetry and syndromes of psychosis-proneness. *International Journal of Psychophysiology* **18**, 217–226. (Special issue on Developmental Psychopathology.)

Gruzelier, J.H., Seymour, K., Wilson, L., Jolley, T. & Hirsch, S. (1988) Impairments on neuropsychological tests of temporo-hippocampal and fronto-hippocampal functions and word fluency in remitting schizophrenia and affective disorders. *Archives of General Psychiatry* **45**, 623–629.

Gruzelier, J., Burgess, A., Stygall, J., Irving, G. & Raine, A. (1995) Patterns of cerebral asymmetry and syndromes of schizotypal personality. *Psychiatry Research* **56**, 71–79.

Gruzelier, J., Richardson, A. & Wilson, L. (1999a) Cognitive asymmetry patterns in schizophrenia: retest reliability and syndrome-related modifiability with recovery. *International Journal of Psychophysiology* **34**, 323–332. (Special issue on Laterality and Psychopathology.)

Gruzelier, J., Kaiser, J., Richardson, A. *et al.* (1999b) Opposite patterns of P300 asymmetry in schizophrenia are syndrome related. *International Journal of Psychophysiology* **34**, 276–282. (Special issue on Laterality and Psychopathology.)

Gruzelier, J., Wilson, L., Liddiard, D., Peters, E. & Pusavat, L. (1999c) Cognitive asymmetry patterns in schizophrenia: active and withdrawn syndromes and sex differences as moderators. *Schizophrenia Bulletin* **25**, 349–362.

Gruzelier, J.H., Jamieson, G.A., Croft, R.J., Kaiser, J. & Burgess, A.F. (2002) Personality Syndrome Questionnaire: reliability, validity and experimental evidence. *International Journal of Psychophysiology*, in press.

Gunderson, J.G., Siever, L.J. & Spaulding, E. (1983) The search for the schizotype: crossing the border again. *Archives of General Psychiatry* **40**, 15–22.

Hain, C., Maier, W., Hoechst-Janneck, S. & Franke, P. (1995) Subclinical thought disorder in first-degree relatives of schizophrenic patients: results from a matched-pairs study with the Thought Disorder Index. *Acta Psychiatria Scandinavica* **92**, 305–309.

Harris, J.G., Adler, L.E., Young, D.A. *et al.* (1996) Neuropsychological dysfunction in parents of schizophrenics. *Schizophrenia Research* **20**, 253–260.

Hazlett, E., Buchsbaum, M.S., Byne, E. *et al.* (1999) Three-dimensional analysis with MRI and PET of the size, shape and function of the thalamus in the schizophrenia spectrum. *American Journal of Psychiatry* **156**, 1190–1199.

Hewitt, J.K. & Claridge, G.S. (1989) The factor structure of schizotypy in a normal population. *Personality and Individual Differences* **10**, 323–329.

Hogg, B., Jackson, H.J., Rudd, R.P. & Edwards, J. (1990) Diagnosing personality disorders in recent-onset schizophrenia. *Journal of Nervous and Mental Disease* **178**, 194–199.

Huber, G. (1997) The heterogeneous course of schizophrenia. *Schizophrenia Research* **28**, 177–185.

Hymowitz, P., Francis, A., Jacobsberg, L.B., Sickles, M. & Hoyt, R. (1986) Neuroleptic treatment of schizotypal personality disorders. *Comprehensive Psychiatry* **27**, 267–271.

Ingraham, L.J. & Kety, S. (2000) Adoption studies of schizophrenia. *American Journal of Medical Genetics* **97**, 18–22.

Jorgensen, A. & Parnas, J. (1990) The Copenhagen high risk study: premorbid and clinical dimensions of maternal schizophrenia. *Journal of Nervous and Mental Disease* **178** (6), 370–376.

Jutai, J.W. (1989) Spatial attention in hypothetically psychosis-prone college students. *Psychiatry Research* **27**, 207–215.

Kaiser, J. & Gruzelier, J.H. (1996) Timing of puberty and EEG coherence during photic stimulation. *International Journal of Psychophysiology* **21**, 135–149.

Kaiser, J. & Gruzelier, J.H. (1999a) Timing of puberty and syndromes of schizotypy: a replication. *International Journal of Psychophysiology* **34**, 237–248. (Special issue on Laterality and Psychopathology.)

Kaiser, J. & Gruzelier, J. (1999b) Effects of pubertal timing on EEG coherence and P3 latency. *International Journal of Psychophysiology* **34**, 225–236. (Special issue on Laterality and Psychopathology.)

Kalus, O., Bernstein, D.P. & Siever, L.J. (1996) Schizoid personality disorder. In: *DSM-IV Sourcebook*, Vol. 2 (eds. T.A. Widiger, A.J. Frances, H.A. Pincus, R. Ross, M.B. First & W.W. Davis), pp. 675–684. American Psychiatric Association, Washington, DC.

Karper, L.P., Freeman, G.K., Grillon, C. et al. (1996) Preliminary evidence of an association between sensorimotor gating and distractibility in psychosis. *Journal of Neuropsychiatry and Clinical Neurosciences* **8**, 60–66.

Katsanis, J., Kortenkamp, S., Iacono, W.G. & Grove, W.M. (1997) Antisaccade performance in patients with schizophrenia and affective disorder. *Journal of Abnormal Psychology* **106**, 468–472.

Kavoussi, R.J. & Siever, L.J. (1992) Overlap between borderline and schizotypal personality disorders. *Comprehensive Psychiatry* **33**, 7–12.

Keefe, R., Lees-Roitman, S. & Dupre, R. (1997) Performance of patients with schizophrenia on a pen and paper visuospatial working memory task with short delay. *Schizophrenia Research* **26**, 9–14.

Keefe, S.R., Silverman, J.M., Roitman, S.E. et al. (1994) Performance of nonpsychotic relatives of schizophrenic patients on cognitive tests. *Psychiatry Research* **53**, 1–12.

Kelly, M.P. & Bakan, P. (1999) Eye tracking in normals: spem asymmetries and association with schizotypy. *International Journal of Neuroscience* **98**, 27–81.

Kelly, M.P. & Coursey, R.D. (1992) Lateral preference and neuropsychological correlates of schizotypy. *Psychiatry Research* **41**, 115–135.

Kendler, K.S. (1985) Diagnostic approaches to schizotypal personality disorder: a historical perspective. *Schizophrenia Bulletin* **11**, 538–553.

Kendler, K.S. (1988) Familial aggregation of schizophrenia and schizophrenia spectrum disorders: evaluation of conflicting results. *Archives of General Psychiatry* **45**, 377–383.

Kendler, K.S. & Hewitt, J.K. (1992) The structure of self-report schizotypy in twins. *Journal of Personality Disorders* **6**, 1–17.

Kendler, K.S., Gruenberg, A.M. & Strauss, J.S. (1981) An independent analysis of the Copenhagen sample of the Danish adoption study of schizophrenia. II. The relationship between schizotypal personality disorder and schizophrenia. *Archives of General Psychiatry* **38**, 982–987.

Kendler, K.S., Ochs, A.L., Gorman, A.M. et al. (1991) The structure of schizotypy: a multitrait twin study. *Psychiatry Research* **36**, 19–36.

Kendler, K.S., McGuire, M., Gruenberg, A.M. et al. (1993a) The Roscommon Family Study. III. Schizophrenia-related personality disorders in relatives. *Archives of General Psychiatry* **50**, 781–788.

Kendler, K.S., McGuire, M., Gruenberg, A.M. et al. (1993b) The Roscommon Family Study. I. Methods, diagnosis of probands and risk of schizophrenia in relatives. *Archives of General Psychiatry* **50**, 527–540.

Kendler, K.S., Gruenberg, A.M. & Kinney, D.K. (1994) Independent diagnosis of adoptees and relatives as defined by DSM-III in the provincial and national samples of the Danish adoption study of schizophrenia. *Archives of General Psychiatry* **51**, 456–468.

Kety, S.S., Rosenthal, D., Wender, P.H. et al. (1975) Mental illness in the biological and adoptive families of adopted individuals who have become schizophrenic: preliminary report based o psychiatric interviews. In: *Genetic Research in Psychiatry* (eds R.R. Fieve, D. Rosenthal & H. Brill), pp. 147–165. Johns Hopkins University Press, Baltimore.

Kim, D., Raine, A., Triphon, N. & Green, M.F. (1992) Mixed handedness and features of schizotypal personality in a nonclinical sample. *Journal of Nervous and Mental Disease* **180**, 133–135.

Kirrane, M., Mitropoulou, V., Nunn, M. et al. (2000) Effects of amphetamine on visuospatial working memory in schizophrenia spectrum personality disorder. *Neuropsychopharmacology* **22**, 14–18.

Klosterkotter, J., Breuer, H., Gross, G. et al. (1992) New approaches to early recognition of idiopathic psychoses. In: *Schizophrenia and Affective Psychoses: Nosology in Contemporary Psychiatry* (eds F.P. Ferro, A.E. Haynal & N. Sartorius), pp. 111–120. J. Libbey, Rome.

Koenigsberg, H.W., Reynolds, D. Goodman, M. et al. (2002) Risperidone in the treatment of schizotypeal personality disorder. *Journal of Clinical Psychiatry* (in press).

Kolachana, B., Saunders, R., Bachevalier, J. & Weinberger, D. (1996) Abnormal prefrontal cortical regulation of striatal dopamine release after neonatal medial temporal-limbic lesions in rhesus monkeys. *Abstracts for the Society for Neuroscience* **22**, 1974.

Kraepelin, E. (1919/1971) *Manic-Depressive Insanity and Paranoia.* Translated by R.M. Barclay. E. & S. Livingstone, Edinburgh.

Kretschmer, E. (1921) *Physique and Character.* Translated 1936. Kegan Paul, London.

Kutcher, S.P., Blackwood, D.H.R., Gaskell, D.F., Muir, W.J. & St. Clair, D.M. (1989) Auditory P300 does not differentiate borderline personality disorder from schizotypal personality disorder. *Biological Psychiatry* **26**, 766–774.

Kwon, J.S., Shenton, M.E., Hirayasu, Y. et al. (1998) MRI study of cavum septum pellucidi in schizophrenia, affective disorder and schizotypal personality disorder. *American Journal of Psychiatry* **155**, 509–515.

Langdon, R. & Coltheart, M. (1999) Mentalising, schizotypy, and schizophrenia. *Cognition* **71**, 43–71.

Lenzenweger, M.E. & Gold, J.M. (2000) Auditory working memory and verbal recall memory in schizotypy. *Schizophrenia Research* **42**, 101–110.

Leonhard, D. & Brugger, P. (1998) Creative, paranormal and delusional thought: a consequence of right hemisphere semantic activation? *Neuropsychiatry, Neuropsychology and Behavioral Neurology* **11**, 177–183.

Lieberman, J.A., Kane, J.M. & Alvir, R. (1987) Provocative tests with psychostimulant drugs in schizophrenia. *Psychopharmacology* **91** (4), 415–433.

Lipp, O.V. & Vaitl, D. (1992) Latent inhibition in human Pavlovian conditioning: effect of additional stimulation after preexposure and relation to schizotypal traits. *Personality and Individual Differences* **13**, 1003–1012.

Lipska, B.K., Jaskiw, G.E. & Weinberger, D.R. (1993) Postpubertal emergence of hyperresponsiveness to stress and to amphetamine after neonatal excitotoxic hippocampal damage: a potential animal model of schizophrenia. *Neuropsychopharmacology* **9**, 67–75.

Lipska, B.K., Swerdlow, N.R., Geyer, M.A. *et al.* (1995) Neonatal excitotoxic hippocampal damage in rats causes post-pubertal changes in prepulse inhibition of startle and its disruption by apomorphine. *Psychopharmacology* **122**, 35–43.

Lubow, R.E., Weiner, I., Schlossberg, A. & Baruch, I. (1987) Latent inhibition and schizophrenia. *Bulletin of the Psychonomic Society* **25**, 464–467.

Lyons, M., Merla, M.E., Young, L. & Kremen, W. (1991) Impaired neuropsychological functioning in symptomatic volunteers with schizotypy: preliminary findings. *Biological Psychiatry* **30**, 424–426.

McCarley, R.W., Shenton, M.E., O'Donnell, B.F. *et al.* (1993) Auditory P300 abnormalities and left posterior superior temporal gyrus volume reduction in schizophrenia. *Archives of General Psychiatry* **50**, 190–197.

McCarley, R.W., Shenton, M.E., O'Donnell, B., Dickey, C.C. & Holinger, R. (1996) Schizophrenia spectrum disorders: electrophysiological and structural MRI features. 20th Annual Collegium Internationale Neuro-Psychopharmalogicum Congress, Melbourne, Australia.

McDowell, J. & Clementz, B. (1997) The effect of fixation condition manipulations on antisaccade performance in schizophrenia: studies of diagnostic specificity. *Experimental Brain Research* **115**, 333–344.

McGlashan, T.H. (1986) Schizotypal personality disorder, Chestnut Lodge follow-up study. VI. Long-term follow-up perspective. *Archives of General Psychiatry* **43**, 329–334.

Maier, W., Lichterman, D., Minges, J. *et al.* (1993) Continuity and discontinuity of affective disorders and schizophrenia: results of a controlled family study. *Archives of General Psychiatry* **50**, 871–883.

Maier, W., Lichterman, D., Minges, J. *et al.* (1994) Personality disorders among the relatives of schizophrenic patients. *Schizophrenia Bulletin* **20**, 481–493.

Mason, O., Claridge, G. & Clark, K. (1997) Electrodermal relationships with personality measures of psychosis-proneness in psychotic and normal subjects. *International Journal of Psychophysiology* **27**, 137–146.

Meehl, P.E. (1962) Schizotaxia, schizotypy, schizophrenia. *American Psychologist* **17**, 827–839.

Mehlum, L., Friis, S., Irion, T. *et al.* (1991) Personality disorders 2–5 years after treatment: a prospective follow-up study. *Acta Psychiatrica Scandinavica* **84**, 72–77.

Merritt, R.D. & Balogh, D.W. (1989) Backward masking spatial frequency effects among hypothetically schizotypal individuals. *Schizophrenia Bulletin* **15**, 573–583.

Michael, C.M., Morris, D.P. & Soroker, E. (1957) Follow-up studies of shy, withdrawn children. II. Relative incidence of schizophrenia. *American Journal of Orthopsychiatry* **27**, 331–337.

Mohr, C., Rohrenbach, C.M., Laska, M. & Brugger, P. (2001) Unilateral olfactory perception and magical ideation. *Schizophrenia Research* **47**, 255–264.

Moritz, S. & Mass, R. (1997) Reduced cognitive inhibition in schizotypy. *British Journal of Clinical Psychology* **36**, 365–376.

Muntaner, C., Garcia-Sevilla, L., Alberto, A. & Torrubia, R. (1988) Personality dimensions, schizotypal and borderline personality traits and psychosis proneness. *Personality and Individual Differences* **9**, 257–268.

Nalcaci, E., Kalaycioglu, C., Cicek, M. & Budanur, O.E. (2000) Magical ideation and right-sided hemispatial inattention on a spatial working memory task: influences of sex and handedness. *Perceptual and Motor Skills* **91**, 883–892.

Obiols, J.E., Serrano, F., Caparros, B., Subira, S. & Barrantes, N. (1999) Neurological soft signs in adolescents with poor performance on the continuous performance test: markers of liability for schizophrenia spectrum disorders? *Psychiatry Research* **86**, 217–228.

O'Donnell, D.F., Swearer, J.M., Smith, L.T. *et al.* (1996) Selective deficits in visual perception and recognition in schizophrenia. *American Journal of Psychiatry* **153**, 687–692.

O'Driscoll, G.A., Lenzenweger, M.F. & Holzman, P.S. (1998) Antisaccades and smooth pursuit eye tracking and schizotypy. *Archives of General Psychiatry* **55**, 837–843.

O'Flynn, K., Koenigsberg, H.W., Abi Dhargam, A. *et al.* (2001) Striatal dopaminergic activity in schizotypal personality disorder. *Abstract of the 56th Annual Meeting of the Society of Biological Psychiatry* **49**, Abstract 424.

Olin, S.S. & Mednick, S.A. (1996) Risk factors of psychosis: Identifying vulnerable populations premorbidly. *Schizophrenia Bulletin* **22**, 223–240.

Olin, S.S., Raine, A., Cannon, T.D. *et al.* (1997) Childhood behavior precursors of schizotypal personality disorder. *Schizophrenia Bulletin* **23**, 93–103.

O'Neal, P. & Robins, L.N. (1958) Childhood patterns predictive of adult schizophrenia: a 30-year follow-up study. *American Journal of Psychiatry* **115**, 385–391.

Park, S. & Holzman, P.S. (1992) Schizophrenics show spatial working memory deficits. *Archives of General Psychiatry* **49**, 975–982.

Park, S., Holzman, P.S. & Lenzenweger, M.F. (1995) Individual differences in spatial working memory in relation to schizotypy. *Journal of Abnormal Psychology* **104**, 355–363.

Parnas, J. & Jorgensen, A. (1989) Pre-morbid psychopathology in schizophrenia spectrum. *British Journal of Psychiatry* **155**, 623–627.

Parnas, J., Schulsinger, F., Schulsinger, H., Mednick, S.A. & Teasdale, T.W. (1982) Behavioral precursors of schizophrenia spectrum. *Archives of General Psychiatry* **39**, 658–664.

Peralta, V., Cuesta, M.J. & de Leon, J. (1991) Premorbid personality and positive and negative symptoms in schizophrenia. *Acta Psychiatrica Scandanavica* **84**, 336–339.

Peters, E.R., Pickering, A.D. & Hemsley, D.R. (1994) 'Cognitive inhibition' and positive symptomatology in schizotypy. *British Journal of Clinical Psychology* **33**, 33–48.

Pickar, D., Labarac, R., Linnoila, M. *et al.* (1984) Neuroleptic-induced decrease in plasma homovanillic acid and antipsychotic activity in schizophrenic patients. *Science* **225**, 954–956.

Pycock, C.J., Kerwin, R.W. & Carter, C.J. (1980) Effects of lesions of cortical dopamine terminals on subcortical dopamine receptors in rats. *Nature* **286**, 74–77.

Raine, A. (1991) The SPQ: a scale for the assessment of schizotypal personality based on DSM-IIIR criteria. *Schizophrenia Bulletin* **17**, 555–564.

Raine, A. & Allbutt, J. (1989) Factors of schizoid personality. *British Journal of Clinical Psychology* **28**, 31–40.

Raine, A. & Lencz, T. (1995) Conceptual; and theoretical issues in schizotypal personality disorder research. In: *Schizotypal Personality* (eds A. Raine, T. Lencz & S. Mednick), pp. 3–15. Cambridge University Press, Cambridge.

Raine, A. & Manders, D. (1988) Schizoid personality, inter-hemispheric transfer, and left hemisphere over-activation. *British Journal of Clinical Psychology* **27**, 333–347.

Raine, A., Sheard, C., Reynolds, G.P. & Lencz, T. (1992) Pre-frontal structural and functional deficits associated with individual differences in schizotypal personality. *Schizophrenia Research* **7**, 237–247.

Raine, A., Lencz, T. & Mednick, S.A., eds. (1995) *Schizotypal Personality*. Cambridge University Press, UK.

Raine, A., Benishay, D., Lencz, T. & Scarpa, A. (1997) Abnormal orienting in schizotypal personality disorder. *Schizophrenia Bulletin* **23**, 75–82.

Richardson, A.J. (1994) Dyslexia, handedness and syndromes of psychosis-proneness. *International Journal of Psychophysiology* **18**, 251–263.

Richardson, A. & Gruzelier, J. (1994) Visual processing, lateralisation and syndromes of schizotypy. *International Journal of Psychophysiology* **18**, 227–240. (Special issue on Developmental Psychopathology.)

Ricks, D.F. & Berry, J.C. (1970) Family and symptom patterns that precede schizophrenia. In: *Life History Research in Psychopathology*, Vol. 1. (eds M. Roff & D.F. Ricks), pp. 3–18. University of Minnesota Press, Minneapolis.

Robins, L.N. (1966) *Deviant Children Grown Up*. Williams & Wilkins, Baltimore.

Roff, J.D., Knight, R. & Wertheim, E. (1976) Disturbed preschizophrenics: childhood symptoms in relation to adult outcome. *Journal of Nervous and Mental Disease* **162**, 274–281.

Roitman, S.E., Cornblatt, B.A., Bergman, A. et al. (1997) Attentional functioning in schizotypal personality disorder. *American Journal of Psychiatry* **154**, 655–660.

Roitman, S.E., Mitropoulou, V., Keefe, R.S. et al. (2000) Visuospatial working memory in schizotypal personality disorder patients. *Schizophrenia Research* **41**, 447–455.

Ross, R.G., Hommer, D., Radant, A., Roath, M. & Freedman, R. (1996) Early expression of smooth-pursuit eye movement abnormalities in children of schizophrenic parents. *Journal of the American Academy of Child and Adolescent Psychiatry* **35**, 941–949.

Ross, R.G., Olincy, A., Harris, J.G. et al. (1998) Anticipatory saccades during smooth pursuit eye movements and familial transmission of schizophrenia. *Biological Psychiatry* **44**, 690–697.

Saykin, A.J., Shtasel, D.L., Gur, R.E. et al. (1994) Neuropsychological deficits in neuroleptic naïve patients with first episode schizophrenia. *Archives of General Psychiatry* **51**, 124–131.

Schuck, J.R. & Lee, R.G. (1989) Backward masking, information processing, and schizophrenia. *Schizophrenia Bulletin* **15**, 491–500.

Schulz, P.M. & Soloff, P.H. (1987) Still borderline after all these years. 140th Annual Meeting of the American Psychiatric Association, Chicago, IL.

Schulz, P.M., Schulz, S.C., Goldberg, S.C. et al. (1986) Diagnoses of the relatives of schizotypal outpatients. *Journal of Nervous and Mental Disorders* **174**, 457–463.

Schwarzkopf, S.B., Lamberti, J.S. & Smith, D.A. (1993) Concurrent assessment of acoustic startle and auditory P50 evoked potential measures of sensory inhibition. *Biological Psychiatry* **33**, 815–828.

Shaw, J., Claridge, G. & Clark, K. (2001) Schizotypy and the shift from dextrality: a study of handedness in a large non-clinical sample. *Schizophrenia Research* **50**, 181–189.

Shelton, R.C. & Weinberger, D.R. (1986) X-ray computerized tomography studies in schizophrenia: a review & synthesis. In: *The Neurology of Schizophrenia* (eds H.A. Nasrallah & D.R. Weinberger), pp. 207–250. Elsevier, New York.

Shihabuddin, L., Buchsbaum, M.S., Hazlett, E. et al. (2001) Striatal size and relative glucose metabolic rate in schizotypal personality disorder and schizophrenia. *Archives of General Psychiatry* **58** (9), 877–884.

Siegel, B.V., Trestman, R.L., O'Flaithbheartaigh, S. et al. (1996) D-amphetamine challenge effects on Wisconsin Card Sort test: performance in schizotypal personality disorder. *Schizophrenia Research* **20**, 29–32.

Siegel, C., Waldo, M., Mizner, G., Adler, L.E. & Freedman, R. (1984) Deficits in sensory gating in schizophrenic patients and their relatives: evidence obtained with auditory evoked responses. *Archives of General Psychiatry* **41**, 607–612.

Siever, L.J. (1991) The biology of the boundaries of schizophrenia. In: *Advances in Neuropsychiatry and Psychopharmacology*, Vol. 1, *Schizophrenia Research* (eds C.A. Tamminga & S.C. Schulz), pp. 181–191. Raven Press, New York.

Siever, L.J., Coursey, R.D., Alterman, I.S., Buchsbaum, M.S. & Murphy, D.L. (1984) Impaired smooth-pursuit eye movement: vulnerability marker for schizotypal personality disorder in a normal volunteer population. *American Journal of Psychiatry* **141**, 1560–1566.

Siever, L.J., Coursey, R.D., Alterman, I.S. et al. (1989) Clinical, psychophysiologic, and neurologic characteristics of volunteers with impaired smooth pursuit eye movements. *Biological Psychiatry* **26**, 35–51.

Siever, L.J., Keefe, R., Bernstein, D.P. et al. (1990a) Eye tracking impairment in clinically identified schizotypal personality disorder patients. *American Journal of Psychiatry* **147**, 740–745.

Siever, L.J., Silverman, J.M., Horvath, T.B. et al. (1990b) Increased morbid risk for schizophrenia-related disorders in relatives of schizotypal personality disordered patients. *Archives of General Psychiatry* **47**, 634–640.

Siever, L.J., Kalus, O.F. & Keeffe, R.S.E. (1993) The boundaries of schizophrenia. *Psychiatry Clinics of North America* **16** (2), 217–244.

Siever, L.J., Rotter, M., Losonczy, M. et al. (1995) Lateral ventricular enlargement in schizotypal personality disorder. *Psychiatry Research* **57**, 109–118.

Siever, L.J., Bernstein, D.P. & Silverman, J.M. (1996) Schizotypal personality disorder. In: *DSM-IV Sourcebook*, Vol. 2 (eds T.A. Widiger, A.J. Frances, H.A. Pincus et al.), pp. 685–701. American Psychiatric Association, Washington.

Siever, L.J., Koenigsberg, H.W., Harvey, P. et al. (2002) Cognitive and brain function in schizotypal personality disorder. *Schizophrenia Research* **54**, 157–167.

Silverman, J.M., Smith, C.J., Guo, S.L. et al. (1998) Lateral ventricular enlargement in schizophrenic probands and their siblings with schizophrenia-related disorders. *Biological Psychiatry* **43**, 97–106.

Simons, R.F. & Katkin, W. (1985) Smooth pursuit eye movements in subjects reporting physical anhedonia and perceptual aberrations. *Psychiatry Research* **14**, 275–289.

Slaghuis, W.L. & Bakker, V.J. (1995) Forward and backward visual masking of contour by light in positive- and negative-symptom schizophrenia. *Journal of Abnormal Psychology* **104**, 41–54.

Squires-Wheeler, E., Skodol, A.E., Friedman, D. & Erlenmeyer-Kimling, L. (1988) The specificity of DSM-III Schizotypal personality traits. *Psychological Medicine* **18**, 757–765.

Squires-Wheeler, E., Skodol, A.E., Bassett, A. & Erlenmeyer-Kimling, L. (1989) DSM-IIIR schizotypal personality traits in offspring of schizophrenic disorder, affective disorder, and normal control parents. *Journal of Psychiatric Research* **23**, 229–239.

Squires-Wheeler, E., Skodol, A.E. & Erlenmeyer-Kimling, L. (1992) The assessment of schizotypal features over two points in time. *Schizophrenia Research* **6**, 75–85.

Squires-Wheeler, E., Friedman, D., Amminger, G.P. *et al.* (1997) Negative and positive dimensions of schizotypal personality disorder. *Journal of Personality Disorders* **11**, 285–300.

Strik, W.K., Dierks, T., Franzek, E. Stober, G., & Maurer, K. (1994) P300 asymmetries in schizophrenia revisited with reference independent methods. *Psychiatry Research: Neuroimaging* **55**, 153–166.

Swerdlow, N.R. & Geyer, M.A. (1998) Using an animal model of deficient sensorimotor gating to study the pathophysiology and new treatments of schizophrenia. *Schizophrenia Bulletin* **24**, 285–301.

Swerdlow, N.R., Filion, D., Geyer, M.A. *et al.* (1995) 'Normal' personality correlates of sensorimotor, cognitive, and visuospatial gating. *Biological Psychiatry* **37**, 286–299.

Szigethy, E.M. & Schulz, S.C. (1997) Risperidone in comorbid borderline personality disorder and dysthymia. *Journal of Clinical Psychopharmacology* **17**, 326–327.

Tien, A.Y., Costa, P.T. & Eaton, W.W. (1992) Couariance of personality, neurocognition, and schizophrenia spectrum traits in the community. *Schizophrenia Research* **7**, 149–158.

Torgersen, S., Onstad, S., Skre, I., Edvardsen, J. & Kringlen, E. (1993) 'True' schizotypal personality disorder: a study of co-twins and relatives of schizophrenic probands. *American Journal of Psychiatry* **150**, 1661–1667.

Trestman, R.L., Keefe, R.S.E., Mitropoulou, V. *et al.* (1995) Cognitive function and biological correlates of cognitive performance in schizotypal personality disorder. *Psychiatry Research* **59**, 127–136.

Trestman, R.L., Horvath, T., Kalus, O. *et al.* (1996) Event-related potentials in schizotypal personality disorder. *Journal of Neuropsychiatry and Clinical Neuroscience* **8**, 33–40.

Trevarthen, C. (1996) Lateral asymmetries in infancy: implications for the development of the hemispheres. *Neuroscience and Biobehavioural Reviews* **20**, 571–586.

Venables, P.H., Wilkins, S., Mitchell, D.A., Raine, A. & Bailes, K. (1990) A scale for the measurement of schzotypy. *Personality and Individual Differences* **11**, 481–495.

Voglmaier, M.M., Seidman, L.J., Salisbury, D. & McCarley, R.W. (1997) Neuropsychological dysfunction in schizotypal personality disorder: a profile analysis. *Biological Psychiatry* **41**, 530–540.

Waldo, M.C., Adler, L.E. & Freedman, R. (1988) Defects in auditory sensory gating and their apparent compensation in relatives of schizophrenics. *Schizophrenia Research* **1**, 19–24.

Waldo, M.C., Carey, G., Myles-Worsley, M. *et al.* (1991) Codistribution of a sensory gating deficit and schizophrenia in multi-affected families. *Psychiatry Research* **39**, 257–268.

Waldo, M.C., Cawthra, E., Adler, L.E. *et al.* (1994) Auditory sensory gating, hippocampal volume, and catecholamine metabolism in schizophrenics and their siblings. *Schizophrenia Research* **12**, 93–106.

Warnken, R.G. & Seiss, T.F. (1965) The use of the cumulative record in the prediction of behavior. *Personnel and Guidance Journal* **31**, 231–237.

Watt, N.F. (1978) Patterns of childhood social development in adult schizophrenics. *Archives of General Psychiatry* **35**, 160–165.

Webb, C.T. & Levinson, D.F. (1993) Schizotypal and paranoid personality disorder in the relatives of patients with schizophrenia and affective disorders: a review. *Schizophrenia Research* **11**, 81–92.

Weintraub, S. & Neal, J.M. (1984) Social behavior of children at risk for schizophrenia. In: *Children at Risk for Schizophrenia: a Longitudinal Perspective* (eds N.F. Watt, E.J. Anthony, L.C. Wynne & J.E. Rolf), pp. 279–285. Cambridge University Press, New York.

White, P.M. & Yee, C.M. (1997) Effects of attentional and stressor manipulations on the P50 gating response. *Psychophysiology* **34**, 703–711.

Williams, G.V. & Goldman-Rakic, P.S. (1995) Modulation of memory fields by dopamine D_1 receptors in prefrontal cortex. *Nature* **376**, 572–575.

Williams, L.M. (1995) Further evidence for a multidimensional personality disposition to schizophrenia in terms of cognitive inhibition. *British Journal of Clinical Psychology* **34**, 193–213.

Course and outcome of schizophrenia

H. Häfner and W. an der Heiden

Introduction

Studies on the natural history of schizophrenia aim at shedding light on the variance in the natural course and outcome, on the spectrum of consequences of the disorder as well as on the factors influencing these dimensions. Kraepelin (1893), preoccupied with the course of dementia praecox throughout his professional life, was believed to have found the basis for this 'disease entity' in the combination of symptomatology and course. Eventually, his belief was shaken when he came to realize the great variety of courses (Kraepelin 1920).

All recent longitudinal studies have, of necessity, examined the treated rather than the natural course of schizophrenia. The only exceptions have been the studies following up placebo controls; unfortunately, all these are limited to highly selected patient groups with a maximum follow-up of 2 years because they have been carried out to assess the efficacy of therapeutic interventions.

Time trends

A selection of first-admission cohorts of patients with schizophrenia from different countries shows that since the turn of the nineteenth century the length of hospital stay has decreased progressively (Fig. 8.1). Decreasing lengths of stay after first admission for schizophrenia have been reported by several authors, for example Ødegård (1964), who compared data from the national Norwegian case register for cohorts of patients discharged in the periods 1936–42, 1945–52 and 1955–59.

Influenced as they are by disease-independent factors, time trends in the frequency and length of hospital stay hardly provide reliable indicators of the course of the illness, an der Heiden *et al.* (1995), in the Mannheim follow-up study covering 15.6 years, demonstrated a widening gap between mean symptom scores, which remained stable, and a continued decrease in days per year spent in inpatient treatment. Simultaneously, outpatient treatment contacts increased, reflecting the change that has taken place in the system of care, while the illness course has remained the same.

More or less comparable outcome indicators are provided by rates of recovery or good outcome. Shepherd *et al.* (1989) reviewed selected twentieth century outcome studies of schizophrenia and found a substantial increase in recovery rates since the 1950s. In contrast, Warner (1985), in his more comprehensive but still selective review, came to the conclusion that the recovery rate had scarcely improved since the early years of the twentieth century.

A meta-analysis (Hegarty *et al.* 1994) of 320 longitudinal studies of a century that fulfilled minimum methodological standards found a recovery rate of 35% for the period 1895–1955 and a clearly higher rate of 49% for 1956–85, possibly indicating the success of neuroleptics. However, in the following period of novel antipsychotics, 1986–92, the rate fell back to 36%.

These data are not reliable enough to allow conclusions on possible time trends of the course of schizophrenia. One reason is that the diagnostic criteria have clearly changed over these periods (Loranger 1990; Stoll *et al.* 1993). Furthermore, Hegarty *et al.* (1994) pointed out that not a single study they reviewed was based on a truly representative cohort.

M. Bleuler (1968) noted that the proportion of good outcomes had remained stable, but the number of 'catastrophic' and chronic cases had decreased since the beginning of the

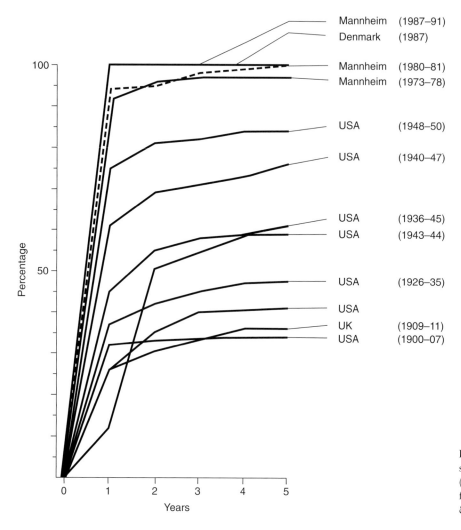

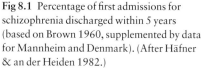

Fig 8.1 Percentage of first admissions for schizophrenia discharged within 5 years (based on Brown 1960, supplemented by data for Mannheim and Denmark). (After Häfner & an der Heiden 1982.)

twentieth century. This sounds plausible considering the fact that psychotic symptoms and episodes can be cured or alleviated by antipsychotic drugs. A gradual disappearance of extremely severe forms of schizophrenia, e.g. life-threatening catatonia, with the improvement in early recognition and the availability of efficacious antipsychotic medication and intensive care has been reported from Germany by Häfner and Kasper (1982). However, the remedies currently available reduce neither predisposition to the illness nor the deficit syndrome in the long term. Since the mid twentieth century the system of care provided for people with schizophrenia, time spent in hospital in particular and, as a result, the social biographies of persons affected have undergone marked changes, as outpatient treatment and complementary care have become more and more widespread.

Methodological aspects of course and outcome research

Systematic studies into the medium- and long-term course of schizophrenia require considerable effort. This explains why only few studies meet the time-consuming methodological requirements.

A review of 44 long-term follow-up studies, over 10 years or more (an der Heiden 1996), shows considerable variance in the proportion of good outcome in schizophrenia (Fig. 8.2). Factors explaining part of the variance are differences in the outcome measures, in the diagnostic criteria and in the study populations.

Methodological requirements for longitudinal studies into schizophrenia have been proposed by several authors (Robins 1979; Ram *et al.* 1992; Jablensky 1995; Gaebel & Frommann 2000; Häfner 2000). To ensure the validity and comparability of the results, the following are the main requirements to observe.

1 The *inclusion criteria* – diagnosis is the most important – determining what will be studied.

2 To define *diagnosis* only cross-sectional criteria should be adopted. Course-related criteria, such as Criterion C1 – persistance of symptoms for at least 6 months – for an American Psychiatric Association DSM-IIIR (1987) or DSM-IV (American Psychiatric Association 1994) diagnosis of schizophrenia, leads

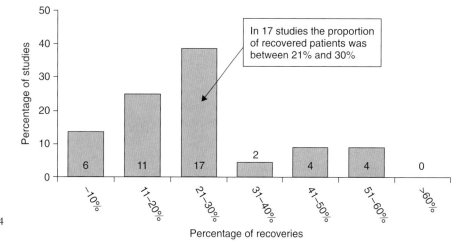

Fig 8.2 Proportion of recovered patients in 44 long-term studies.

to the exclusion of acute cases with predominantly good outcomes.

3 Only if the cohort at entry into a longitudinal study is *representative* of all cases diagnosed with schizophrenia in a given population or of a precisely defined subgroup of these cases, e.g. late-onset schizophrenia, will the study results be valid for all cases of the disorder or for the subgroup in question.

Because of an annual incidence rate of as low as 1–2 cases per 10 000 population it is impractical to try to reach first episodes of schizophrenia in large enough numbers by door-to-door surveys. For this reason, index cases are usually recruited from treatment services. It remains a controversial question whether a treated incidence calculated from inpatient data is a valid estimate of the true incidence. According to the few comparative studies addressing this question, the risk for persons with schizophrenia of coming in contact with inpatient services ranges from 50% to 100% (Link & Dohrenwend 1980; Engelhardt *et al.* 1982; von Korff *et al.* 1985; Goldacre *et al.* 1994; Geddes & Kendell 1995; Thornicroft & Johnson 1996). As the proportion of cases in inpatient care decreases with the increasing proportion of patients cared for in outpatient services, case recruitment should be extended to outpatient services as well. In countries with a hospital-centred system of mental health care, a practical alternative to a field study is to recruit first admissions for schizophrenia from all the mental hospitals serving a defined population or from case registers.

However, the representativeness of samples is bound to be limited if probands are recruited from hospitals not seeing the entire spectrum of schizophrenic illness. Some of the famous US long-term follow-up studies (Table 8.1) recruited their samples from among long-stay inpatients (Breier *et al.* 1991) 'who had not improved sufficiently with chlorpromazine' (Harding *et al.* 1987a) or from among wealthy long-stay inpatients of a private mental hospital (McGlashan 1984a).

Of great importance for the external validity of study results is the question of whether the samples assessed at follow-up are representative of the initial samples. This requirement is difficult to fulfil, particularly in studies covering long periods of time (Riecher-Rössler & Rössler 1998; Häfner & an der Heiden 2000).

In pure outcome studies an initial assessment is compared with a follow-up. Follow-up studies try either to identify trends from at least three cross-sectional assessments or to analyse changes between at least two cross-sections by using a retrospective approach (Robins 1979; Ram *et al.* 1992; Häfner & an der Heiden 2000). A criterion of the quality of follow-up studies that has been paid only little attention, as the great variation in the follow-up periods in Table 8.1 shows (an der Heiden 1996), is that follow-up periods should be identical in length for all the individuals included in a study. If changes are expected to occur in the illness course, and this is a basic hypothesis of all follow-up studies, designs not paying attention to this rule are bound to produce distorted results.

For this same reason, entering subjects at different stages of illness progression should be avoided (Jablensky 1995). In short-term follow-up studies looking into the early stages of illness, rapid changes and much variability can be expected so great care should be taken to avoid variation in the early follow-up periods. Only recently have the requirements of commencing studies at identical stages of illness and of using identical follow-up periods become fulfilled in a few longitudinal studies, e.g. WHO Determinants of Outcome of Severe Mental Disorders Study: 2 and 5 years (Jablensky *et al.* 1992), WHO Disability Study: 13–15 years (Schubart *et al.* 1986; an der Heiden *et al.* 1995; Mason *et al.* 1996; Sartorius *et al.* 1996; Wiersma *et al.* 1998; Häfner *et al.* 1999b).

In studies on the natural course of schizophrenia, the follow-up period ideally begins with the onset of the disorder. As it is not yet possible to predict the onset of schizophrenia with certainty, the first hospital admission is usually chosen as the starting point. Usually triggered by psychotic episodes, first and subsequent admissions take place at illness stages with maximum symptom presentation (Häfner *et al.* 1995). When an initial assessment conducted on hospital admission is compared with a

Table 8.1 Studies on long-term course of schizophrenia (after an der Heiden 1996).

Source	Study/subjects	Design	Diagnosis	N: beginning /end	Follow-up	Course/outcome dimensions; main instruments	Course	Outcome
Bleuler (1972)	Burghölzli study; hospital patients; 31.5% with first admissions	'Real-time' prospective study	Schizophrenia according to Bleuler criteria	216/208 (205)	>20 years	Psychopathological status; social and occupational development; assessment of 'end state' (during the last 5 years)	Eight course types: 4 simple courses – acute or chronic with severe end states, 13%; acute or chronic with mild end states, 25%; 3 undulating courses – severe end states, 9%; mild end states, 27%; recovery, 22%; atypical courses – 4%	(In 152 patients) severe end states, 24%; moderate end states, 24%; mild end states, 33%; recovery, 20%
Bottlender et al. (1999)	Inpatients with first admission to a psychiatric hospital	'Catch-up' prospective study; single follow-up assessment	Diagnosis according to ICD-9: 295, 297, 298.39	245/145	15 years after first hospital admission	AMDP: paranoid-hallucinatory syndrome, depressive syndrome, negative syndrome, 'deficit'-syndrome GAS	–	Average GAS-score, 55.8; negative symptoms, 52.4%; 'deficit' syndrome, 26.2%
Breier et al. (1991)	NIMH Longitudinal Study of Chronic Schizophrenia; 'chronically ill' hospital population	'Catch-up' prospective study; single follow-up assessment	Chronic/ subchronic schizophrenia or schizoaffective disorder according to RDC	74/58	On average 13 years after illness onset, resp. 2–12 years after index treatment	Symptomatology; functioning; treatment history BPRS, SANS; LOFS, GAS, WCS	No reduction in symptomatology, instead of this increase during the first 10 years	GAS-score: poor 35%; moderate 62%; good 3% BPRS-total score: poor 38%; moderate 53%; good 10% SANS total score: poor 48%; moderate 36%; good 15% Global outcome: poor 42%; moderate 38%; good 21%
Carpenter & Strauss (1991)	Washington IPSS cohort; hospital population (no evidence of continuous psychosis for longer than 3 years)	'Real-time' prospective study; 3 follow-up assessments: 2, 5 and 11 years	At least one psychotic symptom; schizophrenia, manic-depressive illness, personality disorder according to DSM-II	131/53 (40 with DSM-II schizophrenia)	11 years after index treatment	Duration of inpatient treatment; social relationships; occupational functioning; severity of symptoms DIS, LOFS	No indication for either significant amelioration or deterioration in the period between 5- and 11-year follow-up; many patients tend to reach a plateau of psychopathology early in the course of the illness	Outcome domains of functioning are only moderately correlated
Changhui et al. (1995)	WHO ISoS Study; epidemiologically defined population irrespective of duration of illness	'Catch-up' prospective study; single follow-up assessment	Schizophrenia according to ICD-9	91/56 (55)	12 years after index assessment	Global functioning; social disability; psychological impairments; positive/negative symptoms DAS, GAF, LCS,PIRS, PSE-9, SANS	Simple course, 51.8%; episodic course, 7.1%; neither episodic nor simple, 7.1%; no psychotic episode during follow-up period, 33.9%	GAF-score: good outcome, 32.1%; fair outcome, 16.1%; poor outcome, 41.1%; very poor outcome, 10.7% SANS total score ≥3: 80% PIRS total score ≥2: 74.5% PSE total score ≥11: 60% DAS total score ≥2: 75%
Ciompi & Müller (1976)	Lausanne study; former hospital patients aged <65 at first admission and ≥65 at follow-up	'Catch-up' prospective study; single follow-up assessment	Definition of schizophrenia according to Kraepelin and E. & M. Bleuler	1642/289	36.9 years (median) after index admission	Course and 'end state' criteria according to Bleuler (1972); social adjustment; global psychological status	Simple-progredient courses, 43%; undulating courses, 50%; uncertain, 7%	(Continuous status during the last 5 years) poor end states, 18%; fair end states, 24%; mild end states, 22%; recovered, 27%; uncertain, 9%

Study	Sample	Design	Diagnosis	N	Follow-up	Measures		
Dube et al. (1984)	Agra IPSS cohort; WHO ISoS study; patients with first contact and illness onset within 1 year before index assessment	'Real-time' prospective study; 3 follow-up assessments: 2, 5 and 13–14 years	Clinical diagnosis of schizophrenia (72.1%), manic-depressive psychosis (20%), psychoneurosis (7.9%)	140/79 (46 = 74.2% with schizophrenia)	13–14 years	Global functioning; symptomatology PSE-9, PPHS	–	(In 46 schizophrenic patients) 'normal', 59%; 'neurotic', 2%; residual states, 20%; schizophrenia, 13%; manic-depressive psychosis, 7%
Eaton et al. (1992a, b)	3 case register cohorts (Victoria, Australia/Denmark/Salford, UK); patients, who received a diagnosis of schizophrenia in a hospital setting during a period of observation of some 23 years	Case register analysis	Schizophrenia according to ICD-8, DSM-I	1850	At least 16 years (Salford: 14 years) after discharge for first hospitalization for schizophrenia	Hospital readmissions	The probability for readmission decreases significantly with the passage of time; risk for readmission is highest in the first month after discharge; as a tendency duration of community tenure during hospital stays seems to lengthen over time	–
Ganev et al. (1998); Ganev (2000)	WHO disability study/WHO ISoS study; schizophrenics in inpatient and outpatient treatment from a defined catchment area; illness onset no longer than 2 years before index treatment; age between 15 and 44 years at index admission	'Real-time' prospective study; 3 follow-up assessments: 2, 5 and 13–14 years	Clinical diagnosis of schizophrenia; Schneiderian first rank symptoms; ICD-9 295, 297, 298.3, 298.4, 298.8, 298.9	60/55	16 years after index treatment	Psychopathology, social disability, psychological impairments PSE-9, PHSD, PIRS, DAS, LCS, GAF	–	Course of psychotic illness during 2 years before long-term follow-up: continuously psychotic, 45.5%; episodic course, 12.7%; no symptoms, 38.2%; negative symptoms, 63%; 64.8% with continuous; 13% with intermittent neuroleptic treatment; 74.5% without inpatient treatment GAF score 31–50: 50.9%
Gmür (1991)	2 cohorts of chronically ill patients: (i) night-clinic patients (average duration of illness 18 years); (ii) hospital patients (average duration of illness 15 years)	'Catch-up' prospective study; single follow-up assessment	Diagnosis of schizophrenia according to Bleuler; PSE-CATEGO diagnosis schizophrenia (based on case history records)	46 night clinic +46 hospital patients/ 39 +44	12 years after index admission (15–18 years after first manifestation)	Psychopathology; social adjustment (among others: work situation; social contacts; sexuality) FBF2	Decline in number and duration of acute episodes, as well as in number and duration of hospital stays; decreasing ability to work; increasing prominence of residual symptoms during quiescent intervals; no differences between the two cohorts	Conspicuous psychopathology: cohort (i), 66.5%; cohort (ii), 64.4%. Work situation: disability pension, 71.8% vs. 62%; employed, 33.3% vs. 35.5%. Relationships: married, 7.7% vs. 20%; living alone, 45.4% vs. 44.4%; no friends or acquaintances, 43.6% vs. 35.6%

Table 8.1 (cont.)

Source	Study/subjects	Design	Diagnosis	N: beginning /end	Follow-up	Course/outcome dimensions; main instruments	Course	Outcome
Harding et al. (1987a); see also Harding et al. (1987b); Harding (1988); Childers & Harding (1990)	Vermont Longitudinal Study; long-stay patients, 'who had not improved sufficiently with chlorpromazine'	'Real-time' prospective study; 2 follow-up assessments: 5–10 years and 20–25 years after discharge from index admission	Chronically ill patients; 79.2% with DSM-I diagnosis schizophrenia	269/168	On average 32 years after index assessment (range: 22–62 years)	Among others: utilization of treatment/social services; residence; work; finances; social support system; competence; community involvement; psychopathology; medication VCQ-L; VCQ-C; GAS; LOFS	–	One-half to two-thirds of the patients achieved considerable improvement/recovery Living conditions: independent housing, 50.3%; boarding home, 39.8%; hospital, 3.1%; nursing homes, 4.3%; other setting, 2.5% Employment status: employed (half of them classified as working in unskilled jobs) 26%; unemployed, 33% GAS score ≥62 (generally functioning pretty well'), 68% Overall functioning (LOFS), slight or no impairment, 55%
an der Heiden et al. (1995, 1996)	WHO Disability Study/WHO ISoS Study; hospital patients from a defined catchment area; illness onset no longer than 1 year before index admission; age at index admission: 15–44 years	'Real-time' prospective study; 9 follow-up assessments: 6, 12, 18, 24 months, 3 years, 5, 14, 14.9, 15.6 years	Clinical diagnosis of schizophrenia; Schneiderian first-rank symptoms	70/56 (14-year follow-up)/ 51 (15.6 years)	14 years +18 months after index admission	Among others: living conditions; social contacts; need for inpatient/outpatient care; work situation; negative symptoms; social disability; psychological impairments PSE-9; DAS-M; PIRS; BPRS; SANS; IRAOS-C	Significant decrease in need for inpatient treatment with the passage of time; no change in the number of patients with significant psychopathology (PSE-DAH) and psychological impairments (PIRS); significant increase in the number of patients with social disability (DAS-M)	(9-month interval after 14-year follow-up) significant positive and/or negative symptoms, 60.7%; clinically inconspicuous with neuroleptic treatment, 12.5%; recovered, 26.8%
Helgason (1990)	Epidemiologically based cohort with first inpatient/ outpatient contacts	'Real-time' prospective study; 2 follow-up assessments: 6–7 years, 21 years	ICD-8/9; Schneiderian first-rank symptoms	107/82	21 years	Mental state; ability to work; social interaction	–	Mental state: no/minor symptoms of psychopathology/ no treatment, 30%; obvious symptoms, inpatient treatment <2 months/year, 50%; severe symptoms, inpatient treatment >2 months/year, 21% Social interaction: normal/few but close friends, 55%;

						tendency towards or social isolation, 45% Employment: employed full-time/<6 months/year, 33%; <6 months/year/unemployed, 67%	Complete remisssion, 22.1%; non-characteristic residual syndromes, 43.2%; characteristic residual syndromes, 34.7%
Huber *et al.* (1979)	Bonn study (67% first admissions)	'Catch-up' prospective study; single follow-up assessment	Criteria of schizophrenia according to K. Schneider and M. & E. Bleuler	758/502	On average 22.4 years (range: 9–59 years) after index admission	Course types considering both the kind of course and psychopathological outcome ('end states') according to M. Bleuler (1972)	12 course types: monophasic course type, 10%; polyphasic course type, 12.1%; chronic pure psychoses, 4.2%, one manifestation to pure residues, 6.2%; phasic-'schubförmig' to pure residues, 10%; 'schubförmig' with second positive bend to pure residues, 5.8%; 'schubförmig/simple to structural deformities, 6.2%; simple to pure residues, 5.4%; 'schubförmig' to pure residues, 12.9%; 'schubförmig' to mixed residues, 9.6%;simple to mixed residues, 7.2%; 'schubförmig'/simple to typically schizophrenic defect psychoses, 10.5%
Leon (1989)	Former IPSS cohort; WHO ISoS study; age of patients at inclusion between 15 and 44 years	'Real-time' prospective study; 3 follow-up assessments: 2, 5 and 10 years	Clinical diagnosis of schizophrenia; diagnosis of schizophrenia according to PSE-9 (ICD-7/8)	101/84 (74)	10 years after index assessment	Psychopathology; social disability; psychological impairments; inpatient treatment DAS, PIRS, PSE-9; SEA, SAF, SPHS, Global outcome assessment: 1 complete recovery (no psychotic symptoms); 2 partial recovery (no psychotic symptoms, but symptoms of neurosis/adaptive problems); 3 covert (inactive) psychosis presence of psychotic characteristics, in a covert way); 4 residual state (usually negative symptoms); 5 overt psychosis (clear presence of psychotic symptoms); 6 deterioration (severe disability of mental functions)	Global course description, based on the analysis of all available clinical information: (1) single episode, 8%; (2) episodic, occasional, 13%; (3) episodic, recurrent, 20%; (4) mixed, with recovery, 8%; (5) recurrent, progressive, 4%; (6) mixed, without recovery, 12%; (7) continuous, stationary, 9%; (8) continuous, fluctuating, 13%; (9) continuous, severe, 13%

Leon (1989) additional outcome column: (1) complete recovery, 43.4%; (2) partial recovery, 7.9%; (3) covert psychosis, 15.8%; (4) residual state, 7.9%; (5) overt psychosis, 14.5%; (6) deterioration, 10.5%

Table 8.1 (cont.)

Source	Study/subjects	Design	Diagnosis	N: beginning/end	Follow-up	Course/outcome dimensions; main instruments	Course	Outcome
Thara et al. (1994)	Madras longitudinal study; first-onset patients	'Real-time' prospective study; 3 follow-up assessments: 2, 5 and 10 years	Schizophrenia according to ICD-9	90/76	10 years after index assessment	Psychopathology; treatment; course types as defined in the IPSS IFS; PSE-9; PPHS	Complete recovery without relapse, 14.5%; no relapses, but with residual symptoms, 2.6%; one or more relapses, complete remissions, 48.7%; one or more relapses, incomplete remissions, 27.6%; continuously psychotic, 6.6%	Status at follow-up: psychotic 22% (7% continuously since inclusion into the study)
Tsoi & Wong (1991)	First admissions to a psychiatric hospital in Singapore; age range: 15–39 years	'Real-time' prospective study; 3 follow-up assessments: 5, 10 and 15 years	Schizophrenia according to ICD-9	330/224	15 years after index treatment	Psychiatric treatment; employment	Treatment and employment; status at 3 points in time: (1) 5 years; (2) 10 years; (3) 15 years after index treatment: in treatment: (1) 45%; (2), 40%; (3) 45%; employed: (1) 55%; (2) 54%; (3) 48%; inpatient treatment: (1) 15%; (2) 17%; (3) 17%; no readmissions in 15, 34%; 1–5 readmission, 45%; 6–10 readmissions, 12%; more than 10 readmission, 11%	–

AMDP, Befundbogen (Arbeitsgemeinschaft für Methodik und Diagnostik in der Psychiatrie 1995); BPRS, Brief Psychiatric Rating Scale (Overall & Gorham 1962); BRS, Broad Rating Schedule (WHO 1992); DAS, Disability Assessment Schedule (WHO 1988); DAS-M, Disability Assessment Schedule – Mannheim Version (Jung et al. 1989); DIS, Diagnostic Interview Schedule (Robins et al. 1981); FBF2, Frankfurt Symptoms Questionnaire (Süllwold 1977); GAF, Global Assessment of Functioning Scale (American Psychiatric Association 1987); GAS, Global Assessment Scale (Endicott et al. 1976); IFS, Interim Follow-up Schedule (Sartorius et al. 1986); IPSS, International Pilot Study of Schizophrenia; IRAOS, Instrument for the Retrospective Assessment of the Onset of Schizophrenia (Häfner et al. 1992); ISoS, International Study on Schizophrenia; Katz and Lyerly Adjustment Scales (Katz & Lyerly 1963); LCS, Life Chart Schedule (WHO 1992); LOFS, Level of Functioning Scale (Hawk et al. 1975); PHSD, Past History and Sociodemographic Description Schedule (WHO 1977); PPHS, Psychiatric and Personal History Schedule (WHO 1978b); PSE-9, Present State Examination (Wing et al. 1974); PIRS, Psychological Impairment Rating Schedule (Biehl et al. 1989); PSE-DAH, Present State Examination – Delusional and Hallucinatory Syndromes; RDC, Research Diagnostic Criteria (Spitzer et al. 1978); SADS, Schedule for Affective Disorders and Schizophrenia (Endicott & Spitzer 1978); SAF, Self-Assessment Form (WHO 1979); SANS, Scale for the Assessment of Negative Symptoms (Andreasen 1989); SEA, Subjective Experience Account (WHO 1979); SPHS, Social and Personal History Schedule (WHO 1979); Strauss–Carpenter Scale (Strauss & Carpenter 1972); VCQ-L, Vermont Community Questionnaire (Harding & Brooks 1984); VCQ-C, Vermont Community Questionnaire – cross-sectional interview (Harding & Brooks 1984); WCS, Wisconsin Card Sorting Test (Berg 1948).

Table 8.2 The 14 most frequent symptoms in a cohort of 811 patients with schizophrenia, examined in the WHO International Pilot Study of Schizophrenia (WHO 1979) (from Jablensky 2000).

Symptom	Frequency (%) in the psychotic index episode	Frequency (%) at 2-year follow-up
Ideas of reference	55.1	18.0
Suspiciousness	60.0	25.2
Delusions of reference	50.3	14.2
Delusions of persecution	48.1	12.7
Presence of auditory hallucinations	43.8	11.6
Presence of verbal hallucinations	37.9	10.7
Voices speak to patient	36.3	9.4
Delusional mood	47.5	10.5
Thought alienation	33.5	7.4
Restricted speech	17.5	12.9
Flatness of affect	51.0	27.1
Apathy	30.4	18.8
Lack of insight	82.7	42.5
Inadequate description	67.2	25.2

later follow-up, the result will show an artefact of improvement or recovery, because in the further course of the disorder only about 20% of the patients are bound to be in psychotic episodes (Biehl *et al.* 1986; Häfner & an der Heiden 1986; Wiersma *et al.* 1996). Table 8.2 illustrates the 14 symptoms most frequently presented by 811 patients with schizophrenia in the International Pilot Study of Schizophrenia (IPSS; WHO 1979). The almost proportional decrease over 2 years is accounted for by an artefact of illness stage. To prevent this mistake from happening, later follow-up assessments should be compared with assessments conducted after remission of the psychotic episode, e.g. 6 months after first admission (Biehl *et al.* 1986; Craig *et al.* 1999; Häfner & an der Heiden 2000).

Ram *et al.* (1992) have described follow-up studies based on utilization data of services as statistical reports on admissions and discharges. These can be conducted with considerably less effort than epidemiological longitudinal studies based on direct standardized assessments of patients. Drawbacks are the problems of lacking or limited generalizability. For this reason their aims are mostly limited to (i) describing treatment careers as a basis for comparisons over space and time; and (ii) under certain preconditions, to reconstructing the illness course in clinical populations, mostly to find out whether and to what extent patients' needs for treatment and care are met. Especially when based on case-register data from defined catchment areas, analyses of this sort provide valuable information for services planning, but are of secondary importance in research on the natural course of schizophrenia.

A follow-up study in which patients are clinically assessed directly at follow-up is termed a catch-up prospective study. In these studies case identification takes place at the beginning of the follow-up period (Robins 1979; Ram *et al.* 1992; Häfner & an der Heiden 2000). The study sample is retrospectively recruited from admission or discharge records and assessed at the beginning of the study, mostly on the basis of case records, then reassessed at follow-up in a clinical interview. This design is also vulnerable to bias, because the representativeness of samples is difficult to ensure. As good cases tend to drop out, chronic cases are usually overrepresented at follow-up (Jablensky 1995). The direct assessment at follow-up makes it possible to reconstruct the illness course retrospectively using suitable instruments.

A retrospective approach with case identification at follow-up (follow-back design) proceeds from an existing study population, e.g. hospital admissions or discharges, and traces illness onset and history from the patients' memory and/or clinical records. This design misses good courses no longer in treatment contact and also leads to a high degree of variability in the lengths of illness courses included. For this reason this design is only rarely used. An example is the investigation of 77 patients with schizophrenia, treated in the course of 1 year, from the Oxford case register in which the lengths of illness varied from 2 to 22 years (Kolakowska *et al.* 1985).

In prospective studies – Robins (1979) calls them 'real-time' studies – the assessment and the study started at the beginning of the illness. Ideally, both the initial examination and the follow-up assessments are conducted on the same cohort by the same investigators using the same instruments.

All longitudinal studies – including prospective ones – as far as they map the timespan between two assessments, have retrospective components. Ciompi and Müller (1976) conducted a follow-up at 36.9 years (median) after index admission. In the Bonn Study (Huber *et al.* 1979) the follow-up assessments took place after an average of 22.4 years, in the Northwick Park Study (Johnstone *et al.* 1992) 3–13 years and in the Chestnut Lodge Study (McGlashan 1984a) an average of 15 years after initial assessment. The Vermont Longitudinal Study comprised two follow-up assessments (Harding *et al.* 1987a), 5–10 years and 20–25 years after discharge from index treatment.

Studies with a still greater number of follow-up assessments are rare: e.g. in the Washington IPSS study (Carpenter & Strauss 1991) patients were reassessed 2, 5 and 11 years after index treatment, in the ABC (Age, Beginning, Course) Study*6 months, 1, 2, 3 and 5 years after first admission (Häfner *et al.* 1999b), and the Mannheim WHO cohort was examined at a total of 10 cross-sections over a period of 15.5 years (an der Heiden *et al.* 1995, 1996).

The ABC Study, to which we will refer in some contexts, was carried out with a population-based sample of 232 patients aged 12–59 years with first illness episodes of broadly defined schizophrenia (ICD-9 diagnoses 295, 297, 298.3, 298.4; WHO 1978a). This sample comprised 84% of all the patients admitted for the first time with a diagnosis of schizophrenia to 10 hospitals serving a semi-rural, semi-urban German population of 1.5 million (Mannheim, Heidelberg and surrounding countryside).

In a retrospective part of the study, data on family background, pre- and perinatal complications, premorbid development, substance and alcohol use, onset and accumulation of symptoms and impairments were collected using the Interview for the Retrospective Assessment of the Onset of Schizophrenia (IRAOS; Häfner *et al.* 1992, 1999a) including a time matrix until first admission. As controls non-schizophrenic individuals drawn from the population register and matched to the probands for age, sex and place of residence were included. Data were collected from three sources: patients, key persons and case records (e.g. from general practitioners) and compared for reliability testing (Maurer & Häfner 1995; for more details see Häfner *et al.* 1993).

At the first cross-section on first admission, patients were assessed using the Present State Examination (PSE: Wing *et al.* 1974), the Scale for the Assessment of Negative Symptoms (SANS: Andreasen 1983), the Psychological Impairments Rating Schedule (PIRS: Biehl *et al.* 1989) and the Psychiatric Disability Assessment Schedule (DAS-M: WHO 1988; Jung *et al.* 1989). The prospective part, conducted in a population-based subsample of 115 patients with first illness episodes, consisted of follow-up assessments at 6 months, 1, 2, 3 and 5 years after first admission using the instruments mentioned above and, additionally, the Follow-up History and Sociodemographic Description Schedule (FU-HSD) (WHO 1980; for more details see Häfner *et al.* 1995, 1998, 1999c). Currently, a controlled 12-year follow-up of the total ABC sample and a study of their children and the non-schizophrenic parents of these children are underway.

Measures for describing course and outcome

The constructs for describing the course and outcome of schizophrenia depend on the issues studied. When the aim is to evaluate treatment measures, standardized illness-course-related indicators of the effectiveness and side-effects of therapies are frequently chosen. In studies on the 'natural' course of schizophrenia, standards are more or less lacking that would allow direct comparisons of the results. One of the reasons is that none of the designs can really do without using retrospective data on varying periods of time (see above).

Most of the instruments used for assessing the course of schizophrenia are cross-sectional in nature. They are aimed at producing data on the current state, usually focusing on periods of 2–4 weeks preceding the interview. For measuring symptoms over several years: (i) information on reliability is scattered (Andreasen *et al.* 1981; Helzer *et al.* 1981; Robins *et al.* 1982; McGuffin *et al.* 1986; Zimmerman *et al.* 1988; Maurer & Häfner 1995); and (ii) information on validity is almost non-existent (an der Heiden & Krumm 1991).

Kraepelin was one of the first who tried to bring some order into the great variety of illness courses in schizophrenia. He proposed only a few categories. The efforts undertaken in his wake on the basis of such – questionably operational – categories as stable, progressing and remittent, or psychosis vs. disability,

have produced typologies of course types whose number ranges from a mere four (Watt *et al.* 1983) to as many as 79 (Huber *et al.* 1979; see also Jansson & Alström 1967; Bleuler 1972; Ciompi & Müller 1976; Leon 1989; Marengo *et al.* 1991; Marneros *et al.* 1991; Thara *et al.* 1994; Changhui *et al.* 1995). Ciompi (1980) added to the two course types – simple and undulatory were used by Kraepelin – two further stages at the beginning and the end: onset (acute, chronic), course type (simple, undulatory) and end state (recovery or mild, moderate or severe). He applied this system to classify 289 patients from the Lausanne study. Attempts to compare the different typologies of the course of schizophrenia (Bleuler 1972; Ciompi & Müller 1976; Harding 1988; Marengo *et al.* 1991) have largely failed to show agreement (Fig. 8.3).

The course of schizophrenia has also been studied on the basis of the need for inpatient treatment (e.g. Daum *et al.* 1977; Engelhardt *et al.* 1982; Gmür 1991; Tsoi & Wong 1991; Eaton *et al.* 1992a,b; Maurer 1995; an der Heiden *et al.* 1995).

Many longitudinal studies focus on outcome. For studies of this type there are approved and reliable instruments available but this approach does not produce comparable results automatically. In Harding *et al.*'s (1987a,b) follow-up study of 269 inpatients with schizophrenia (at follow-up 168) over a period of 32 years, 68% had a good global outcome (Global Assessment Score, GAS ≥61; Endicott *et al.* 1976). In comparison, Breier *et al.*'s (1991) study of 74 (at follow-up 58) chronic patients with schizophrenia over 13 years on average, using the same instrument and measure (GAS score ≥61), yielded a good outcome in only 3%.

The most important clinical indicators of the course of schizophrenia are symptoms, socio-occupational and cognitive functioning, social impairment and disability, demographic and socioeconomic status, illness behaviour and quality of life. Strauss and Carpenter (1972, 1974) distinguish four domains of outcome in schizophrenic illness, which are only loosely connected with one another ('open-linked systems'): social relations, occupational status, treatment and symptomatology. Whether these domains really are more or less independent remains to be clarified. Several studies (Stephens *et al.* 1980; Breier *et al.* 1991; an der Heiden *et al.* 1996) report pronounced associations between symptom measures, negative symptoms in particular, and domains of functioning, while others have failed to show any correlation between changes on different symptom-related or functional dimensions over the illness course (Loebel *et al.* 1992; Tohen *et al.* 1992; Gupta *et al.* 1997). The various domains show great differences in stability, e.g. positive symptoms, which have mainly an episodic course, vs. negative symptoms, occupational and marital status, so that cross-sectional analyses are bound to yield low correlations.

The categories of 'florid' (Kraepelin) or 'acute' (positive–productive) and 'chronic' (primarily negative–unproductive) symptoms have a special role in the description of the course of schizophrenia. They are presumed to be produced by different psychopathological processes (Crow 1980a,b; Andreasen &

	Onset	Course type	End state	Lausanne study	Burghölzli study	Vermont study	Chicago study	ISoS study*
1	Acute	Undulating	Recovery/mild	25.4	30–40 / 25–35	7	10.8	29.4
2	Chronic	Simple	Moderate/severe	24.1	10–20	4	36.5	14.4
3	Acute	Undulating	Moderate/severe	11.9	5	4	9.5	4.9
4	Chronic	Simple	Recovery/mild	10.1	5–10	12	4.1	10.4
5	Chronic	Undulating	Recovery/mild	9.6	–	38	6.8	22.6
6	Acute	Simple	Moderate/severe	8.3	5–15	3	13.5	9.1
7	Chronic	Undulating	Moderate/severe	5.3	–	27	12.2	4
8	Acute	Simple	Recovery/mild	5.3	5	5	6.8	5.3

Fig 8.3 Course types in schizophrenia. On the right, each of the five columns represents a study. The numbers indicate the percentage of patients with the course type depicted on the left, e.g. 7% of the patients in the Vermont Study demonstrated an acute onset, an undulating course and a recovered mild end state (type 1), in contrast to the ISoS Study in which 29.4% of the patients belonged to this course type (based on Harding 1988; data from Chicago and ISoS studies have been added by the authors). *Incidence cohorts only. Lausanne study, Ciompi and Müller (1976); Burghölzli study, Bleuler (1972); Vermont study, Harding *et al.* (1987); Chicago study, Marengo *et al.* (1991); ISoS study, Harrison *et al.* (2001).

Olsen 1982). Besides these symptoms more or less characteristic anomalies are observed ('impairments'). While the diagnosis is mainly based on symptoms, the psychological impairments (e.g. of attention, cognition, affect, speech) are less specific, because they are also encountered in other disorders, e.g. in major depressive disorder, where they show less severe presentations, and may to some extent result from external factors, e.g. investigator's attitude. Like symptoms and premorbid personality, the behavioural anomalies are classified as disease-inherent factors, i.e. factors characteristic of the disorder and its course (Schubart *et al.* 1986).

To a greater extent than in the origin of 'impairment', external factors – especially patients' social and occupational status – have a role in the emergence of disabilities. Disability is defined as disordered or deficient functioning in the social roles and domains (work, family, social group, etc.) regarded as normal in that society, by the family or social group or by the person affected (DAS; WHO 1988; Jablensky 1978).

For purposes of clinical and rehabilitative practice, additional measures for assessing the course and outcome of schizophrenia are needed, especially because there are methods of therapy and training available that help to reduce symptoms, cognitive and social impairment and to improve the patients' level of social functioning. As a result, there is a growing demand for tools that, in addition to measuring global outcome, allow a differential assessment of indicators of course and outcome and effects of treatment.

Diagnosis, clinical subtypes, empirical symptom dimensions and their course

Without an identifiable aetiology, and a distinct underlying pathophysiology still rather obscure, the disease concept of schizophrenia is currently based on tradition, clinical experience and the operational definitions of the diagnosis derived from this experience (see Chapters 1, 2, 3 and 12). The symptom patterns conventionally diagnosed as schizophrenia and regarded as reliable produce a rather heterogeneous spectrum of illness courses. The few stable patterns of symptoms or functional deficits from the schizophrenia spectrum nourish hopes that they could soon be linked to brain dysfunctions. Perhaps in this way and with increasing clarification of the role of genes it might become possible to break what is currently known as schizophrenia down into definable subentities of dysfunctioning (Jablensky 2000). However, for the time being there is no alternative to an operationally defined disease concept of schizophrenia in studies into the course and outcome of schizophrenia (see Chapter 12).

The international classification systems divide the diagnosis of schizophrenia into subtypes. The subtypes given in the ICD classification (WHO 1993) follow the clinical tradition, whereas those included in DSM-IV (American Psychiatric Association 1994) to some extent take account of symptom dimensions generated by factor analysis. The subtypes are distinguished mainly by their type of early illness course and outcome.

Of the clinically defined subtypes, 'simple type' and 'hebephrenia' mostly have a poor social prognosis, and 'acute catatonia' and 'paranoid psychosis' the most favourable prognosis. Fenton and McGlashan (1991a,b) used three DSM-III-based subtypes in their follow-back study of 187 patients over an average of 19 years: hebephrenia had an insidious onset and a poor prognosis – in accordance with the definition; undifferentiated schizophrenia occupied an intermediate position; and the paranoid subtype tended to a remittent course and minimum disability. In the IPSS (WHO 1979) the ICD-9 subtypes were subjected to empirical testing on the basis of discriminant function analysis. The result was a considerable degree of overlap, particularly between the simple and hebephrenic type on the one hand and paranoid schizophrenia on the other hand (see Chapter 3).

The most simple distinction between subtypes is based on acute vs. insidious onset (Jablensky et al. 1992). A detailed subtyping is yielded by Leonhard's (1966, 1999) classification of 32 symptomatological course units. However, the data available do not provide enough evidence for regarding these subtypes as discrete entities. In clinical practice some of the clinical subtypes can be helpful, despite the occurrence of continuous transitions between the categories, because they provide therapeutic and prognostic information. Jablensky (2000), however, doubts their prognostic power because of the 'scarcity of well-designed longitudinal studies'.

Positive and negative symptoms

An early attempt to divide the symptoms of schizophrenia into dichotomous categories was undertaken by Emil Kraepelin (1893). In the 1970s the terms 'negative' and 'positive' came into use (Jablensky 2000). These stem from Reynolds (1858), the underlying concepts from Jackson's (1887) hierarchical model, according to which deficit symptoms are classified as primary or lower level nervous dysfunctions and secondary symptoms as reflecting responses from a higher level of the central nervous system (for a detailed description of the history of positive and negative symptoms see Chapter 3). This dichotomous distinction of schizophrenic symptoms is clinically useful. It gives the complex psychopathology a simple order and is reflected in different course types, outcomes and therapy responses.

New interest in the positive and negative symptom dimensions was awakened by the speculative model of causality proposed by T. Crow (1980a,b; see also Chapter 3). Crow described a type I (positive) schizophrenia as characterized by hallucinations, delusions and formal thought disorder. He presumed that the underlying cause was a dopaminergic dysfunction and that for this reason type I as a pure type involved no deficits and responded well to antidopaminergic neuroleptic therapy. Type II (negative) schizophrenia was described by Crow as a clinical poverty syndrome (Wing & Brown 1970) involving social withdrawal, avolition, affective blunting and poverty of content and production of thought and speech. He interpreted it as caused by embryonal or perinatal brain lesions. The persistence of these symptoms and their poor therapy response seemed to point to a stable neurodevelopmental deficit.

According to Crow, type I and II were expressions of co-existing, but independent pathophysiological processes, but he did not specify how they were related to one another. Actually, neither cross-sectionally nor over the course of the disorder have these two types turned out to be mutually exclusive (Lindenmayer et al. 1984; Pogue-Geile & Harrow 1985; Biehl et al. 1986; Gross et al. 1986; Deister et al. 1990; Addington & Addington 1991; Häfner & Maurer 1991; Maurer & Häfner 1991; Peralta et al. 1992; Rey et al. 1994; Marneros et al. 1995; Eaton et al. 1995).

A further effort to classify the symptoms of schizophrenia by the positive–negative dichotomy was made by Andreasen and Olsen (1982) by means of factor analysis. They studied a heterogeneous clinical sample comprising first-admitted patients in psychotic episodes and patients with long histories of illness. As expected, replications of their results in homogeneous samples have failed both cross-sectionally and longitudinally over the course of the disorder (Maurer & Häfner 1991; Tandon & Greden 1991). Andreasen and Olsen (1982) posited one single symptom dimension. At the one extreme end of this dimension the authors identified patients with severe purely negative symptoms and at the other extreme patients with purely positive symptoms and they claimed that these extremes were negatively correlated with each other. The negative type was associated with poor premorbid adjustment, low level of social functioning, cognitive impairment and local brain anomalies, and the positive type with less impairment, absence of neuropsychological changes in the brain and a good outcome. In between, the authors believed, there was a mixed group presenting symptoms from both categories. When the results of a follow-up study of 10 first episodes of schizophrenia over 4 years became available, the model was finally abandoned (Andreasen 1990).

A transphenomenal approach to applying the positive–negative dichotomy is the severity–liability model (Gottesman et al. 1987). On a continuum of genetic liability, patients with negative symptoms occupy significantly more unfavourable rankings than patients with purely positive symptoms (Kendler et al. 1983, 1984, 1985; McGuffin et al. 1987; Tsuang et al. 1991; Lenzenweger & Dworkin 1996). Most studies trying to cluster schizophrenic symptoms or to analyse their dimensionality have produced more than two clusters or factors (Liddle &

Barnes 1990; Lenzenweger *et al.* 1991; Löffler & Häfner 1999; see below).

Negative symptoms are a frequent and fairly persistent characteristic of schizophrenia. Mostly emerging at the prodromal stage long before the first psychotic episode (Häfner *et al.* 1995, 1999b), they cannot be just a residuum of a psychotic episode. Carpenter *et al.* (1988) distinguish between primary and secondary negative symptoms. The primary or deficit syndromes, the authors believe, are a persisting environmentally determined characteristic which precedes psychosis onset and frequently persists between the episodes. These syndromes neither respond to traditional antipsychotic treatment nor do they vary with depressive symptoms, anxiety or dosage of medication. Carpenter *et al.* (1988) classify in this primary group anhedonia, flattening and narrowing of affect, poverty of speech, avolition and reduced social activity. For diagnosing the deficit syndrome they developed the Schedule for the Deficit Syndrome (SDS: Kirkpatrick *et al.* 1989). In patients with the deficit syndrome the authors found poor premorbid adjustment, an increased frequency of neurological soft signs and low depression scores (Buchanan *et al.* 1990; Kirkpatrick *et al.* 1996a,b; see also Chapter 3). Jablensky (2000) contends that these authors have failed to validate the existence of the core deficit syndrome. In his opinion it is more plausible to presume a continuum of negative symptomatology with two extremes: a severe deficit syndrome at the one end and a mild negative syndrome, encountered in borderline cases and in character variants, at the other end.

Primary negative symptoms by definition are traits, stable over time and largely independent of environmental factors (Carpenter *et al.* 1988). In contrast, the course and amount of secondary negative symptoms, such as psychomotor poverty/slowness, anergia, social withdrawal and lack of perseverence, are presumed to fluctuate with psychotic episodes, depression, side-effects of medication, substance abuse and physical morbidity (Whiteford & Peabody 1989; Carpenter *et al.* 1991). An attempt to prove the validity of this model in an epidemiological sample of first episodes of schizophrenia over 3 years failed (Maurer & Häfner 1991). All the five SANS sections (Andreasen 1983) – affective flattening, alogia/paralogia, abulia/apathy, anhedonia/asociality and attentional impairment – showed high proportions of both fluctuating and persistent courses (Fig. 8.4). Nevertheless, the picture that emerged from the mean score for each measure of the SANS and the six cross-sectional assessments was one of limited stability. Anhedonia turned out to be the most stable syndrome, showing a persistent course across the six cross-sections in 30%. The course of the secondary or 'non-deficit syndrome' could not be shown to depend on extrinsic factors, as originally expected. In contrast, the subgroup of 'primary' negative symptoms showed significant correlations with these factors (Häfner & Maurer 1997). The authors interpreted this result according to Jablensky's (2000) model: patients with a deficit syndrome are more severely ill than patients presenting 'milder' non-deficit negative symptoms. For this reason they are also more sensitive to adversity.

Course of negative symptoms and cognitive impairment

In the last few years a growing body of evidence has emerged indicating that negative symptoms might have a pathophysiological basis distinct from that of positive symptoms. In this context especially their association with cognitive impairment and brain dysfunctions has been explored (Addington & Addington 1991; Arndt *et al.* 1995; Maziade *et al.* 1996; Tamminga *et al.* 1998).

It can be regarded as an established fact that schizophrenia is frequently associated with neurocognitive dysfunctions. In persons with schizophrenia, compared with healthy controls, typically impairment in attention, working and episodic memory and executive functions occur (Saykin *et al.* 1994; Goldberg *et al.* 1998; Gold *et al.* 1999; Weickert *et al.* 2000). A small proportion of patients, however, independently of their illness stage, exhibit a broad range of severe impairment – of vigilance, neuromotor skills, abstract and conceptual thinking, etc. – in the sense of overall cognitive impairment (see Chapter 10). The amount of cognitive and functional impairment shows a high degree of interindividual variance, ranging from absence of any impairment to presence of severe cognitive deficits.

Patients with schizophrenia usually show 0.5–2 SD below the values for the general population (Lubin *et al.* 1962; Schwartzman & Douglas 1962; Hoff *et al.* 1999). While in most studies an association between positive symptoms and cognitive functioning has failed to emerge (Goldberg *et al.* 1993; Weickert & Goldberg 2000), weak to medium-sized positive correlations have been found between negative symptoms and cognitive deficits. However, these associations explain less than half of the variance in cognitive functioning (Bilder *et al.* 1985, 1995; Shtasel *et al.* 1992; Goldberg & Gold 1995; Paulsen *et al.* 1995; Censitis *et al.* 1997; Norman *et al.* 1997; Sobizack *et al.* 1999; Weickert & Goldberg 2000).

Saykin *et al.* (1994) demonstrated that the profiles of cognitive impairment in 37 new untreated cases of schizophrenia hardly differed from those of a group of unmedicated formerly treated patients with long histories of illness. A similar result has been reported by Albus *et al.* (1996). Sobizack *et al.* (1999) compared 66 first-episode patients and 49 chronic cases of schizophrenia with 40 healthy controls with regard to memory functions, speech and cognitive flexibility/abstraction by administering a comprehensive neuropsychological test battery. They too found no differences in cognitive performance between the first-episode and the previously treated group, but both patient groups differed highly significantly from healthy controls. According to an overview given by Rund (1998) of 15 studies with follow-up periods of at least 1 year, deficits in verbal skills (word meaning, word association, verbal fluency), memory (long- and short-term, spatial and visual) and attentional span are fairly stable over time. Characteristic profiles of cognitive impairment at early stages of schizophrenia indicate fairly reliably – as long as we lack the means of treating them effectively – that cognitive and functional deficits are going to persist

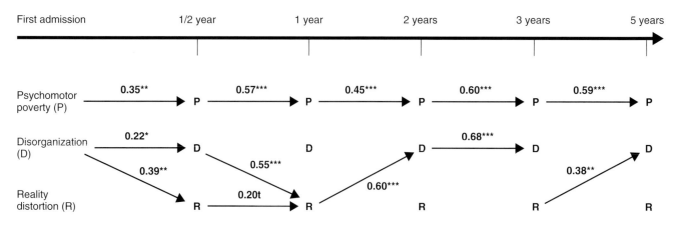

Fig 8.5 Correlations within and between syndrome ratings at 6 points in time over 5 years. The factors were tested by explorative orthogonal factor analysis at each of the five follow-ups – ABC subsample of 115 first illness episodes. Pearson correlations: t $P < 0.1$; *$P < 0.05$; **$P < 0.01$; ***$P < 0.001$. (From Löffler & Häfner 1999.)

ring between the three factors tested by explorative orthogonal factor analysis at each of the five follow-up assessments. As expected, the factor 'negative symptoms' remained stable and independent of the other factors over the total 5-year period showing highly significant coefficients. The factors 'disorganization' and 'positive symptoms' showed low correlations at the follow-ups. Four of the 10 possible correlations attained significance. Contrary to the two other factors, which showed no prognostic power with respect to social outcome, the presence of negative symptoms at the second follow-up, 6 months after first admission, was a highly significant predictor of the patients' social status up until 3-year follow-up.

The dimensions 'positive symptoms' and 'disorganization' seem not to be separable as two independent and stable factors in the medium-term course. Negative symptoms, stable over time and associated with overall functional impairment and the consequences of the disorder, constitute the only factor that might reflect an independent brain dysfunction persisting at stable values after the first illness episode.

Studying the same sample and the same period of illness, but applying a different methodological approach, Häfner and Maurer (1991) obtained slightly different results: the sum scores for positive and negative symptoms, classified according to the clinical tradition (PSE) and measured on a yearly basis before first admission and in the year preceding first admission on a monthly basis, showed significant positive correlations attaining medium-sized to small coefficients. Similar results have also been reported by Cechnicki and Walczewski (1999) from a controlled prospective investigation with follow-ups at 1, 3 and 7 years and by Biehl et al. (1986), who studied a sample of first-admission patients with schizophrenia (PSE-8: 295) prospectively at seven cross-sections over 5 years. Lenzenweger et al. (1991) and Löffler and Häfner (1999) have suggested how these seemingly discrepant results might be explained: the two modes of operationalizing positive and negative symptoms differ not only in the underlying methodological procedures. The two-dimensional models differ in how the symptoms pertaining to

the disorganization factor in Liddle's and the other three factor models are classified in the positive and the negative symptom clusters or with the corresponding dimensions. Inadequate affect and bizarre behaviour are usually classified in the positive, positive formal thought disorders in the negative cluster.

Lenzenweger et al. (1991) were able to demonstrate that the significant correlations shown by the positive and negative dimensions in Crow's two-factor model are accounted for by this fact. Hence, Fenton and McGlashan (199lb) conclude that the correlations sometimes found between positive and negative symptoms can be explained by their covariation with disorganization symptoms. These findings once more underscore that both the clinical symptom clusters and the latent symptom dimensions are merely heuristic representations of specific patterns of dysfunctioning and impairment and their underlying brain dysfunctions. In contrast, positive symptoms and the disorganization syndrome have been found to show hardly any association with cognitive deficits in the course of the disorder.

Early course of schizophrenia (prodromal stage and first psychotic episode)

In current clinical practice, the first treatment contact is preceded by increasing psychotic symptomatology of a mean duration of about 1 year or more and a prodromal stage of several years. The duration of pretreatment illness is determined by the onset of the disorder, patients' help-seeking behaviour and the availability of care. Prodromal symptoms and behaviours may include mood symptoms (e.g. depression, anxiety, dysphoria and irritability), cognitive symptoms (e.g. distractibility and difficulty concentrating), social withdrawal, obsessive behaviours and attenuated positive symptoms (e.g. illusions, ideas of reference and magical thinking) to name but a few (Yung & McGorry 1996; Davidson & McGlashan 1997; Maurer & Häfner 1997). The duration of untreated psychosis (DUP) or duration of untreated illness (DUI) is seen, although not consistently, as a predictor of an unfavourable illness course (see Table 8.1; Crow *et al.* 1986; Loebel *et al.* 1992; McGorry *et al.* 1996; Wyatt & Henter 1998). The proponents of this hypothesis presume that untreated psychosis may constitute 'an active morbid process' 'toxic' to the brain. If this disease process is not treated with antipsychotics, it might become chronic (Loebel *et al.* 1992; Craig *et al.* 1999; Ho *et al.* 2000).

McGlashan and Johannessen (1996) presume that the plasticity of the brain can be preserved and the condition prevented from deteriorating if the persons affected receive both medication and simultaneous social stimulation at a 'sensitive' stage of the illness. As neuroleptic medications affect only symptom expression and not the underlying biological predisposition, their effects will be limited to the period of their administration. Hence, a positive correlation between a reduced DUP and medium- to long-term outcome might depend on maintenance medication after the end of the period of untreated psychosis (Linszen *et al.* 1998).

In one of the earliest studies Loebel *et al.* (1992), examining 70 patients with a Research Diagnostic Criteria (RDC) diagnosis of schizophrenia or schizoaffective disorder, demonstrated a negative correlation between DUP, time until remission and quality of remission. Bottlender *et al.* (2000) studied, in a sample of 998 first admissions for schizophrenia, how DUP influences various outcome parameters, positive and negative symptoms at discharge from index admission, global level of functioning and length of inpatient treatment. The expected association was observable with all these outcome measures: the longer the DUP, the more pronounced the amount of persisting symptoms and the longer the inpatient treatment.

The expected association was also demonstrated in a study conducted by Haas *et al.* (1998). In 103 patients – of whom 77 had a DSM-IIIR diagnosis of schizophrenia – a significant association was found between DUP (<1 year vs. ≥1 year) and poverty syndrome or reality distortion at discharge from index treatment. Linszen *et al.*'s (1998) study of 63 patients, who had received a combination of inpatient and outpatient treatment, showed that a delay in treatment by more than a year was associated with a poor prognosis (delayed remission of symptoms). Szymanski *et al.* (1996), studying 36 first-episode patients, most of whom had a DSM-IIIR diagnosis of schizophrenia or schizophreniform disorder, demonstrated that an increased DUP was associated with less reduced positive symptoms after 6 months of treatment. McEvoy *et al.* (1991) found in 106 patients – of whom only 32 had not been previously treated with neuroleptics – significant correlations between time to therapy response and length of active illness before hospitalizatton.

The results on the association between DUP and medium-term outcome are less clear-cut. McGorry *et al.* (1996), in their investigation of 200 patients (of whom more than half were patients with schizophrenia or schizophreniform disorder), demonstrated a positive association between DUP on the one hand and positive and negative symptoms, global functioning and quality of life on the other hand 12 months after index assessment. In contrast, three studies found no such association: Craig *et al.* (2000) could not demonstrate any association

between illness course and clinical outcome 24 months after first assessment, nor could Ho *et al.* (2000) and Robinson *et al.* (1999a,b). Overall, the studies tend to show that patients with short DUPs respond better to treatment in the first schizophrenic episode, but evidence for a lasting effect on the medium- or long-term illness course has so far refused to emerge.

The findings of significant associations between DUP and short-term effects of therapy are also liable to alternative explanations, because they might have been influenced by third factors. An indication that such influences could be at work is provided by the correlation reported between DUP and negative symptoms (Waddington *et al.* 1995; Scully *et al.* 1997; Binder *et al.* 1998; Haas *et al.* 1998; Larsen *et al.* 1998; Bottlender *et al.* 2000; de Haan *et al.* 2000). An insidious illness onset and an early occurrence of negative symptoms are – regardless of treatment – predictors of a poor course (Ciompi & Müller 1976; Müller *et al.* 1986; Sartorius *et al.* 1986) and an acute onset is a predictor of a favourable illness course, as shown by numerous studies conducted before neuroleptic medications became available (Sartorius *et al.* 1977). Whether it is the duration of the active disease process before the beginning of an efficacious treatment or an unfavourable form of the disorder indicated by an insidious onset that actually determines the poor illness course (Crow *et al.* 1986), could only be shown in controlled intervention trials in early illness. However, such studies are not yet possible for lack of means of sufficiently early case identification. Norman and Malla (2001) thus conclude that it is not yet possible to pass final judgement on the causal relationship between belated treatment onset as a determinant of DUP or DUI and outcome. Hope exists that early detection and early intervention will enable us to reduce at least the pronounced social consequences of the disorder, mostly emerging at this early stage of illness (Häfner *et al.* 1996, 1999b; McGorry *et al.* 1996; McGlashan 1998).

The pretreatment illness course of several years' duration has implications for the interpretation of results from studies that have used first admission as the definition of illness onset. This is the case, for example, with the reports of a significant excess of first admissions for schizophrenia from the lowest social class and their interpretation along the lines of the social causation hypothesis (Faris & Dunham 1939; Kohn 1969; Eaton 1999).

To study the onset of schizophrenia, the transformation from health or from premorbid signs into the prodromal stage in prospective population studies is not practical because of the low incidence rate, the rather poor predictive power of developmental antecedents (Malmberg *et al.* 1998; Jones 1999) and the fact that in about 75% of cases schizophrenia onset occurs with non-specific signs or negative symptoms (Häfner *et al.* 1993). There are two studies that have attempted to investigate this question and with considerable success.

A Swedish conscript study (Malmberg *et al.* 1998) among 50 087 young men aged 18–20 years showed that deficits in socializing are a crucial indicator: the four items 'having fewer than two friends', 'preference for socializing in small groups', 'feeling more sensitive than others' and 'not having a steady girlfriend' were associated with a high relative risk (odds ratio 30.7)* for developing schizophrenia in a period of risk of 13 years. In the total sample, a positive response to all four items predicted psychosis only in 3%, because of the high prevalence of these features in the general population. Davidson *et al.* (1999) and Rabinowitz *et al.* (2000) conducted a similar study of 16- to 17-year-old Israeli male conscripts born during a 7-year period in Israel. Using the National Hospitalization Psychiatric Case Register, the authors identifed 692 individuals who had been hospitalized for schizophrenia for the first time in a 9-year period following the initial testing. The results on these persons, who were compared with the entire conscript population and matched controls, pointed in the same direction as the results of the Swedish study. With effect sizes[†] ranging from 0.40 to 0.58, the young males later diagnosed with schizophrenia faired significantly worse in cognitive and behavioural functioning. As in the Swedish study, it was poor social functioning with an effect size difference of 1.25 that turned out to be the main indicator of risk.

First attempts at systematically assessing prodromal signs were made in the context of a targeted antipsychotic therapy of relapses of schizophrenia (Carpenter & Heinrichs 1983; Birchwood *et al.* 1989; Cutting & Done 1989: Hirsch & Jolley 1989; Gaebel *et al.* 1993). However, the results were inconsistent, mainly as a result of: (i) differences in the type of prodromal signs included and in the definitions of a psychotic relapse; and (ii) insufficient monitoring of their development over time. Nevertheless, various items from the early scales for psychotic relapses have been incorporated into subsequent instruments for the assessment of onset and early course (Häfner *et al.* 1992; Maurer & Häfner 1995; Yung *et al.* 1998; Miller *et al.* 1999).

The difficulty in generating biological indicators of the onset and early stages of the disorder lies in the fact that current knowledge of the neurobiological disease process is still limited. Most of the biological findings associated with the risk of psychosis are trait factors that appear to be indicators of lifetime risk that may not be causally involved in onset (Cornblatt & Keilp 1994; Cornblatt *et al.* 1998; Isohanni *et al.* 1999).

For these reasons psychosis onset is currently depictable only at the level of self-experienced symptoms and observable behaviour. None the less, the monitoring of the neuropsychological and neurophysiological indicators of the disorder from the earliest possible timepoint on is a highly promising approach to modelling the early course of schizophrenia (McGorry *et al.* 1996; Klosterkötter *et al.* 1997; Bilder 1998; Cornblatt *et al.* 1998; Salokangas *et al.* 1999).

The most frequent initial symptoms mainly belong to two dimensions: a depressive and a negative syndrome. Among these, indicators of cognitive impairment, such as trouble with thinking and concentration and loss of energy, point to early consequences of the disorder (Häfner *et al.* 1999b,c).

Arranging the earliest symptoms in a time matrix, Häfner *et al.* (1999c) found, on the basis of IRAOS data collected in the ABC cohort of 232 first episodes of schizophrenia (Häfner *et al.* 1992), that depressed mood, suicide attempt, loss of self-confidence and feelings of guilt tended to occur 3–5 years before first admission with odds ratios ranging from 3 to 5 compared with controls. In the second time window, 2–4 years before first admission, all the negative symptoms appeared, and it was only in the last year before first admission that positive symptoms emerged. After the first psychotic symptom had appeared, all three symptom categories accumulated rapidly. The climax of the first episode was followed by an almost parallel decrease on all symptom dimensions.

The data were derived from a German population-based sample of 232 first illness episodes of broadly defined schizophrenia (84% of first admissions; Häfner *et al.* 1993). The prodromal stage, from onset to first psychotic symptom, had a mean duration of 5 years (median: 2.33 years), and the psychotic prestage, from the first positive symptom to the maximum of positive symptoms, of 1.1 years (median: 0.8 years). First admission took place some 2 months later, mostly precipitated by the full-blown psychosis. All the milestones of the early illness course show a significant age difference, widely reported and crucial for the further course of illness, of 3–4 years between the sexes (Hambrecht *et al.* 1992; Häfner *et al.* 1995).

The distribution of the durations of early illness course is markedly skewed to the left: 33% of the broadly defined schizophrenias took less than 1 year to develop. Only 18% had an acute type of onset of 4 weeks or less and 68% a chronic type of onset of 1 year or more. Only 6.5% started with positive symptoms, 20.5% presented both positive and negative symptoms within the same month, and 73% had negative or non-specific symptoms, thus experiencing a prodromal stage.

Stages in the development of schizophrenia

Conrad (1958), studying 107 young German soldiers, distinguished four stages of developing schizophrenia.

1 *Trema*, characterized by depression, anxiety, tension, irritability and mysterious experiences.

2 The transition from trema to *apopheny*, which corresponds to the transition from the non-specific prodromal phase to incipient psychosis, is characterized by phenomena occurring without a visible cause.

3 In the third phase, which he called *anastrophae*, these new

---

* The odds ratio (OR) is a measure of the relative risk, i.e. the risk of having a certain characteristic in the index group divided by the risk of having this characteristic in the reference group. If **a** is the number of people falling ill with schizophrenia in the index group scoring high on the four items defining socializing; and **b** is the number of people not falling ill with schizophrenia in this group; and if **c** is the number of people falling ill with schizophrenia in the reference group scoring low on the four items; and **d** is the number of people not falling ill with schizophrenia in this group, then OR = a : b / c : d.

[†] The effect size (ES) is a measure of the magnitude of an effect; it can be measured as the standardized difference between the means of the index group and the reference group.

experiences are attributed to external causes: delusions and hallucinations. Reality control and insight into illness will be lost.

4 With full-blown psychosis, the stage of *apocalypse* has begun, which refers to the complete loss of structure in perception, experience and thought.

After this psychotic stage the episode may remit in mental consolidation, with patients showing various degrees of functional impairment and residual symptoms. A rare outcome is a further increase in the severity of the psychosis and a transition of the apocalyptic into an often final stage called *catastrophae*, e.g. febrile catatonia, but modern treatment is capable of preventing this stage and its lethal course.

Following Conrad, Docherty *et al.* (1978) proposed four stages of progressive decompensation, which they believed to explain how both first episodes and relapses evolve:

1 overextension;
2 restricted consciousness;
3 disinhibition; and
4 psychotic disorganization.

Hambrecht and Häfner (1993) tested Conrad's phase model on IRAOS data from the ABC Schizophrenia Study. In 73% of the cases trema preceded apopheny, i.e. a prodromal stage and incipient psychosis. Significant transitions from apopheny to the other phases could not be shown to occur.

Both Conrad and Docherty *et al.* proceeded from the assumption that all cases of incipient schizophrenia run through these presumed regular sequences of stages, but this has not been shown to be the case. Nevertheless, quite a number of studies are being conducted with the aim of improving our means of early recognition and prediction of psychosis onset as a basis for early intervention.

Selections of patients with mental disorder in need of treatment and suspected to suffer from schizophrenia (Klosterkötter *et al.* 2001) improve the chances for correct predictions, but reduce the generalizability of the results and their applicability in population-based risk assessments. Applying the concept of self-perceived 'basic disturbances' (Huber 1983) and assessing a sample of 160 such persons using the Bonn Scale for the Assessment of Basic Symptoms (BSABS: Gross *et al.* 1987) – almost 50% of the probands developed a full-blown psychosis during the follow-up period with a mean length of 9.6 years – Klosterkötter *et al.* (2001) demonstrated a high sensitivity (=0.98) but a rather low specificity (=0.59), especially with self-experienced cognitive changes and attenuated positive symptoms.

Enriching the psychosis risk in this way may be sensible in individual intervention studies, provided that precise and reproducible information is given on the high-risk persons studied. However, the 'state approach' (Yung *et al.* 1998) used in many past studies reflects another crucial issue: if the aim is to predict an imminent psychosis onset, as an indication for early intervention, and not only the lifetime risk, a distinction must be drawn between persistent trait markers and truly prodromal signs. This might be possible by mapping symptom accumulation and func-

tional decline (Maurer & Häfner 1995; Cornblatt *et al.* 1998; Yung *et al.* 1998). Applying a series of indicators of an imminent psychosis onset, including a rapid decline in global functioning (a 15-point decrease in the GAF score in 6 weeks), Yung *et al.* (1998) were able to predict psychosis onset in young high-risk individuals (aged 18–30 years) over a period of 1 year in 40% of their cohort.

Early and later course of depressive symptoms

One of the main symptoms of schizophrenia, besides positive, negative and disorganization, is the depressive syndrome. Its frequency naturally depends on the inclusion of the schizoaffective–depressive syndrome. Knights and Hirsch (1981) studied depressive symptoms in the first psychotic episode in a population-based sample with schizophrenia-like disorder. Of all these first admissions, almost all patients had been discharged at 3-month follow-up. On admission depressive and affective symptoms had been as prevalent as psychotic symptoms, whereas at follow-up only depressive and affective symptoms persisted with little reduction, while psychotic symptoms had clearly remitted. The authors concluded that depression is revealed in schizophrenia because, although evident on admission, the symptoms were masked by psychotic symptoms which responded more than the neurotic symptoms. Of the IPSS (WHO 1973) cohort with an ICD-8 diagnosis of schizophrenia (295) who had experienced psychotic symptoms or relapses, 17% experienced clear-cut depressive episodes in a period of 2 years and 15% in a period of 5 years (Sheldrick *et al.* 1977; Leff *et al.* 1992). In a Munich study (Dobmeier *et al.* 2000) conducted among 76 patients with an ICD-10 diagnosis of schizophrenia, assessed at first admission, discharge and 15-year follow-up, depressive symptoms measured by the Calgary Depression Scale (Addington *et al.* 1992) were most frequent in acute psychotic episodes. With remitting psychosis the depression scores fell from about 70% to below 20% and more or less remained at that level without any substantial change in the symptom profile at 15-year follow-up.

In the population-controlled ABC study (Häfner *et al.* 1999c) the maximum of patients with depressive mood, also over 70%, was found in the first psychotic episode, which was in agreement with the findings of Knights and Hirsch (1981) and Dobmeier *et al.* (2000). In the following 5 years a fairly stable proportion of about 20% of the patients were in depressive episodes (according to ICD-10). From their comparable first-episode studies, Biehl *et al.* (1986) and Koreen *et al.* (1993) reported that about 75% of patients presented depressive symptoms in the first psychotic episode and showed a clear tendency to their remission (Hamilton and/or syndrome criteria). At 5-year follow-up, 26% of the patients with psychotic symptoms were rated as concurrently depressed; of the ~8% of patients without psychotic symptoms only 4% (Koreen *et al.* 1993).

Depressive symptoms frequently appear long before the first positive symptoms (McGorry *et al.* 1996; Davidson & McGlashan 1997; Häfner *et al.* 1999b,c). They are the most frequent initial symptoms in schizophrenia, appearing, on aver-age, 5 years before the climax of the first episode. In the ABC co-hort, the lifetime prevalence for depressive mood of 2 or more weeks' duration until first admission was 70.2% vs. 19.3% for age- and sex-matched controls from the general population, for feelings of guilt 33.3% vs. 10.5% for controls and for a poor self-confidence 59.4% vs. 12.3% for controls (the symptoms had to persist for at least 2 weeks). The odds ratios for these sin-gle symptoms, presumed not to overlap negative symptoms, ranged from 2 to 5. The frequency of attempted suicide at this early illness stage showed an excess of some 40% (Häfner et al. 1999b,c; see above).

From these patterns of symptom presentation over time Häfner et al. (1999b,c) conclude that the depressive syndrome is, for the most part, a pattern of response of the brain to fairly mild degrees of dysfunction. It seems to be produced by the same neurobiological processes that at a later stage bring forth the characteristic schizophrenic symptoms.

Fenton and McGlashan (1992), looking at a longer period of illness, also found affective and negative symptoms that they did not classify as belonging to the core symptoms of the two main dimensions; e.g. feelings of insufficiency, hopelessness, social withdrawal and rigidity of affect. It is not clear whether these symptoms can be interpreted as expressions of the disorder or as reactions to it. In the course of schizophrenia, reactive depres-sive symptoms can indeed occur, especially in patients with full insight into their illness (Selten et al. 2000) and with unfavourable life situations. Subdepressive symptoms can also result from stressful experiences of acute or chronic life events in the medium-term course of schizophrenia, while no change occurs in the core symptoms of paranoid schizophrenia (Danielyan & Danielyan 1999).

The constructs of a postpsychotic depression (McGlashan & Carpenter 1976), pharmacogenic depression (Helmchen & Hippius 1967) or postremissive depression (Heinrich 1967) have only secondary roles in explaining the occurrence of de-pressive symptoms in the course of schizophrenia. This was made clear by an early study conducted by Knights and Hirsch (1981) into the course of depressive symptoms before and after the treatment of psychotic episodes. Two plausible explanations have been proposed by Koreen et al. (1993): 'Depressive symp-toms in schizophrenia may represent a core part of the acute illness or may occur as a subjective reaction to the experience of psychotic decompensation'.

The prognostic value of depression occurring at the initial ill-ness stage is limited to a few clinical variables. Initial depression predicts a greater severity of symptoms in the first episode (CATEGO total score and depression score) (Häfner et al. 1999c), but has no effect on depression or on positive symptoms in the further course – which, in the main, tend to show plateaus. In contrast, early-course depression is a significant predictor of reduced negative symptoms, affective flattening in particular, in the medium-term course (Häfner et al. 1999c). This is also reflected in the more favourable course of schizoaffective disorder of the depressive type (Johnson 1988).

Depressive symptoms also seem to have an important role as a prodromal stage of relapses. In studies looking at signs that might predict exacerbations during the course of the illness, be-tween 30% and 75% of the patients as well as family informants experienced depressive or dysphoric symptoms as part of the process of schizophrenic decompensation (Herz & Melville 1980; Heinrichs et al. 1985; Birchwood et al. 1989; Hirsch & Jolley 1989; Kumar et al. 1989; Tarrier et al. 1991).

Less frequent in schizophrenia than depressive symptoms are manic and hypomanic symptoms. Studies on the course of schiz-ophrenia are consistent in reporting frequencies ranging from 3% to 10% of cases, depending on the definition of these symp-toms. They are in part associated with bipolar symptoms (mostly bipolar II) and are primarily episodic or remittent in type. Like bipolar mania, they are associated with the risk of severe social consequences because of ideas of grandeur, disinhibition and reduced impulse control (Marneros et al. 1986), but as regards a chronic course with negative symptoms and social impairment, they seem to have a better prognosis than 'pure' schizophrenia.

The catatonic syndrome, one of Kraepelin's subtypes, which was rather frequent before the advent of neuroleptics and still is in some developing countries, has become rare in western Europe and the USA (Häfner & Kasper 1982; Jablensky et al. 1993). For this reason, studies looking into this syndrome are rare (Mahendra 1981). Only recently have catatonic features started to attract renewed interest both as aetiologically unspecific symptoms and, first and foremost, as subtypes of Leonhard's nosology (Pfuhlmann & Stöber 2001) comprising motility psychosis, periodic catatonia and systematic catatonia (Stöber & Ungvari 2001). These diagnoses have been found to be both reliable and stable over a 5-year course of illness at one university hospital (Würzburg/Germany) (Franzek & Beckmann 1992). Stöber et al. (2000) have even described a susceptibility locus on chromosome 15q15 for periodic catatonia but this finding requires replication.

The only systematic long-term study looking into the stability of the catatonic syndrome within the spectrum of schizophrenic disorders and into the clinical variables involved has been conducted in Croatia. Mimica (1996) and Mimica et al. (2001) studied a representative case-register sample of 402 patients with a diagnosis of schizophrenia over a period of 18 years. Of these patients 14.7% received a clinical diagnosis of schizophre-nia of the catatonic type (ICD-9: 295.2) at least once in this peri-od. This diagnosis, associated with a significantly lower age at onset and a higher familial loading than the other subtypes of schizophrenia, turned out to be extremely unstable with fre-quent transitions into other diagnoses. Aggressive behaviour and, hence, hospital admissions were overrepresented in young patients with the catatonic subtype.

Given the scarcity of systematic long-term studies, it is impos-sible to give a conclusive appraisal of the validity of one or several catatonic subtypes of schizophrenia. The low stability of the syndrome demonstrated in the only large-scale epidemio-logical long-term study suggests that catatonic symptoms are best interpreted as nosologically unspecific signs.

Suicide in the course of schizophrenia (see also Chapter 12)

It has long been known that schizophrenia is associated with an enhanced risk for both natural and unnatural death (Drake *et al.* 1985; Roy 1986). According to follow-up studies the proportion of patients who have died from suicide – depending on the length of the period studied – ranges from about 5% to about 10% on average. Sartorius *et al.* (1987) found at 5-year follow-up in the WHO Determinants of Outcome Study that nearly 4% of the patients with a diagnosis of schizophrenia had committed suicide. Wilkinson (1982) reported a rate of 8% for suicide from a retrospective case-register-based analysis covering 10–15 years. Of the patients of the Chestnut Lodge Study, 6.4% committed suicide over a mean period of 19 years (Fenton *et al.* 1997). Krausz *et al.* (1995) reported a proportion of 13.5%. Recent long-term studies of first episodes of schizophrenia covering 14–16 years of illness have found proportions ranging from 3–4% (Mason *et al.* 1995; Ganev 2000) to 10% (an der Heiden *et al.* 1996; Wiersma *et al.* 1998). Factors contributing to these differences are missed cases and varying basic risk rates of suicide in the general populations.

On the basis of a meta-analysis of 18 publications, Brown (1997) calculated a crude mortality rate (CMR) of 189 deaths per 10 000 population a year, an aggregate standard mortality rate (SMR) of 151 and a 10-year survival rate of 81%. According to his estimates, 28% of the excess mortality is accounted for by suicide and 12% by accidents. The remaining 60% are attributable to the same causes as in the general population. For suicide alone, Brown reported an SMR of 838. The SMR for unnatural causes of death was significantly higher for men than women and showed a tendency to decrease with age (see also Krausz *et al.* 1995). Similar results have recently been reported by Osby *et al.* (2000) from a linkage study based on the inpatient register and the national cause-of-death register of Stockholm County, Sweden. SMRs, calculated by 5-year age classes and 5-year calendar time periods, were at their highest for suicide as a single cause of death. In this study, though, the rates for women at 19.7 were slightly higher than those for men at 15.7. Baxter and Appleby (1999), combining data from the Salford Psychiatric Case Registers and the NHS Central Registers, also found an excess rate of 11.4 for men and of 13.7 for women.

In their attempt to find out indicators for predicting the risk of suicide, Fenton *et al.* (1997), studying patients from the Chestnut Lodge Study (McGlashan 1984a,b), demonstrated a significant association between a low score for negative symptoms at index admission and death from suicide. Conversely, being classified as belonging to the paranoid schizophrenia subtype was associated with an excess risk of 12% for suicide. Similar results were also reported by Kaplan and Harrow (1996) from their comparison of 70 patients with schizophrenia with 97 depressed patients. While psychotic symptoms, such as delusions and hallucinations, were correlated with a later attempt of suicide, deficit symptoms (psychomotor retardation, concreteness) had

prognostic relevance only in depressed patients. The risk for suicide seems to be highest for patients with the best chances for a good outcome (Fenton 2000). Life events appear to enhance the risk for suicide (Heila *et al.* 1999a), whereas appropriate antipsychotic medication reduces it (Heila *et al.* 1999b).

The excess risk for suicide in schizophrenia seems to decrease exponentially with age (Brown 1997), which can mainly be explained by the high rate of suicide among young patients. The study by Harkavy-Friedman *et al.* (1999) is an exception. The authors found that the risk for suicide was associated neither with demographic factors nor with disease variables, such as length of illness, depression or substance abuse. In contrast, Bartels *et al.* (1992) demonstrated an association between alcohol abuse, depression and an increased risk for suicide: 80% of the variance in suicidal behaviour could be explained by depressive symptoms. Two other reviews (Caldwell & Gottesman 1990; Miles 1997) also came to the conclusion that depressive symptoms are a powerful risk factor for suicide.

Short- and medium-term social course of schizophrenia

Indicators of the social course of schizophrenia are social competence and functioning on the one hand, and social impairment, disability and social disadvantage (e.g. socioeconomic status) on the other. The latter factors are to some extent codetermined by the sociocultural environment. In studies into the social course of schizophrenia, comparisons with controls from the general population are necessary, and the results are expressed as comparing patients with schizophrenia to age- and sex-matched controls.

At first admission, persons with schizophrenia already show a considerable degree of social impairment (Häfner *et al.* 1999b) when compared with age- and sex-matched controls from the population of origin (Table 8.3). As expected, impairment is most pronounced in cases diagnosed by restricted criteria (DSM-IIIR and DSM-IV). Patients with schizophrenia do not show significantly inferior social development, as based on the proportion of probands fulfilling the six major social roles characteristic of the main age of risk for schizophrenia (Häfner *et al.* 1999b; Table 8.3).

Both the ABC study (Häfner *et al.* 1999b) and Salokangas's (1978) first admission study found that in patients diagnosed by broad criteria, the mild retardation or abnormality in neuromotor, cognitive and social development exhibited in childhood and youth (Jones & Done 1997) do not lead to serious social disadvantage before illness onset.

Most of the social impairment in people with schizophrenia occurs between illness onset and the end of the early illness stage (McGorry *et al.* 1996; Häfner *et al.* 1999b; see above for explanation of methodology). The impairments in social functioning and social role performance measured by the DAS (WHO 1988) emerge after the illness onset but between 2 and 4 years before the first admission (Häfner *et al.* 1999b). Most severely affected

Table 8.3 Social role performance at the emergence of the first sign of mental disorder and at first admission for schizophrenia (percentage) in an ABC subsample ($n = 57$) compared with 57 population controls matched for age and sex (after Häfner *et al.* 1999b).

	Subjects (%) fulfilling social role at age by first sign of mental disorder (24.0 years)			Subjects (%) fulfilling social role at age by first admission (30.0 years)		
	Patients ($n = 57$)	Controls ($n = 57$)	P	Patients ($n = 57$)	Controls ($n = 57$)	P
School education	65	61	NS	93	95	NS
Occupational training	37	44	NS	63	65	NS
Employment	33	42	NS	44	58	t
Own income	37	42	NS	49	74	**
Own accommodation	46	51	NS	63	75	NS
Marriage or stable partnership	47	58	NS	25	68	***

NS, not significant; t: $P < 0.1$; ** $P < 0.01$; *** $P < 0.001$.

are marriage and partnerships. In the ABC sample, 52% of the women and 28% of the men were married or lived in a stable partnership at illness onset, but by the first admission the corresponding figures were 33% for women, compared with 78% for healthy controls, and 17% for men, compared with 60% for controls. These results coincide with findings from the retrospective studies of the early course of schizophrenia conducted by McGorry *et al.* (1996), Yung *et al.* (1998) and McGlashan (1998). Jablensky and Cole (1997) have speculated that marriage might be a factor protecting against the onset of schizophrenia; because of the larger proportion of married women than men, this might account for older age of illness onset for women, but this assumption has found no support in other studies (Jennen-Steinmetz *et al.* 1997). In the main, causality appears to run the other way around (Häfner *et al.* 1999b).

In most cases of schizophrenia, social disability becomes manifest with accumulating negative symptoms and increasing cognitive impairment in the most active phase of the disorder long before the first psychiatric contact (Bilder 1998). According to the few prospective epidemiological studies on the course of schizophrenia extending over up to 5 years after first admission (Biehl *et al.* 1986; Salokangas *et al.* 1987; Shepherd *et al.* 1989; Leary *et al.* 1991; Jablensky *et al.* 1992; Leff *et al.* 1992; Vázquez-Barquero *et al.* 1995; Monking *et al.* 1996; Häfner *et al.* 1999b), the scores and profiles of social disability remain more or less stable after remission of the first episode, i.e. between 6 months and 1.5 years after first admission, as do negative symptoms and cognitive impairment. The studies are also consistent in showing significantly poorer social outcomes for men than women, whereas the symptom-related outcomes show no difference (Häfner *et al.* 1999b).

In almost all studies, a poor premorbid social functioning, the most powerful predictor of social course and outcome in schizophrenia, is contaminated with the prodromal illness stage

(Drues *et al.* 1978; Childers & Harding 1990; Haas & Sweeney 1992; Bailer *et al.* 1996; Maziade *et al.* 1996; Rakfeldt & McGlashan 1996; Asarnow 1999). When the illness starts to interfere with the social biography, it leads to social consequences that depend on the individual's level of social development at illness onset, which is the baseline that the social course is measured against. An early illness onset hits at a low level of social development and presumably cognitive development as well. The disorder impairs further social development and leads to stagnation at this low level. In contrast, a late illness onset at a high level of social development results in social decline (Fig. 8.6). Women, at onset on average 4 years older than men, have attained a higher level of social development than men before falling ill with schizophrenia under the precondition that the educational and occupational chances are the same for both sexes in the population.

In addition, population studies have consistently shown that adolescent and young adult males with schizophrenia show a significantly higher frequency of socially adverse behaviour (e.g. alcohol and drug abuse, self-neglect, aggressive behaviour, lack of interest in a job, reduced leisure activity, poor personal hygiene, etc.) than their female counterparts. Women show a significantly greater social adaptiveness at the early illness stage (Häfner *et al.* 1999b). This difference in illness behaviour reflects a characteristic, age-dependent sex difference in social behaviour. It leads to a reduced compliance with treatment, poor coping behaviour and poor social adjustment in male patients in the course of the disorder. Applying a regression model, Häfner *et al.* (1999b,c) demonstrated that the ability to earn a living 5 years after first admission was significantly predicted by the level of social development at the onset of the psychosis and by illness behaviour in the first episode rather than by age, gender, symptomatology or type of illness onset. Age and gender for their part are significant determinants of sex-specific social behaviour and of the level of social development

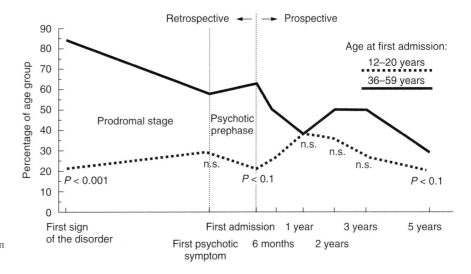

Fig 8.6 The social course of schizophrenia: the ability to earn one's living in two age-of-onset groups (ABC subsample of 115 first illness episodes). The *P*-values test the significance of the difference between the early- and the late-onset group at each point in time.

that patients have attained at illness onset, and it is through these variables that the influence of age and gender on the course and outcome comes about.

Consequently, the significantly poorer social course of schizophrenia in men results from their socially adverse illness behaviour and their lower level of social development at the onset of their illness. Except for the delayed onset in women, probably because of the protective effect of oestrogens, the disorder is similar in core symptoms and course in men and women. As the protective effect of oestrogens in women disappears after menopause and socially adverse male behaviour becomes less frequent with age, women show poorer illness courses in later age while men have milder symptoms and a significantly more favourable course of illness (Opjordsmoen 1998; Häfner *et al.* 1999b,c, 2001).

Further prognostic indicators of the social course are negative symptoms and cognitive impairment. These directly influence social functioning and, hence, the outcome of psychosocial strategies of rehabilitation as well as community outcome (Green 1996). Such patient-related outcome criteria are not the only factors determining community outcome. It also depends on the patients' acceptance in the community, for example on the prevalence of stigma and discrimination, on the availability of good quality care, on the patients' acceptance by their families and, finally, on certain behaviours and personality factors on the patients' part, such as a high communicability versus aggressive behaviour. Most of these factors, again, are associated with gender and more favourable in women than men (Leff 1997; Dörner 1998).

Table 8.4 illustrates the most important variables of social outcome at 5-year follow-up for men and women in an epidemiological sample of 115 first episodes of schizophrenia (cf. Häfner 1999; for sample and design see p. 112). The table makes plain that schizophrenia still is a disorder that entails social loss, even if studied on the basis of a broad definition of

diagnosis including cases of a favourable prognosis and despite the availability of modern methods of treatment.

A radical change for the better in the environment, e.g. by discharge from long-term inpatient treatment into good community care, may even bring about a slight but significant reduction in negative symptoms in the medium-term course (Leff 1997). In fact, it cannot be ruled out that these might be symptoms of institutionalism, described by Wing (1962) as secondary disabilities, which can be brought to remission by resettling the patients in normal stimulating environments. These observations underline the importance of the type of care provided and of the patients' living conditions for course and outcome in schizophrenia.

Short- and medium-term symptom-related course of schizophrenia

Frequency of readmissions or number of days spent in inpatient treatment are no longer regarded as reliable indicators of the course of schizophrenia. According to first-episode studies, the proportion of patients who improve and have no relapses over a 5-year period varies from 21% (Bland & Orn 1978) to 25% (Biehl *et al.* 1986; Maurer & Biehl 1988; Vázquez-Barquero *et al.* 1995) to 30% (Scottish Schizophrenia Research Group 1992). In the WHO cohort (Leff *et al.* 1992) 22% of the patients diagnosed as suffering from schizophrenia according to ICD-9 (295) at entry into the study had experienced no psychotic relapses. A meta-analysis (Hegarty *et al.* 1994) estimates the overall mean proportion of less restrictively defined favourable outcomes at 40% after an average of 6 years of illness.

The proportion of less precisely defined unfavourable outcomes with non-remitting or frequently recurring psychotic symptoms shows more marked variation, ranging from 22% in the WHO cohort to 60% in an der Heiden *et al.*'s study (1996).

Table 8.4 Social outcome in men and women 5 years after first admission for schizophrenia – ABC first-episode subsample ($n = 115$).

Domain	Men (%)	Women (%)	Domain	Men (%)	Women (%)
Marital status[t]			Occupational status[t]		
Married	9	28	Regularly employed	31	42
Single	78	45	Unemployed	43	27
			In rehabilitation/ Occupational therapy	20	9
Living situation: Patient lives[t]					
Alone	15	24	Financial situation*		
With a partner	17	45	Patient earns his or her living	35	58[†]
With parents	53	24			
In sheltered accommodation	11	4			

t: $P < 0.1$; * $P < 0.05$.
[†] Including housewives capable of fulfilling their tasks.

Other investigators have reported proportions varying between these extremes (Salokangas 1978; Carpenter & Kirkpatrick 1988; McGlashan 1988; Schmid *et al.* 1991; Davidson & McGlashan 1997; Mueser & Tarrier 1998).

Prognostic indicators

Prognostic indicators are studied for two reasons. First, to obtain good prognostic tools for the clinical practice. Such indicators are predominantly characteristics that reflect the disease process because, as a rule, it is possible to predict the further course of a disease from its early stages. The second reason is to generate aetiologically relevant predictors. These predictors must be independent of the disease process. Some of them, e.g. age and gender, are also predictors of the illness onset.

Some prognostic factors are predictive only of certain course and outcome domains. This is the case for example with negative and positive symptoms, which, for the most part, predict only these same dimensions (Strauss & Carpenter 1977; Möller *et al.* 1982; Pietzcker & Gaebel 1983; Löffler & Häfner 1999). Their predictive power usually decreases with increasing length of illness.

Acute and transient psychoses, which according to Wig and Parhee (1989) show rapid remissions in developing countries (Varma *et al.* 1996; Craig *et al.* 1997), have a particularly favourable short- and medium-term prognosis regarding symptomatology, cognitive impairment and social course. That this is also the case in industrialized countries has been shown by Marneros *et al.* (1991) in a controlled prospective study, the only difference being that these acute syndromes have a considerably lower incidence in the industrialized world. Psychotic symptoms are relevant for the social prognosis only in special cases, e.g. when psychotic episodes are extremely frequent or the

persisting psychotic symptoms particularly severe (Carpenter & Kirkpatrick 1988; McGlashan 1988).

The traditional subtypes, as already mentiond, are only of limited prognostic value (Hargreaves *et al.* 1977; Strauss & Carpenter 1977; Brockington *et al.* 1978). In a prospective follow-up study conducted after remission of acute symptoms (6 months after first admission), Ohta *et al.* (1990) identified three clusters of patients as empirical subtypes on the basis of PANSS data using cluster analysis: 31% with negative symptoms, 32% with persisting delusions and hallucinations and 37% in full remission. As expected, the two symptom-related clusters allowed a fairly reliable prognosis of an elevated relapse rate, higher symptom scores and impaired attention 2 years later.

Poor premorbid functioning (prior to first contact), insidious onset, young age at onset, male gender and not being married have consistently been related to a poor medium-term prognosis of overall outcome (Harrison *et al.* 1996; Malmberg *et al.* 1998; Wiersma *et al.* 2000). Hence, irrespective of their association with the disease process, these factors can be regarded as powerful indicators of the clinical outcome.

With the aim of providing data on all key predictors of 5-year outcome, Möller *et al.* (1986) studied a sample of hospitalized patients with a diagnosis of schizophrenia according to ICD-9 (295). Of the 17 predictors that the authors tested prospectively only five explained 10–20% of the variance in the general level of functioning (GAS score <50): the duration of occupational disintegration (5 years before admission), impaired working ability (1 year before admission), personality change (1 year before admission), poor psychopathological state at discharge and paranoid tendencies.

A number of predictors have been impossible to replicate. Furthermore, the well-known predictors have rarely explained more than 30% of the total outcome variance (Strauss &

Carpenter 1977; Möller *et al.* 1986). Therefore, attempts have been made to enhance the accuracy of predictions by pooling various predictors. However, such complex predictor patterns are difficult to use in practice and so they have been incorporated into prognostic scales. Möller and von Zerssen (1995) and Möller *et al. (*1982, 1984, 1986, 1988) compared six prognostic scales on five dimensions on the basis of product–moment correlations with outcome criteria in their own and in a replication sample at 5-year follow-up. The highest degree of the variance was explained by the Stephens scale and the Strauss–Carpenter scale (Möller *et al.* 1982, 1984).

Jablensky (2000) has given an overview of the clinically practical, sufficiently validated prognostic indicators, which we have supplemented and adapted to the results of recent predictor studies.

1 Sociodemographic characteristics (gender, age or level of social and cognitive development at psychosis onset.

2 Premorbid personality (schizothymic, schizoid or paranoid).

3 Level of social and occupational functioning prior to illness onset.

4 Past psychotic episodes and successful treatments (rapid remission vs. persisting symptoms).

5 Type of illness onset (acute vs. chronic) and duration of untreated illness.

6 Severe negative symptoms, cognitive and social impairment at the initial illness stage and in the first episode.

7 Illness behaviour (socially adverse behaviour, poor compliance).

8 Cortical atrophy at first admission (Vita *et al.* 1991; Gattaz *et al.* 1995).

9 Alcohol and drug abuse, pre- and comorbidly.

Comorbidity with alcohol and drug abuse

The prevalence of alcohol and drug abuse in patients with schizophrenia at the first treatment contact is two- to threefold higher than among controls from the same populations (Mueser *et al.* 1990, 1992a,b; Addington & Addington 1998; Bühler *et al.* 2002). Because of an overrepresentation of men among comorbid patients, alcohol and drug abuse has a compounding effect on the sex difference in the social course of schizophrenia. In the short- and medium-term course comorbidity aggravates psychotic symptoms – delusions, hallucinations and thought disorder – increases psychotic relapses but decreases negative symptoms, affective flattening and indifference in particular (Addington & Addington 1998; Bühler *et al.* 2002). As persons affected appear to suffer less from positive symptoms than from a lack of emotional intensity and pleasure, substance abuse is to some extent also practised as a dysfunctional way of coping with the illness.

Substance abuse leads to reduced compliance with care measures (rehabilitation) and antipsychotic drug treatment (Bühler *et al.* 2002). In the long term there is an increased risk for social consequences, such as divorce, unemployment and crime

(Mueser *et al.* 1990, 1992a,b; Addington & Addington 1998; Angermeyer *et al.* 1998; Brennan *et al.* 2000).

Long-term course of schizophrenia

The first publications on the long-term course of schizophrenia on the basis of Kraepelin's and Bleuler's diagnostic concept appeared in the 1930s. Mayer-Gross (1932) reports on a 16–17 year follow-up study of 294 patients originally diagnosed with schizophrenia at the psychiatric university hospital in Heidelberg. At follow-up, about 30% were found to be 'practically cured, living at home, socially adjusted', 5% were 'living at home, employed, but poorly socially adjusted', 3.5% were 'living at home, but manifestly ill', 19% were 'in institutions' and, of those, 42.5% of the patients were no longer alive; a majority had died in institutions. Examples of other early studies on the long-term course are those conducted by Langfeldt (1937), Rennie (1939), Hutter (1940), Rupp and Fletcher (1940) and Silverman (1941). All confirm the heterogeneity of illness courses but, because of differences in the diagnostic definitions and study design, valid conclusions cannot be drawn on the proportion with a good outcome or the factors influencing the course of illness (for greater detail see an der Heiden 1996).

In his review published in 1970 Stephens included 31 studies with follow-up periods of at least 5 years. In most cases the clinical diagnosis of schizophrenia was not further specified. Numerous studies have followed. Three large-scale follow-up studies were conducted in German-speaking countries in the 1970s.

Ciompi and Müller (1976) were able to trace from 1642 first admissions in one hospital 289 patients surviving on average 37 years and diagnosed as schizophrenic by Kraepelin's and Bleuler's criteria: 27% of these patients were found to be in full remission and 22% showed only mild impairment, so that in about half the course of the illness and outcome was considered favourable.

Huber *et al.* (1979) conducted a follow-up investigation of 502 patients from a total of 758 cases with first-rank symptoms admitted to the university psychiatric hospital in Bonn in the period 1945–59. Of these patients 67% were first admissions. At follow-up, an average of 22.4 years later, 22% had remitted, 43% showed, on the basis of the authors' definition, 'uncharacteristic' symptoms and 35% showed 'characteristic' residual syndromes.

Bleuler (1972) re-examined, after an average of 22 years, 208 patients with schizophrenia (66 first admissions) who had been admitted into his Zurich hospital in 1942–43. Bleuler had himself been responsible for these patients' treatment and had stayed in contact with them for over 22 years. His outcome categories are not clear-cut. He considered that about one-half to three-quarters of the patients showed more or less stable conditions after 10 years or more of illness as judged by their overall state of health, their need for treatment in hospital and their social status. One-quarter to one-third Bleuler judged to be fully recovered and between 10% and 20% he classed as having the most severe chronic psychotic symptoms.

All these results are based on interviews conducted by the investigators themselves. The samples were not controlled or representative and had marked variation in their lengths of illness; neither the inclusion diagnoses, the outcome variables nor the assessment instruments were standardized.

The most famous US long-term studies are the Chestnut Lodge Follow-up Study (McGlashan 1984a,b), the Vermont Longitudinal Study (Harding *et al.* 1987a) and the Washington International Pilot Study (Carpenter & Strauss 1991). In the Chestnut Lodge Follow-up Study, 446 patients were included of whom 163 had a diagnosis of schizophrenia. The patients had all been admitted to a very expensive private hospital which emphasized psychodynamic treatment. The patients were reassessed on average 15 years (range 2–32 years) after discharge. They were rated on global functioning at follow-up as showing continued severe impairment (41%), severe impairment (23%), moderate impairment (23%), mild impairment (8%) and no impairment (6%). On average, the patients had spent 25% of the observation period in a 'supervised setting' and had been in work for about 20% of this time. They had 'experienced symptomatic expressions of illness for about 75% of the time'. Broadly, neither significant improvement nor substantial deterioration occurred during the observation period but, as the sample were chronically hospitalized in an expensive psychoanalytically orientated setting, they cannot be regarded as representative.

In the Vermont Longitudinal Study, Harding *et al.* included 168 chronic long-term admissions of whom 72.9% were originally diagnosed as schizophrenic by DSM-I, an unreliable criterion by today's standards. The average follow-up period was 32 years (range 22–62 years). At the end of the observation period about one-half to two-thirds of the patients were rated as 'considerably improved' or 'recovered'. In a later analysis, Harding *et al.* (1987b) and Childers and Harding (1990) rediagnosed schizophrenia for 82 patients by DSM-III; 68% showed no positive or negative (GAS $\geq$ 61) symptoms at follow-up. The methodological bases of these studies are less rigorous than in the European studies.

In their Washington-based study, Carpenter and Strauss (1991) conducted follow-ups at 2, 5 and 11 years after index assessment in 53 patients from the original sample of 131 patients in the WHO IPSS, of whom 40 had received a DSM-II diagnosis of schizophrenia. These authors, too, found no indication of either improvement or deterioration from 5 to 11-year follow-up. In several cases symptomatology settled on a plateau in the first years following index admission.

In his review of these three and seven other long-term studies from the USA, McGlashan (1988) concludes – as did Bleuler (1972), Huber *et al.* (1979) and Ciompi and Müller (1976) – that, on average, schizophrenia is not a progressive illness. Rather, it frequently reaches a plateau in symptoms after 5–10 years. Over the illness course, even after several years of illness, there is a high degree of interindividual heterogeneity. Part of this heterogeneity is accounted for by differences in the samples studied and the definitions used (psychopathology, sociodemographic characteristics, dimensions of chronicity, etc.). Differences in the systems of care and forms of treatment may also have influenced the results, but these questions are still matters for investigation. There seems to be consensus on the observation that even after several years of illness decisive change may occur in the illness presentation (Harding 1988; Kendell 1988; McGlashan 1988).

In his review, an der Heiden (1996) analysed 59 long-term studies of schizophrenia that covered follow-up periods of 10 years or more on average and were published in the years 1932–96. The overarching finding is the heterogeneity of course and outcome. Given the differences in the study designs, patient samples, timespans covered, course and outcome criteria and lengths of follow-up periods, it is impossible to draw any generally valid conclusions from these results. This was already shown by Fig. 8.2, illustrating the variance in the proportion of recovered patients.

As far as comparisons are feasible, there is only rough agreement between the earlier US and European studies on the long-term course of schizophrenia. Comparing the results of their two studies (Bleuler 1972; Huber *et al.* 1979) Bleuler *et al.* (1976) came to the conclusion that 'statistically over decades of illness, from about the fifth year on, no deterioration, but, rather, improvement in the patients' state occurs'. No improvement was found by Breier *et al.* (1991) in the National Institute of Mental Health Longitudinal Study of Chronic Schizophrenia in the 58 patients of the original 74 patients who were followed up after an average of 13 years. At follow-up there was an increase in symptoms over the first 10 years with an extremely low proportion (3%) of recovery (GAS $\geq$ 61). On the basis of these results the authors drew a trajectory of the course of schizophrenia, which showed an early stage of deterioration, an intermediate stage of relative stability and an end stage of gradual improvement. Neither the low proportion of good outcomes nor the trajectory of the illness course has been confirmed in recent, methodologically more solid, long-term studies.

Since 1990 prospective long-term studies of schizophrenia have started appearing, some fairly sophisticated in their methodologies. The first was the International Study of Schizophrenia (ISoS; Sartorius *et al.* 1996), co-ordinated by the WHO. Fifteen- and 25-year follow-ups have been conducted on the cohorts of the former IPSS (WHO 1973), the WHO Collaborative Study on the Assessment and Reduction of Social Disability (Jablensky *et al.* 1980) and the Determinants of Outcome of Severe Mental Disorders Study (DOSMED: Sartorius *et al.* 1986). A total of 19 research centres in 16 countries participated in these studies. The results from these studies confirm the heterogeneity of course and outcome (Hopper *et al.* 2000), but demonstrate no early tendency to deterioration after first admission, which is in line with the results of the studies into the medium-term course of schizophrenia.

Ganev (2000) is the only investigator who, reassessing the Sofia sample of the WHO Disability Study ($n = 55$ at follow-up), has reported a favourable long-term outcome of psychotic symptoms: 55% of the patients improved over the first 10 years before follow-up and only 20% deteriorated. Mason *et al.* (1996) from Nottingham (13-year follow-up) and Wiersma *et al.* (1998) from Groningen found no indication of a late recovery. The Groningen study rather showed that chronicity (continued positive or persisting negative symptoms) increased slightly on average and also the length of episodes grew with each episode.

Possibly the most thorough prospective long-term study of population-based first admissions of schizophrenia (ICD-9: 295) has been conducted in the Mannheim cohort (an der Heiden *et al.* 1995), with 10 cross-sections over a period of 15.5 years. The symptom-related course did not show improvement. Social disability deteriorated slightly, but significantly in the final stage (an der Heiden *et al.* 1995; an der Heiden & Häfner 2000). Of the cohort 25% was free of symptoms and, as a result, needed no treatment in the last 9 months before the 15.5-year follow-up; 60% were rated as chronic because of the presence of substantial positive and/or negative symptoms in that same period; 15% were on neuroleptic medication and free of symptoms. Only the patients rated as chronic showed a slight trend towards an increase in positive and negative symptoms over the period studied. The main indicators of social outcome at 15.5-year follow-up in the Mannheim cohort, compared with matched controls, is shown in Table 8.5.

Geographical variation of course and outcome in schizophrenia

The prospective WHO studies (WHO 1973, 1979; Jablensky *et al.* 1992; Leff *et al.* 1992), conducted with culture-independent methods and identical study designs, are consistent in showing that the course of schizophrenia is more favourable at the centres in developing than industrialized countries. This difference proved stable irrespective of the follow-up period. This difference emerged with all the main characteristics of the illness course, e.g. proportion of full recovery vs. that of persisting or episodic symptoms, proportion of time spent with psychotic symptoms vs. time spent without symptoms and social impairment.

Attempts have not succeeded in explaining differences in course and outcome by a more favourable family environment in developing countries and a higher degree of Expressed Emotion (EE) in the industrialized world. Leff *et al.* (1992) and Craig *et al.* (1997) analysed data for 1056 probands of the DOSMED study, for whom sufficient information at 2-year follow-up was available, by applying the recursive partitioning technique for identifying groups of patients with similar outcomes. The authors found that of the centres in industrialized countries, Prague and Nottingham showed fairly favourable profiles of outcome resembling those reported from the centres in developing countries. The second most powerful predictor was type of onset or the proportion of cases with highly acute initial illness.

The first predictor analysis of the long-term course (over 15 and 25 years) on data for the 1633 patients of the ISoS study (Harrison *et al.* 2001) confirmed the relative stability of the differences over any period of illness studied. The most powerful predictor turned out to be type of illness course in the first 2 years after entry into the study. A shorter overall duration of psychotic episodes in this early period of illness predicted lower symptom and disability scores at the long-term follow-up and, as a result, a more favourable overall course of the illness. In the stepwise regression analysis applied in this study, the individual centres

Table 8.5 Sociodemographic outcome indicators of the long-term course of schizophrenia: comparison of 48 (30 male, 18 female) patients with schizophrenia (PSE CATEGO 295) 15.5 years after first admission and 48 controls matched for age, sex and place of residence from the same population of origin (after Weber 1997).

Domain	Patients with schizophrenia (*n* = 48)		Controls (*n* = 48)
Marital status/ partnership	52.1	Never married	14.6
	29.2	Married	66.7
	35.4	Lives with a spouse/partner	81.3
	20.8	Lives in a home	–
Employment/financial independence	29.2	No occupational training	10.4
	23.1	Employed	83.5
	62.5	Unemployed	8.4
	73.0	Unable to earn a living	10.5

PSE, Present State Examination (Wing *et al.* 1974).

no longer contributed to the rates of recovery. The only conclusion that can be drawn from this result is that early individual illness course constitutes one of the main factors that determine the course of schizophrenia at later illness stages. Consequently, the transcultural differences in the course of schizophrenia are largely accounted for by differences in the type and severity of cases included in the samples of first-onset patients and only to a lesser extent by differences in environmental factors, which affect the course of schizophrenia only in fully developed illness in the long term.

Quality of life

Besides the classical indicators, constructs such as quality of life (QOL) or life satisfaction have attained special importance in the assessment of the social and clinical outcome of schizophrenia and the evaluation of treatment measures (WHO 1998; Becker *et al.* 1999).

Because quality of life depends not only on the disorder but also on the individual, economic and sociocultural conditions that the patients live in, its assessment requires comparisons with controls from the general population, with people with other illnesses and, more rarely, with the goals and expectations of the patients themselves (Michaelos 1980) or their baseline in the social context (Campbell *et al.* 1976).

Evaluating community-based psychiatric services in the US state of New York, Baker and Intagliata (1982) found out that the persons interviewed, compared with a representative general population sample, were less satisfied particularly with their financial situation and their health. Bigelow *et al.* (1982), studying the effectiveness of the treatment and care provided by community psychiatric services, compared quality of life between psychiatric patients and healthy controls. The authors came to the conclusion that mental health programmes do improve quality of life, but their success varies with the domain as well as type and severity of the problems in question. Lehman (1983) and Lehman *et al.* (1986) compared psychiatric patients in residential care with patients living in the community – of whom one-quarter to one-half had been diagnosed with schizophrenia. Irrespective of the setting, these patients were dissatisfied with their financial situation, and also with the domains of work and security. Nevertheless, psychiatric patients living in the community were generally more satisfied than patients in residential care. Satisfaction depended on the patients' objective situation, and here availability of amenities and comforts in the individual setting played a decisive part.

Subjective quality of life also determines to a high degree how patients rate their experience of their symptoms. Comparable studies have been conducted by von Zerssen and Hecht (1987), who studied the associations between mental health, happiness and life satisfaction; by Huber *et al.* (1988), who compared quality of life between persons with psychiatric illness and healthy individuals; and by Malm *et al.* (1981), Oliver and Mohamad (1992), Mechanic *et al.* (1994) and Priebe *et al.* (1995).

Weber's (1997) investigation of patients from the Mannheim WHO Disability Study cohort at 15.5 years after first admission underlines the importance of individual aspirations and their achievement or non-achievement for the QOL construct. She assessed not only the patients' global life satisfaction, but also the importance of their aspirations in different domains of life and their achievements and their expectations. The age- and gender-matched controls from the general population were clearly more satisfied than the patients with schizophrenia, both overall and in the various life domains studied. The controls had better starting conditions than the patients for attaining their aspirations, they were more confident that the conditions would continue to be favourable in the future and that they would be able to influence the achievement of their goals. Aspirations were equally important to patients and controls.

In summary, there is evidence that the quality of life of people with schizophrenia is impaired, on both subjective and objective criteria, including their work and financial situation (Bengtsson-Tops & Hansson 1999). Their quality of life is reduced by the time of first contact with professional services (Browne *et al.* 2000), but the later outcome depends on their symptoms, the duration of untreated psychosis, and their adjustment preadmission. However, Ho *et al.*'s study (2000) failed to confirm most of these findings.

Becker *et al.* (1998) studied how the size of social network influences quality of life and found that a medium number of social contacts was associated with the highest degree of quality of life.

Assessing 58 patients with schizophrenia in outpatient treatment Rudnick and Kravetz (2001) found that social support seeking may influence outcome favourably, but does not correlate with quality of life. The role of medication was assessed in a survey of 565 patients with schizophrenia in Germany (Angermeyer & Matschinger 2000). The authors came to the conclusion that side-effects of medications such as extrapyramidal motor symptoms affect the patients' quality of life. These results coincide with Sullivan *et al.*'s findings (1992) that the quality of life varies with depressive symptoms, family interaction and side-effects of medications. In contrast, Larsen and Gerlach (1996) found no correlation with the side-effects of neuroleptic depot medication in their sample of 53 chronic cases of schizophrenia, but such results may be accounted for by the type and dosage of medication and the amount of undesirable side-effects.

Conclusions

The last few years of research into the course and outcome of schizophrenia have led us to bid farewell to the traditional long-term studies and their heterogeneous results. Progress in research methods, including precisely defined inclusion criteria (diagnosis without selective course criteria), epidemiological first-episode samples, standardized assessment procedures and prospective, in part controlled, study designs, has yielded increasingly consistent data on the trajectory of the course of schizophrenia. The average course of schizophrenia shows neither progressive deterioration of the type of the Kraepelinean dementia praecox nor pronounced improvement in symptoms and impairments at later stages of the illness. After remission of the first episode, neurocognitive impairments and negative symptoms exhibit a surprising degree of intraindividual stability.

In contrast with the traditional view, schizophrenia now has a life-long perspective. It first appears as subtle deviations in the childhood developmental milestones with mild cognitive, social and emotional anomalies as antecedents of the disorder. The most active part of the disease process occurs in the period from illness onset until the climax of the first psychotic episode, marked by the accumulation of symptoms and of cognitive and social impairment. Even today, treatment usually begins only after most of the social consequences have become reality.

The course of schizophrenia is highly heterogeneous: there are cases that show prodromal stages of several years' duration with increasingly severe negative symptoms, functional impairment and subsequent persisting disability. There are other cases which begin with an acute psychotic episode without any negative symptoms, followed by a sustained remission. There is a small extreme group which shows gradual progression over time. Some of these patients seem to prematurely develop dementia of old age. At present the division of this dimensional spectrum into various diagnoses is of relevance in clinical practice, but not in nosology.

The advance in course and outcome research was made by controlled prospective first-admission studies with data on symptomatology, neuropsychological functioning and morphological changes visible on magnetic resonance tomography (MRT). MRT findings have shown that atrophy appears to progress over time in some patients who have had particularly pronounced cognitive deficits in the first episode. The underlying association with changes in symptoms and neuropsychological functioning and the causal mechanism of these processes, although perhaps not yet sufficiently clarified, are described in many of the chapters which follow.

References

Addington, J. & Addington, D. (1991) Positive and negative symptoms of schizophrenia. Their course and relationship over time. *Schizophrenia Research* 5, 51–59.

Addington, J. & Addington, D. (1998) Effect of substance misuse in early psychosis. *British Journal of Psychiatry* 172 (Suppl. 33), 134–136.

Addington, D., Addington, J., Maticka-Tyndale, E. & Joyce, J. (1992) Reliability and validity of a depression rating scale for schizophrenics. *Schizophrenia Research* 6, 201–208.

Albus, M., Hubmann, W., Ehrenberg, C. *et al.* (1996) Neuropsychological impairment in first-episode and chronic schizophrenic patients. *European Archives of Psychiatry and Clinical Neuroscience* 246, 249–255.

American Psychiatric Association (1987) *DSM-IIIR: Diagnostic and Statistical Manual of Mental Disorders*. American Psychiatric Association, Washington, DC.

American Psychiatric Association (1994) *DSM-IV: Diagnostic and Statistical Manual of Mental Disorders, 4th edition*. American Psychiatric Association, Washington, DC.

Andreasen, N.C. (1983) *The Scale for the Assessment of Negative Symptoms (SANS)*. University of Iowa, Iowa City, IA.

Andreasen, N.C. (1984) *The Scale for the Assessment of Positive Symptoms (SAPS)*. University of Iowa, Iowa City, IA.

Andreasen, N.C. (1989) Scale for the Assessment of Negative Symptoms (SANS). *British Journal of Psychiatry* 155 (Suppl. 7), 53–58.

Andreasen, N.C. (1990) Positive and negative symptoms: historical and conceptual aspects. In: *Schizophrenia: positive and negative symptoms and syndromes* (ed. N.C. Andreasen), pp. 1–42. Karger, Basel.

Andreasen, N.C. & Olsen, S.A. (1982) Negative vs. positive schizophrenia. *Archives of General Psychiatry* 39, 789–794.

Andreasen, N.C., Grove, W.M., Shapiro, R.W. *et al.* (1981) Reliability of lifetime diagnosis. *Archives of General Psychiatry* 38, 400–405.

Angermeyer, M.C. & Matschinger, H. (2000) Neuroleptika und Lebensqualität: Ergebnisse einer Patientenbefragung. *Psychiatrische Praxis* 27, 64–68.

Angermeyer, M.C., Cooper, B. & Link, B.G. (1998) Mental disorder and violence: results of epidemiological studies in the era of deinstitutionalization. *Social Psychiatry and Psychiatric Epidemiology* 33, 1–6.

Arbeitsgemeinschaft für Methodik und Diagnostik in der Psychiatrie (1995) *Das AMDP-System: Manual zur Dokumentation psychiatrischer Befunde, 5. Auflage*. Springer, Berlin, Heidelberg, New York.

Arndt, S., Andreasen, N.C., Flaum, M., Miller, D. & Nopoulos, P. (1995) A longitudinal study of symptom dimensions in schizophrenia: prediction and patterns of change. *Archives of General Psychiatry* 52, 352–360.

Arora, A., Avasthi, A. & Kulhara, P. (1997) Subsyndromes of chronic schizophrenia: a phenomenological study. *Acta Psychiatrica Scandinavica* 96, 225–229.

Asarnow, R.F. (1999) Neurocognitive impairments in schizophrenia: a piece of the epigenetic puzzle. *European Child and Adolescent Psychiatry* 8 (Suppl. 1), 5–8.

Bailer, J., Brauer, W. & Rey, E.R. (1996) Premorbid adjustment as predictor of outcome in schizophrenia: results of a prospective study. *Acta Psychiatrica Scandinavica* 93, 368–377.

Baker, F. & Intagliata, J. (1982) Quality of life in the evaluation of community support systems. *Evaluation and Program Planning* 5, 69–79.

Bartels, S.J., Drake, R.E. & McHugo, G.J. (1992) Alcohol abuse, depression, and suicidal behavior in schizophrenia. *American Journal of Psychiatry* 149, 394–395.

Baxter, D. & Appleby, L. (1999) Case register study of suicide risk in mental disorders. *British Journal of Psychiatry* 175, 322–326.

Becker, T., Leese, M., Clarkson, P. *et al.* (1998) Links between social network and quality of life: an epidemiologically representative study of psychotic patients in south London. *Social Psychiatry and Psychiatric Epidemiology* 33, 229–304.

Becker, T., Knapp, M., Knudsen, H.C. *et al.* (1999) The EPSILON study of schizophrenia in five European countries: design and methodology for standardising outcome measures and comparing patterns of care and service costs. *British Journal of Psychiatry* 175, 514–521.

Bengtsson-Tops, A. & Hansson, L. (1999) Subjective quality of life in schizophrenic patients living in the community: relationship to clinical and social characteristics. *European Psychiatry* 14, 256–263.

Berg, E.A. (1948) A simple objective treatment for measuring flexibility in thinking. *Journal of General Psychology* 39, 15–22.

Biehl, H., Maurer, K., Schubart, C., Krumm, B. & Jung, E. (1986) Prediction of outcome and utilization of medical services in a prospective study of first onset schizophrenics. *European Archives of Psychiatry and Neurological Sciences* **236**, 139–147.

Biehl, H., Maurer, K., Jablensky, A., Cooper, J.E. & Tomov, T. (1989) The WHO Psychological Impairments Rating Schedule (WHO/PIRS). I. Introducing a new instrument for rating observed behaviour and the rationale of the psychological impairment concept. *British Journal of Psychiatry* **155** (Suppl. 7), 68–70.

Bigelow, L.B., Brodsky, G., Stewart, L. & Olson, M. (1982) The concept and measurement of quality of life as a dependent variable in the evaluation of mental health services. In: *Innovative approaches to mental health evaluation* (eds G.J. Stahler & W.R. Tash), pp. 345–366. Academic Press, New York.

Bilder, R.M. (1998) The neuropsychology of schizophrenia: what, when, where, how? In: *Schizophrene Störungen: State of the Art II* (eds V.W. Fleischhacker, H. Hinterhuber & U. Meise), pp. 155–171. Verlag Integrative Psychiatrie, Innsbruck.

Bilder, R.M., Mukherjee, S., Rieder, R.O. & Pandurangi, A.K. (1985) Symptomatic and neuropsychological components of defect status. *Schizophrenia Bulletin* **11**, 409–419.

Bilder, R.M., Reiter, G., Bates, J.A., Willson, D.F. & Lieberman, J.A. (1995) Neuropsychological profiles of first-episode schizophrenia. *Schizophrenia Research* **15**, 109.

Binder, J., Albus, M., Hubmann, W. *et al.* (1998) Neuropsychological impairment and psychopathology in first-episode schizophrenic patients related to the early course of illness. *European Archives of Psychiatry and Clinical Neuroscience* **248**, 70–77.

Birchwood, M.J., Smith, J., Macmillan, F. *et al.* (1989) Predicting relapse in schizophrenia: the development and implementation of an early signs monitoring system using patients and families as observers, a preliminary investigation. *Psychological Medicine* **19**, 649–656.

Bland, R.C. & Orn, H. (1978) 14-year outcome in early schizophrenia. *Acta Psychiatrica Scandinavica* **58**, 327–338.

Bleuler, M. (1968) A 23-year longitudinal study of 208 schizophrenics and impressions in regard to the nature of schizophenia. In: *The Transmission of Schizophrenia* (eds D. Rosenthal & S.S. Kety), pp. 3–12. Pergamon Press, Oxford.

Bleuler, M. (1972) *Die schizophrenen Geistesstörungen im Lichte langjähriger Kranken- und Familiengeschichten.* Thieme, Stuttgart.

Bleuler, M., Huber, G., Gross, G. & Schüttler, R. (1976) Der langfristige Verlauf schizophrener Psychosen. *Nervenarzt* **47**, 477–481.

Bottlender, R., Wegner, U., Wittmann, J., Strauß, A. & Möller, H.-J. (1999) Deficit syndromes in schizophrenic patients 15 years after their first hospitalization: preliminary results of a follow-up study. *European Archives of Psychiatry and Clinical Neuroscience* **249** (Suppl. 4), 27–36.

Bottlender, R., Strauss, A. & Möller, H.-J. (2000) Impact of duration of symptoms prior to first hospitalization on acute outcome in 998 schizophrenic patients. *Schizophrenia Research* **44**, 145–150.

Breier, A., Schreiber, J.L., Dyer, J. & Pickar, D. (1991) National Institute of Mental Health longitudinal study of chronic schizophrenia: prognosis and predictors of outcome. *Archives of General Psychiatry* **48**, 239–246.

Brennan, P.A., Mednick, S.A. & Hodgins, S. (2000) Major mental disorders and criminal violence in a Danish birth cohort. *Archives of General Psychiatry* **57**, 494–500.

Brockington, I.F., Kendell, R.E. & Leff, J.P. (1978) Definitions of schizophrenia: concordance and prediction of outcome. *Psychological Medicine* **8**, 387–398.

Brown, G.W. (1960) Length of hospital stay and schizophrenia: a review of statistical studies. *Acta Psychiatrica et Neurologica Scandinavica* **35**, 414–430.

Brown, S. (1997) Excess mortality of schizophrenia: a meta-analysis. *British Journal of Psychiatry* **171**, 502–508.

Browne, S., Clarke, M., Gervin, M. *et al.* (2000) Determinants of quality of life at first presentation with schizophrenia. *British Journal of Psychiatry* **176**, 173–176.

Buchanan, R.W., Kirkpatrick, B., Heinrichs, D.W. & Carpenter, W.T. (1990) Clinical correlates of the deficit syndrome of schizophrenia. *American Journal of Psychiatry* **147**, 290–294.

Bühler, B., Hambrecht, M., Löffler, W., an der Heiden, W. & Häfner, H. (2002) Precipitation and determination of the onset and course of schizophrenia by substance abuse: a retrospective and prospective study of 232 population-based first illness episodes. *Schizophrenia Research* **54**, 243–251.

Caldwell, C.B. & Gottesman, I.I. (1990) Schizophrenics kill themselves too: a review of risk factors for suicide. *Schizophrenia Bulletin* **16**, 571–589.

Campbell, A., Converse, R.E. & Rodgers, W.L. (1976) *The Quality of American Life: Perception, Evaluations, and Satisfactions.* Russell Sage Foundation, New York.

Carpenter, W.T. & Heinrichs, D.W. (1983) Early intervention, time-limited, targeted pharmacotherapy of schizophrenia. *Schizophrenia Bulletin* **9**, 533–542.

Carpenter, W.T. & Kirkpatrick, B. (1988) The heterogeneity of the long-term course of schizophrenia. *Schizophrenia Bulletin* **14**, 645–652.

Carpenter, W.T. & Strauss, J.S. (1991) The prediction of outcome in schizophrenia. IV. Eleven-year follow-up of the Washington IPSS cohort. *Journal of Nervous and Mental Disease* **179**, 517–525.

Carpenter, W.T., Heinrichs, D.W. & Wagman, A.M.I. (1988) Deficit and nondeficit forms of schizophrenia: the concept. *American Journal of Psychiatry* **145**, 578–583.

Carpenter, W.T., Buchanan, R.W., Kirkpatrick, B., Thaker, G. & Tamminga, C. (1991) Negative symptoms: a critique of current approaches. In: *Negative Versus Positive Schizophrenia* (eds A. Marneros, N.C. Andreasen & M.T. Tsuang), pp. 126–133. Springer, Berlin, Heidelberg, New York.

Cechnicki, A. & Walczewski, K. (1999) *Dynamic of positive and negative syndrome in schizophrenia: prospective study.* In: *Psychiatry on new thresholds. Abstracts of the XI World Congress of Psychiatry, Hamburg, August 6–11, 1999* (eds J. López-Ibor, N. Sartorius, W. Gaebel & C. Haasen).

Censitis, D.M., Ragland, J.D., Gur, R.C. & Gur, R.E. (1997) Neuropsychological evidence supporting a neurodevelopmental model of schizophrenia: a longitudinal study. *Schizophrenia Research* **24**, 289–298.

Changhui, C., Weixi, Z. & Shuren, L. (1995) Clinical features and outcome of schizophrenia at 12-years follow-up: a report from Chinese partner of the WHO Coordinated Study on the Long-term Course and Outcome of Schizophrenia. Paper presented at the 3rd Meeting of Investigators of ISoS, Bologna, Italy, September 25–27, 1995.

Childers, S.E. & Harding, C.M. (1990) Gender, premorbid social functioning, and long-term outcome in DSM-III schizophrenia. *Schizophrenia Bulletin* **16**, 309–318.

Ciompi, L. (1980) Catamnestic long-term study on the course of life and aging of schizophrenics. *Schizophrenia Bulletin* **6**, 606–618.

Ciompi, L. & Müller, C. (1976) *Lebensweg und Alter der Schizophrenen.* Springer, Berlin.

Conrad, K. (1958) *Die beginnende Schizophrenie.* Thieme, Stuttgart.

Cornblatt, B.A. & Keilp, J.G. (1994) Impaired attention, genetics, and the pathophysiology of schizophrenia. *Schizophrenia Bulletin* **20**, 31–46.

Cornblatt, B., Obuchowski, M., Schnur, D.B. & O'Brian, J. (1998) Hillside study of risk and early detection in schizophrenia. *British Journal of Psychiatry* **172** (Suppl. 3), 26–32.

Craig, T.J., Siegel, C., Hopper, K., Lin, S. & Sartorius, N. (1997) Outcome in schizophrenia and related disorders compared between developing and developed countries: a recursive partitioning re-analysis of the WHO DOSMeD data. *British Journal of Psychiatry* **170**, 229–233.

Craig, T.J., Fennig, S., Tanenberg, K.M. & Bromet, E.J. (1999) Six-month clinical status as a predictor of 24-month clinical outcome in first-admission patients with schizophrenia. *Annals of Clinical Psychiatry* **11**, 197–203.

Craig, T.J., Bromet, E.J., Fennig, S. *et al.* (2000) Is there an association between duration of untreated psychosis and 24-month clinical outcome in a first-admission series? *American Journal of Psychiatry* **157**, 60–66.

Crow, T.J. (1980a) Molecular pathology of schizophrenia: more than one disease process. *British Medical Journal* **260**, 66–68.

Crow, T.J. (1980b) Positive and negative schizophrenic symptoms and the role of dopamine. *British Journal of Psychiatry* **137**, 383–386.

Crow, T.J., MacMillan, J.F., Johnson, A.L. & Johnstone, E.C. (1986) The Northwick Park Study of first episodes of schizophrenia. II. A randomized controlled trial of prophylactic neuroleptic treatment. *British Journal of Psychiatry* **148**, 120–127.

Cutting, J. & Dunne, F. (1989) Subjective experience of schizophrenia. *Schizophrenia Bulletin* **15**, 217–231.

Danielyan, A. & Danielyan, K. (1999) *Paranoid schizophrenia and chronic stressful experience.* In: *Psychiatry on new thresholds. Abstracts of the XI World Congress of Psychiatry, Hamburg, August 6–11, 1999* (eds J. López-Ibor, N. Sartorius, W. Gaebel & C. Haasen).

Daum, C.M., Brooks, G.W. & Albee, G.W. (1977) Twenty year follow-up of 253 schizophrenic patients originally selected for chronic disability: pilot study. *Psychiatric Journal of the University of Ottawa* **2**, 129–132.

Davidson, L. & McGlashan, T.H. (1997) The varied outcomes of schizophrenia. *Canadian Journal of Psychiatry* **42**, 34–43.

Davidson, M., Reichenberg, A., Rabinowitz, J. *et al.* (1999) Behavioral and intellectual markers for schizophrenia in apparently healthy male adolescents. *American Journal of Psychiatry* **156**, 1328–1335.

Deister, A., Marneros, A., Rohde, A., Staab, B. & Jünemann, H. (1990) Long-term outcome of affective, schizoaffective and schizophrenic disorders: a comparison. In: *Affective and schizoaffective disorders* (eds A. Marneros & M.T. Tsuang), pp. 157–167. Springer, Berlin, Heidelberg, New York.

DeLisi, L.E., Sakuma, M., Tew, W. *et al.* (1997) Schizophrenia as a chronic active brain process: a study of progressive brain structural change subsequent to the onset of schizophrenia. *Psychiatry Research* **74**, 129–140.

DeLisi, L.E., Sakuma, M., Ge, S. & Kushner, M. (1998) Association of brain structural change with the heterogeneous course of schizophrenia from early childhood through 5 years subsequent to a first hospitalization. *Psychiatry Research* **84**, 75–88.

Dobmeier, P., Bottlender, R., Wittmann, J. *et al.* (2000) Depressive Symptome bei schizophrenen Erkrankungen: Ergebnisse der Münchner 15-Jahres-Katamnese. In: *Methodik von Verlaufs- und Therapiestudien in Psychiatrie und Psychotherapie* (eds W. Maier, R.R. Engel & H.-U. Möller), pp. 179–188. Hogrefe, Göttingen.

Docherty, J.P., van Kammen, D.P., Siris, S.G. & Marder, S.R. (1978) Stages of onset of schizophrenic psychosis. *American Journal of Psychiatry* **135**, 420–426.

Dörner, K. (1998) *Ende der Veranstaltung: Anfänge der Chronisch-Kranken-Psychiatrie.* Verlag Jakob von Hoddis, Gütersloh.

Drake, R.E., Gates, C., Whitaker, A. & Cotton, P.G. (1985) Suicide among schizophrenics: a review. *Comprehensive Psychiatry* **26**, 90–100.

Drues, J., Hargreaves, W.A., Glick, I.D. & Klein, D.F. (1978) Premorbid asocial adjustment and outcome in schizophrenia. *Journal of Nervous and Mental Disease* **166**, 881–884.

Dube, K.C., Kumar, N. & Dube, S. (1984) Long term course and outcome of the Agra cases in the International Pilot Study of Schizophrenia. *Acta Psychiatrica Scandinavica* **70**, 170–179.

Eaton, W.W. (1999) Evidence for universality and uniformity of schizophrenia around the world: assessment and implications. In: *Search for the Causes of Schizophrenia.* Vol. IV. *Balance of the Century* (eds W.F. Gattaz & H. Häfner), pp. 21–33. Steinkopff Verlag, Darmstadt.

Eaton, W.W., Bilker, W., Haro, J.M. *et al.* (1992a) Long-term course of hospitalization for schizophrenia. II. Change with passage of time. *Schizophrenia Bulletin* **18**, 229–241.

Eaton, W.W., Mortensen, P.B., Herrman, H. *et al.* (1992b) Long-term course of hospitalization for schizophrenia. I. Risk for rehospitalization. *Schizophrenia Bulletin* **18**, 217–227.

Eaton, W.W., Thara, R., Federman, B., Melton, B. & Liang, K.Y. (1995) Structure and course of positive and negative symptoms in schizophrenia. *Archives of General Psychiatry* **52**, 127–134.

Endicott, J. & Spitzer, R.L. (1978) A diagnostic interview: the schedule for affective disorders and schizophrenia. *Archives of General Psychiatry* **35**, 837–844.

Endicott, J., Spitzer, R.L., Fleiss, J.L. & Cohen, J. (1976) The Global Assessment Scale: a procedure for measurement overall severity of psychiatric disturbance. *Archives of General Psychiatry* **33**, 766–771.

Engelhardt, D.M., Rosen, B., Feldman, J., Engelhardt, J.A.Z. & Cohen, P. (1982) A 15-year follow-up of 646 schizophrenic outpatients. *Schizophrenia Bulletin* **8**, 493–503.

Faris, R.E.L. & Dunham, H.W. (1939) *Mental Disorders in Urban Areas: An Ecological Study of Schizophrenia and Other Psychosis.* University of Chicago Press, Chicago.

Fenton, W.S. (2000) Depression, suicide, and suicide prevention in schizophrenia. *Suicide and Life Threatening Behaviour* **30**, 34–49.

Fenton, W.S. & McGlashan, T.H. (1991a) Natural history of schizophrenia subtypes. I. Longitudinal study of paranoid, hebephrenic, and undifferentiated schizophrenia. *Archives of General Psychiatry* **48**, 969–977.

Fenton, W.S. & McGlashan, T.H. (1991b) Natural history of schizophrenia subtypes. II. Positive and negative symptoms and long-term course. *Archives of General Psychiatry* **48**, 978–986.

Fenton, W.S. & McGlashan, T.H. (1992) Testing systems for assessment of negative symptoms in schizophrenia. *Archives of General Psychiatry* **49**, 179–184.

Fenton, W.S., McGlashan, T., Victor, B.J. & Blyler, C.R. (1997) Symptoms, subtype, and suicidality in patients with schizophrenia spectrum disorders. *American Journal of Psychiatry* **154**, 199–204.

Franzek, E. & Beckmann, H. (1992) Reliability and validity of the Leonhard classification tested in a 5-year follow-up study of 50 chronic schizophrenics. In: *Schizophrenia and Affective Psychoses: Nosology in Contemporary Psychiatry* (eds F.P. Ferrero, A.E. Haynal & N. Sartorius), pp. 67–72. John Libbey CIC, New York.

Gaebel, W. & Frommann, N. (2000) Long-term course in schizophrenia: concepts, methods and research strategies. *Acta Psychiatrica Scandinavica* **102** (Suppl. 407), 49–53.

Gaebel, W., Frick, U., Kopke, W. *et al.* (1993) Early neuroleptic intervention in schizophrenia: are prodromal symptoms valid predictors of relapse? *British Journal of Psychiatry* **163** (Suppl. 23), 8–12.

Ganev, K. (2000) Long-term trends of symptoms and disability in schizophrenia and related disorders. *Social Psychiatry and Psychiatric Epidemiology* **35**, 389–395.

Ganev, K., Onchev, G. & Ivanov, P. (1998) A 16-year follow-up study of

Neuropsychologische Defizite bei ersterkrankten schizophrenen Patienten. *Nervenarzt* **70**, 408–415.

Spitzer, R.L., Endicott, J. & Robins, E. (1978) Research Diagnostic Criteria – rationale and reliability. *Archies of General Psychiatry* **35**, 773–782.

Stephens, J.H. (1970) Long-term course and prognosis in schizophrenia. *Seminars in Psychiatry* **2**, 464–485.

Stephens, J.H., Ota, K.Y. & Carpenter, W.T. (1980) Diagnostic criteria for schizophrenia: prognostic implications and diagnostic overlap. *Psychiatry Research* **2**, 1–12.

Stoll, A.L., Tohen, M., Baldessarini, R.J. *et al.* (1993) Shifts in diagnostic frequencies of schizophrenia and major affective disorders at six North American psychiatric hospitals, 1972–88. *American Journal of Psychiatry* **150**, 1668–1673.

Stöber, G. & Ungvari, G.S. (2001) Catatonia: a new focus of research. *European Archives of Psychiatry and Clinical Neruoscience* **251** (Suppl. 1).

Stöber, G., Saar, K., Rüschendorf, F. *et al.* (2000) Splitting schizophrenia: periodic catatonia-susceptibility locus on chromosome 15q15. *American Journal of Human Genetics* **67**, 1201–1207.

Strauss, J.S. & Carpenter, W.T. (1972) The prediction of outcome in schizophrenia. I. Characteristics of outcome. *Archives of General Psychiatry* **27**, 739–746.

Strauss, J.S. & Carpenter, W.T. (1974) Characteristic symptoms and outcome in schizophrenia. *Archives of General Psychiatry* **30**, 429–434.

Strauss, J.S. & Carpenter, W.T. (1977) The prediction of outcome in schizophrenia. III. Five-year outcome and its predictors. *Archives of General Psychiatry* **34**, 159–163.

Sullivan, G., Wells, K.B. & Leake, B. (1992) Clinical factors associated with better quality of life in a seriously mentally ill population. *Hospital and Community Psychiatry* **43**, 794–798.

Süllwold, L. (1977) *Symptome Schizophrener Erkrankungen.* Springer, Berlin.

Szymanski, S.R. Cannon, T.D., Gallacher, F., Erwin, R.J. & Gur, R.E. (1996) Course of treatment response in first-episode and chronic schizophrenia. *American Journal of Psychiatry* **153**, 519–525.

Tamminga, C.A., Buchanan, R.W. & Gold, J.M. (1998) The role of negative symptoms and cognitive dysfunction in schizophrenia outcome. *International Clinical Psychopharmacology* **13** (Suppl. 3), 21–26.

Tandon, R. & Greden, J.F. (1991) Negative symptoms of schizophrenia: the need for conceptual clarity. *Biological Psychiatry* **30**, 321–325.

Tarrier, N., Barraclough, C. & Bamrah, J.S. (1997) Prodromal signs of relapse in schizophrenia. *Social Psychiatry and Psychiatric Epidemiology* **26**, 157–161.

Thara, R., Henrietta, M., Joseph, A., Rajkumar, S. & Eaton, W.W. (1994) Ten-year course of schizophrenia: the Madras longitudinal study. *Acta Psychiatrica Scandinavica* **90**, 329–336.

Thornicroft, G. & Johnson, S. (1996) True versus treated prevalence of psychosis: the Prism Case Identification Study. *European Psychiatry* **11** (Suppl. 4), 185.

Tohen, M., Stoll, A.L., Strakowski, S.M. *et al.* (1992) The McLean First-Episode Psychosis Project: six-month recovery and recurrence outcome. *Schizophrenia Bulletin* **18**, 273–282.

Toomey, R., Kremen, W.S., Simpson, J.C. *et al.* (1997) Revisiting the factor structure for positive and negative symptoms: evidence from a large heterogeneous group of psychiatric patients. *American Journal of Psychiatry* **154**, 371–377.

Tsoi, W.F. & Wong, K.E. (1991) A 15-year follow-up study of Chinese schizophrenic patients. *Acta Psychiatrica Scandinavica* **84**, 217–220.

Tsuang, M.T., Gilbertson, M.W. & Faraone, S.V. (1991) Genetic transmission of negative and positive symptomes in the biological relatives of schizophrenics. In: *Negative Versus Positive Schizophrenia* (eds A.

Marneros, N.C. Andreasen & M.T. Tsuang), pp. 265–291. Springer, Berlin, Heidelberg, New York.

Varma, V.K., Malhotra, S. & Yao, E.S. (1996) Course and outcome of acute non-organic psychotic states. *Indian Psychiatric Quarterly* **67**, 195–207.

Vazquez-Barquero, J.L., Cuesta-Nunez, M.J., de la Varga, M. *et al.* (1995) The Cantabria first episode schizophrenia study: a summary of general findings. *Acta Psychiatrica Scandinavica* **91**, 156–162.

Vita, A., Dieci, M., Giobbio, G.M. *et al.* (1991) CT scan abnormalities and outcome of chronic schizophrenia. *American Journal of Psychiatry* **148**, 1577–1579.

von Korff, M., Nestadt, G., Romanoski, A. *et al.* (1985) Prevalence of treated and untreated DSM-III schizophrenia: results of a two-stage community survey. *Journal of Nervous and Mental Disease* **173**, 577–581.

von Zerssen, D. & Hecht, H. (1987) Gesundheit, Glück, Zufriedenheit im Lichte einer katamnestischen Erhebung an psychiatrischen Patienten und gesunden Probanden. *Psychotherapie und Medizinische Psychologie* **37**, 83–96.

Waddington, J.L., Youssef, H.A. & Kinsella, A. (1995) Sequential cross-sectional and 10 year prospective study of severe negative symptoms in relation to duration of initially untreated psychosis in chronic schizophrenia. *Psychological Medicine* **25**, 849–857.

Warner, R. (1985) *Recovery from Schizophrenia: Psychiatry and Political Economy.* Routledge & Kegan Paul, London, Boston, Henley.

Watt, D.C., Katz, K. & Shepherd, M. (1983) The natural history of schizophrenia: a 5-year prospective follow-up of a representative sample of schizophrenics by means of a standardized clinical and social assessment. *Psychological Medicine* **13**, 663–670.

Weber, I. (1997) *Die Lebenszufriedenheit einer Kohorte Schizophrener 15, 5 Jahre nach stationärer Erstaufnahme.* Doctoral dissertation, Fakultät für Klinische Medizin Mannheim der Ruprecht-Karls-Universität Heidelberg.

Weickert, T.W. & Goldberg, T.E. (2000) Neuropsychologie der Schizophrenie. In: *Psychiatrie der Gegenwart. Vol 5, 4th edn* (eds H. Helmchen, F. Henn, H. Lauter & N. Sartorius), pp. 163–180. Springer, Berlin, Heidelberg, New York.

Weickert, T.W. Goldberg, T.E. Gold, J.M., Bigelow, L.B., Egan, M.F. & Weinberger, D.R. (2000) Cognitive impairments in patients with schizophrenia displaying preserved and compromised intellect. *Archives of General Psychiatry* **57**, 907–913.

Weinberger, D.R. (1995) Schizophrenia as a neurodevelopmental disorder. In: *Schizophrenia* (eds S.R. Hirsch & D.R. Weinberger) pp. 293–323. Blackwell, Oxford.

White, L., Harvey, P.D., Opler, L. & Lindenmayer, J.P. (1997) Empirical assessment of the factorial structure of clinical symptoms in schizophrenia: a multisite, multimodel evaluation of the factorial structure of the Positive and Negative Syndrome Scale. The PANSS Study Group. *Psychopathology* **30**, 263–274.

Whiteford, H.A. & Peabody, C.A. (1989) The differential diagnosis of negative symptoms in chronic schizophrenia. *Australian and New Zealand Journal of Psychiatry* **23**, 491–496.

WHO (1973) *The International Pilot Study of Schizophrenia. Vol. 1.* WHO, Geneva.

WHO (1977) *Past History and Sociodemographic Description Schedule (PHSD), 3rd draft.* WHO, Geneva.

WHO (1978a) *Mental Disorders: Glossary and Guide to Their Classification in Accordance with the Ninth Revision of the International Classification of Diseases.* WHO, Geneva.

WHO (1978b) *Psychiatric and Personal History Schedule.* WHO 5365 MNH (10/78), Geneva.

WHO (1979) *Schizophrenia: An International Follow-Up Study.* Wiley, New York.

WHO (1980) *Follow-up History and Sociodemographic Description Schedule (FU-HSD).* WHO, Geneva.

WHO (1988) *Psychiatric Disability Assessment Schedule (WHO/DAS).* WHO, Geneva.

WHO (1992) *Life Chart Schedule.* WHO, Geneva.

WHO (1993) *The ICD-10 Classification of Mental and Behavioural disorders: Diagnostic Criteria for Research.* WHO, Geneva.

WHO (1998) The World Health Organization Quality of Life Assessment (WHOQOL): development and general psychometric properties. *Social Science and Medicine* **46**, 1569–1585.

Wiersma, D., Giel, R., de Jong, A., Nienhuis, F.J. & Slooff, C.J. (1996) Assessment of the need for care 15 years after onset of a Dutch cohort of patients with schizophrenia, and an international comparison. *Social Psychiatry and Psychicatric Epidemiology* **31**, 114–121.

Wiersma, D., Nienhuis, F.J., Slooff, C.J. & Giel, R. (1998) Natural course of schizophrenic disorders: a 15-year followup of a Dutch incidence cohort. *Schizophrenia Bulletin* **24**, 75–85.

Wiersma, D., Wanderling, J., Dragomirecka, E. *et al.* (2000) Social disability in schizophrenia: its development and prediction over 15 years in incidence cohorts in six European centres. *Psychological Medicine* **30**, 1155–1167.

Wig, N.N. & Parhee, R. (1989) Acute and transient psychoses: a view from the developing countries. In: *International Classification in Psychiatry: Unity and Diversity* (eds J.E. Mezzich & M. Cranach), pp. 115–121. Cambridge University Press, Cambridge.

Wilkinson, D.G. (1982) The suicide rate in schizophrenia. *British Journal of Psychiatry* **140**, 138–141.

Wing, J.K. (1962) Institutionalism in mental hospitals. *British Journal of Social and Clinical Psychology* **1**, 38–51.

Wing, J.K. & Brown, G.W. (1970) *Institutionalism and Schizophrenia: A Comparative Study of Three Mental Hospitals 1960–1968.* Cambridge University Press, London.

Wing, J.K., Cooper, J.E. & Sartorius, N. (1974) *Measurement and Classification of Psychiatric Symptoms.* Cambridge University Press, London.

Woods, B.T. (1998) Is schizophrenia a progressive neurodevelopmental disorder? Toward a unitary pathogenetic mechanism. *American Journal of Psychiatry* **155**, 1661–1670.

Wyatt, R.J. & Henter, I.D. (1998) The effects of early and sustained intervention on the long-term morbidity of schizophrenia. *Journal of Psychiatric Research* **32**, 169–177.

Yung, A.R. & McGorry, P.D. (1996) The prodromal phase of first-episode psychosis: past and current conceptualizations. *Schizophrenia Bulletin* **22**, 353–370.

Yung, A.R. Phillips, L.J., McGorry, P.D. *et al.* (1998) Prediction of psychosis: a step towards indicated prevention of schizophrenia. *British Journal of Psychiatry* **172** (Suppl. 33), 14–20.

Zimmerman, M., Coryell, W., Pfohl, B. & Stangl, D. (1988) The reliability of the Family History Method for psychiatric diagnosis. *Archives of General Psychiatry* **45**, 320–322.

9 Depression and schizophrenia

S.G. Siris and C. Bench

Kraeplin's astute separation, over 100 years ago, of what we now know as mood disorders from what we now know as schizophrenia forms the conceptual basis of much of modern psychiatric nosology. Nevertheless, the fact remains, and has been noted for many years, that a substantial proportion of patients with schizophrenia, no matter how defined, suffer from 'depression-like' symptomatology during the longitudinal course of their disorder.

Early on, Bleuler noted that symptoms of depression often occur during the course of schizophrenia (Bleuler 1950). Later, in the middle years of the twentieth century, the concept of depression in schizophrenia became largely steeped in psychoanalytically influenced writings. Mayer-Gross discussed depression in schizophrenia as being a denial of the future or a reaction of despair to the psychotic experience (McGlashan & Carpenter 1976a). Others found themes of loss to be central to the dynamics of depressed schizophrenic patients (Semrad 1966; Roth 1970; Miller & Sonnenberg 1973). Semrad (1966) also considered that these patients' depressions represented important progress out of a more pathological narcissistic regressed state which more immediately followed the florid psychosis, although he also considered this state to be influenced by pain and/or the despair of an 'empty ego.' Both he and Eissler (1951) were of the opinion that the occurrence of depression in schizophrenia represented a moment of psychotherapeutic opportunity, with the possibility of insight and mastery which would attend the less primitive defensive state which was then manifest. In this regard, depression was interpreted as having positive prognostic significance.

Later, however, more data-based research was conducted documenting the course, frequency and intensity of depression in schizophrenia (Bowers & Astrachan 1967; McGlashan & Carpenter 1976b; Siris 1991; Siris *et al.* 2001). As the definitions of both depression and schizophrenia became progressively operationalized over time, and as the medication treatment of the subjects involved in studies became more highly controlled, investigations began to indicate that the outcomes are often less favourable in those schizophrenic patients who manifest depression during the longitudinal course of their disorders. Such depressions were noted to be associated with higher risks of relapse or rehospitalization (Mandel *et al.* 1982; Roy *et al.* 1983; Johnson 1988; Birchwood *et al.* 1993), as well as with an increased rate of suicide (Roy *et al.* 1983; Drake & Cotton 1986; Caldwell & Gottesman 1990; Siris 2001a).

Through the years, various descriptors have been applied to states of depression occurring in the course of schizophrenia, and nosological agreement has been difficult to come by. Although the designation is controversial and may even be misleading, a full depressive syndrome presenting in the longitudinal course of schizophrenia has often come to be called 'postpsychotic depression'. Indeed, despite the problems with its name, 'postpsychotic depression' has been listed as a diagnosis in ICD-10, and is also included in the appendix of DSM-IV. Previously, although 'postpsychotic depression' *per se* had not been discussed in either ICD or DSM manuals, 'depression superimposed on residual schizophrenia' was included as a diagnostic category in the Research Diagnostic Criteria (RDC) (Spitzer *et al.* 1978).

However named, depressive-like symptomatology has clearly played a part in the devastating long-term character of schizophrenia. The subjective state involved leads to great personal suffering, both for afflicted patients and for their families. No doubt the mood state, loss of energy, impairment in concentration and diminution of self-confidence also contribute materially to the tremendous loss of social and vocational capacity which these individuals experience, and which become such an important component of the morbidity with which they suffer.

Incidence and prevalence of 'depression' in schizophrenia

Over three dozen studies have been published and reviewed concerning the occurrence of depression-like symptomatology over the longitudinal course of schizophrenia (Siris 1991, 2000; Andreasen *et al.* 1995; Lindenmayer *et al.* 1995; Müller & Wetzel 1998; Norman *et al.* 1998). These studies vary substantially in a number of characteristics, including the definition employed for schizophrenia, the definition of depression, the observational interval and the treatment situation of the patients. One thing that is remarkable is that no matter what the definitions or conditions, all studies found at least some meaningful rate of depression in the course of schizophrenia.

The rate of depression described in all these studies varied substantially. The lowest rates were 6% (in a cross-sectional assessment carried out with the Hamilton Depression Rating Scale (HAM-D) of chronically hospitalized 'Kraepelinian' schizophrenic patients; Tapp *et al.* 1994) and 7% (in a cross-sectional assessment study of chronically hospitalized DSM-III schizophrenic patients, which nevertheless emphasized postpsychotic depression's distinct nature from 'negative symptoms'; Hirsch *et al.* 1989). The highest rates were 65% (in a study which followed 'Feighner criteria' schizophrenic patients for whom an effort had been made to exclude neuroleptic-induced akinesia, with ratings at least every 3 months, for 3 years after they had been free of acute psychotic symptoms; Johnson 1988) and 75% (in a study which followed 'first break' schizophrenic patients with repeated prospective assessments for as long as 5 years and counted them as being depressed if they met either of two definitions for depression; Koreen *et al.* 1993). The apparent large difference between these figures is ascribable, at least in part, to the fact that the first two studies represented a determination of point prevalence while the latter two studies involved a cumulative prevalence over 3 and 5 years, respectively.

The modal rate for the occurrence of depression in schizophrenia for all these various investigations was approximately 25%, a rate which has consistently seemed to be a benchmark in such reports over the course of time (Winokur 1972; McGlashan & Carpenter 1976a; Johnson 1981a; Mandel *et al.* 1982; Siris 1991, 2000). Table 9.1 describes the studies that have reported incidence or prevalence figures for episodes of depression in the course of schizophrenia as defined by recent common criteria such as DSM-III, DSM-IIIR, DSM-IV, RDC, ICD, Present State Examination (PSE), International Pilot Study of Schizophrenia (IPSS), New Haven Index, Feighner, CATEGO or Schneiderian First Rank. The very diversity of diagnostic criteria for schizophrenia and depression, and the variety of patient settings and means of observation, support the broad generalizability of the concept that some form or forms of phenotypic 'depression' occur in the longitudinal course of a substantial proportion of patients with schizophrenia.

These studies of rates of occurrence of depression in schizophrenia in study populations are complemented by the findings of a recent wide survey of practising psychiatrists (Siris *et al.* 2001). That study described a 33% rate of depression in first admission schizophrenic patients, a 38% rate in acute relapse schizophrenic patients and a 29% rate in chronic stable schizophrenia.

Additionally of interest is that women have often been described as being more likely than men to manifest depression (McGlashan & Bardenstein 1990; Emsley *et al.* 1999), depressed mood (Goldstein & Link 1988) or dysphoria (Goldstein *et al.* 1990) in the course of schizophrenia. Other reports, however, have not found a difference between the sexes when such issues are examined (Haas *et al.* 1990; Shtasel *et al.* 1992; Häfner *et al.* 1994; Addington *et al.* 1996a).

Differential diagnosis of depression in schizophrenia

Organic factors

There are many potential aetiologies for depression, or a phenocopy of depression, in schizophrenia (Bartels & Drake 1989). The first potential origin which needs to be considered is the set of organic causes for a depressive syndrome (Bartels & Drake 1988; Siris 2000). Organic aetiologies of a depressive syndrome can arise from medical conditions, such as anaemias, carcinomas, endocrinopathies, metabolic abnormalities, infectious diseases, autoimmune, cardiovascular or neurological disorders. Commonly prescribed medications such as sedative hypnotics, β-blockers, various other antihypertensive medications, antineoplastic agents, barbiturates, non-steroidal anti-inflammatory agents, sulphonamides and indometacin, or from the discontinuation of certain other prescribed medications, such as corticosteroids or psychostimulants, can also predispose to a depression syndrome. Substances of abuse can also have a role in the creation of depressed states, either through their acute use, chronic use or discontinuation. Alcohol can contribute to a depression-like state through either acute or chronic use. Chronic cannabis use can lead to an anergic state which shares many features with depression; the withdrawal state from cocaine involves well-described depressive phenomenology. Withdrawal from two commonly used legal substances, caffeine or nicotine (both often used to excess by schizophrenic patients), can also lead to dysphoric states which can be confused with depression (Griffiths & Mumford 1995; Dalack *et al.* 1998).

Neuroleptic-induced dysphoria

One relevant and frequently asked question concerns whether or not neuroleptic medications themselves can contribute to a 'depressed' state in schizophrenic patients (Awad 1993), and impairments in quality of life related to neuroleptic-induced dysphoria have, indeed, been reported (Browne *et al.* 1998). This is a plausible question on a theoretical level because neuroleptic medications blockade dopamine receptors, and dopamine receptors are known to be involved in brain pathways

Table 9.1 Studies reporting incidence or prevalence of secondary depression in cases of schizophrenia diagnosed by popular criteria. (Modified and supplemented after Siris 1991.)

Study (n)	Definition of psychosis	Definition of 'postpsychotic' interval	Definition of depression	Percentage depressed	Comment
McGlashan & Carpenter (1976b) n = 30	IPSS: more than 90% chance of schizophrenia	Cross-sectional assessment at discharge and at 1-year follow-up	'Depression' as per PSE	43% at discharge 50% cummulative as per 1-year follow-up	Depression dimension of PSE had a bimodal distribution
Weissman et al. (1977) n = 50	Outpatients with New Haven Schizophrenia Index diagnosis of schizophrenia	Point prevalence	Raskin Scale score of 7 or more	28%	No differences in demography of depressed group
Van Putten & May (1978) n = 94	Newly admitted patients with Feighner criteria for schizophrenia	Length of acute hospital stay	Increase in BPRS depression scale rating	38%	57% for patients with akinesia 22% for patients without akinesia
Knights et al. (1979) n = 37	CATEGO criteria: 87% = unequivocal schizophrenia	6 months or until relapse while on depot neuroleptic	PSE-based depression rating scale	54%	43% had onset or increase in depression ratings during interval
Roy (1980) n = 100	DSM-III chronic paranoid schizophrenia	Chart review for mean of 6 years	DSM-III for major depressive disorder, secondary type	30%	Depressed mood as assessed by PSE: 9% depressed at follow-up
Johnson (1981a) Cohort A: n = 41	Schizophrenia diagnosis based on Schneiderian first-rank symptoms	Cohort A: 2 months prospective prevalence study	Cohort A: HAM-D and/or BDI = 15 or more	Cohort A: 24%	The risk of an episode of depression was three times the risk of an episode of psychosis for patients maintained on depot neuroleptic
Cohort B: n = 100	Outpatients free of acute symptoms for at least 3 months	Cohort B: Cross-sectional prevalence	Cohort B: Nurses' rating and self-rating	Cohort B: 26%	

Study	Diagnostic criteria	Assessment timing	Depression measure	Result	Comments
Cohort C: n=30	Patients maintained on depot neuroleptic	Cohort C: 2-year follow-up	Cohort C: HAM-D and/or BDI=15 or more	Cohort C: 50% excluding episodes associated with psychotic relapse	
Siris et al. (1981) n=50	Acutely admitted inpatients diagnosed by RDC	Duration of hospitalization after resolution of flagrant psychotic symptoms	RDC for major or minor depression by chart review of symptoms	6% major depression 22% minor depression	34% appeared depressed to staff 40% manifested subjective sadness
Roy (1981) n=100	DSM-III for schizophrenia	Chart review: 4–10 years	Treated for depression by antidepressants or ECT	39%	More early parental loss among patients with depression
Möller & von Zerssen (1982) n=81	Inpatients with schizophrenia (77%) or paranoid psychosis (23%) by ICD criteria	Point prevalence at hospital discharge	3 consecutive Actual Mood Scores at or above 21	23%	17% developed new episodes of depression
Guze et al. (1983) and Martin et al. (1985) n=44	Feighner criteria for schizophrenia	Retrospective survey at 6–12 year follow-up point	Feighner criteria for depression	57%	Criteria were not exactly those of Feighner, but were extremely close to those
Summers et al. (1983) Cohort A: n=161	RDC for schizophrenia Cohort A: chronic	Cohort A: at admission to aftercare	Cohort A: SCL-90 scales	Cohort A: as a group, schizophrenics more depressed than normals	Acute and chronic patients found to have comparable depression symptoms after hospitalization
Cohort B: n=72	Cohort B: acute	Cohort B: past month assessment (average 2.13 year post discharge)	Cohort B: two composite depression scales from KAS	Cohort B: 37% poor 68% poor or equivocal	
Watt & Shepherd (1983) (as reported in Roy 1986) n=121	Chronic schizophrenia (PSE criteria)	PSE at admission and 1 month, 1 year, and 5 years after discharge	PSE assessment of depression syndrome	40% at 1 month and 1 year ('severe' in 1/4 of these) 19% at 5 years	Prospective epidemiological study

Table 9.1 (cont.)

Study (n)	Definition of psychosis	Definition of 'postpsychotic' interval	Definition of depression	Percentage depressed	Comment
Munro et al. (1984) n = 100	Outpatients with DSM-III for schizophrenia	Clinic cross-sectional prevalence	Carroll Rating Scale	41%	10% severe depression 18% moderate depression 13% mild depression
Leff et al. (1988) n = 31	Newly admitted patients with PSE/CATEGO definition of schizophrenia	Until discharged or until 6 months	Depressed mood as assessed by PSE	45%	Patients were not on neuroleptics Correlation between improvement in depressive symptoms and in psychosis suggested depression was an 'integral part' of these cases
Johnson (1988) n = 80	Feighner criteria for schizophrenia Presence of Schneiderian first-rank symptoms	Period began when patients were free of all acute symptoms Period A: 0–12 months Period B: 12–36 months (ratings at least every 3 months)	Altered mood state lasting at least 7 days with HAM-D and BDI each more than 15 Meet DSM-III for depression	13–30% for period A 65% for period B	Akinesia excluded by physical examination for parkinsonism Risk of psychotic relapse was significantly higher for patients depressed in 2nd or 3rd year, than for patients depressed 1st year or not depressed
Kulhara et al. (1989) n = 95	Outpatients with ICD-9 diagnosis of schizophrenia	Cross-sectional assessment	Finding of depressed mood on PSE instrument	32%	Only 12 patients had no depressive symptoms as assessed by the BPRS and/or PSE
Hirsch et al. (1989)	DSM-III for schizophrenia Also:				Depressive symptoms are less common in chronic schizophrenic inpatients than would be predicted if they were a manifestation of negative symptoms or neuroleptic-induced parkinsonism
Cohort A: n = 46	Cohort A: thought by nurses to be 'depressed'	Cohort A & B: cross-sectional assessment	Cohort A: HAM-D & BDI	Cohort A: 7%	Depressed patients had more auditory hallucinations in Cohort B

Study	Population / Diagnosis	Method	Criteria	Prevalence	Comments
Cohort B: $n=196$ (also Barnes et al. 1989) Cohort C: $n=44$	Cohort B: long-stay inpatients; Cohort C: outpatients with no florid symptoms in previous 6 months	Cohort C: repeated bimonthly assessments for 1 year while randomly assigned to depot neuroleptic or placebo	Cohort B: item 23 ('depression') of PSE; Cohort C: depression item =2 or more on Manchester Scale	Cohort B: 13% Cohort C: 73% of psychotic relapses were preceded prodromal symptoms which included depression	
Bandelow et al. (1990) $n=364$	ICD-9 and RDC for schizophrenia	Point prevalence 3 months after discharge and stabilization on neuroleptic medication for an acute psychotic episode	BPRS anxious depression scale equal to or greater than 10	19.5%	Two other scales for depression rated between 26.6% and 42.8% of patients as depressed, depending on cut-off scores. 35.7% of patients were rated as depressed when a milder BPRS cut-off was employed
Addington & Addington (1990) $n=50$	Schizophrenia by DSM-III criteria	Point prevalence among consecutive admissions	'Depressive episode' by DSM-III criteria, based on PSE interview	24%	Statistically significant, but weak, correlations between depression rating scales and presence of major depressive episode
Brier et al. (1991) $n=58$	RDC diagnosis of schizophrenia ($n=42$) or schizoaffective disorder (mostly schizophrenic) ($n=16$, of whom 12 were depressed type)	Average follow-up period $=6\pm3$ years	Episode of major depression as diagnosed by RDC	24%	38% of the sample had made at least one suicide attempt
Lindenmayer et al. (1991) $n=240$	Inpatients (mostly chronic) with a diagnosis of schizophrenia by DSM-III criteria	Point-prevalence study	'Severe' PANSS depression component ≥19; 'mild to moderate' 11–18	5% severe depression 52% mild to moderate	Patients rated high in depression tended also to exhibit greater amounts of positive symptoms
Birchwood et al. (1993) $n=49$	CATEGO class 's' for schizophrenia	Randomly selected from urban outpatient 'depot' treatment clinic	Score of at least 15 on the BDI	29%	Patients with lesser sense of control concerning their illness were more likely to manifest depression
Koreen et al. (1993) $n=70$	'First break', RDC for schizophrenia (77%) or schizo-affective disorder (23%)	Repeated prospective assessment at weekly intervals during acute treatment, and monthly intervals thereafter up to 5 years	Syndromal criteria for depression and/or Extracted Hamilton Rating Scale for Depression based on a SADS interview	75% (met one or the other criteria at some point) 22% (met both criteria concurrently at some point)	26% of ratings for patients who were psychotic noted concurrent depression vs. 4% concurrent depression for patients noted to be non-psychotic at that rating point

Table 9.1 (cont.)

Study (n)	Definition of psychosis	Definition of 'postpsychotic' interval	Definition of depression	Percentage depressed	Comment
Tapp et al. (1994) n = 91	DSM-IIIR and RDC by SADS for schizophrenia	Not stated	HAM-D rating (not further specified)	37% (for 'non-Kraepelinian') 6% (for 'Kraepelinian')	More depression in non-Kraepelinian than in Kraepelinian group
Harrow et al. (1994) n = 54	RDC diagnosis of schizophrenia	Prevalence during 1 year preceding follow-up interview Follow-up interview was an average of 4.5 years after hospital discharge for index psychotic episode	Presence of a full depressive syndrome by RDC	37%	Patients receiving neuroleptics were more likely to have depression (P < 0.01) or experience anhedonia (P < 0.001). Depression finding remains when psychosis was controlled for
Mauri et al. (1995) n = 43	Chronic schizophrenic inpatients (DSM-IIIR criteria) during an acute exacerbation phase	Prevalence at baseline and after 6 weeks of neuroleptic treatment	BPRS depression subscale HAM-D	16.3% for moderate symptoms of depression 23.2% for mild symptoms of depression	All patients were medication-free for at least 3 weeks. All patients then treated with haloperidol with no other psychotropic or anticholinergic drug allowed
Markou (1996) n = 94	Schizophrenia (DSM-IIIR criteria) 50 inpatients and 44 outpatients of a chronic hospital	Point-prevalence assessment	'Significant depression' was a HAM-D score > 17; 'mild to moderate depression' was a HAM-D between 10 and 17	Inpatients: 10% – significant 42% – mild to moderate Outpatients: 4.5% – significant 48% – mild to moderate	A significant correlation was found between the negative subscale of the PANSS and the measure of depression (r = 0.301, P = 0.003)
Wassink et al. (1997, 1999) n = 62	Recent onset schizophrenia (DSM-III, R or DSM-IV criteria)	Point-prevalence at presentation	DSM-IV criteria for major depressive episode	35%	Patients with depression had more severe initial symptoms, but were not different on premorbid, demographic, or outcome variables

Study	Sample	Assessment	Criteria	Prevalence	Comments
Müller & Wetzel (1998) n = 132	Acute schizophrenia diagnosed by DSM-IIIR criteria	Point-prevalence assessment	Score of 14 or more on the BRMES	42%	Data analysis suggest three factors: retardation, depressive core symptoms, and accessory depressive symptoms
Sands & Harrow (1999) n = 70	RDC for schizophrenia	Follow-up assessment 7.5 years after hospital discharge. Assessment covers the previous year	Full depressive syndrome or subsyndromal by RDC (subsyndromal is depressed mood and two or three other depressive symptoms or four or more depressive symptoms without depressed mood)	36% (full depressive syndrome or subsyndrome 14% (subsyndromal depression)	Only 35% of a cohort of 46 patients among whom the evaluation had been performed were free of the depression syndrome or subsyndrome for the years preceding a 4.5-year evaluation and the 7.5-year evaluation
Zisook et al. (1999) n = 60	Outpatients with schizophrenia (DSM-IIIR or DSM-IV criteria) between the ages of 45 and 79	Point-prevalence study	Score of 17 or more on the HAM-D	20% of the women 7% of the men	Note that, in this sample, 15 patients (25%) were taking adjunctive antidepressant medication. 63% of the men and 60% of the women had HDRS scores from 7 to 16
Baynes et al. (2000) n = 120	Stable outpatients with chronic schizophrenia by DSM-IIIR criteria	Point prevalence	A score of 17 or more on the BDI	13.3% (24.2% had a BDI score 10–16)	If patients already on antidepressants or lithium were excluded, depression rate rose to 14.8%

BDI = Beck Depression Inventory; BPRS = Brief Psychiatric Rating Scale; BRMES = Bech-Rafaelsen Melancholia Scale; DSM = Diagnostic and Statistic Manual; HAM-D = Hamilton Depression Rating Scale; ICD = International Classification of Diseases; IPSS = International Pilot Study of Schizophrenia; KAS = Katz Adjustment Scale; n = number of subjects in the study; PANSS = Positive and Negative Symptom Scale; PSE = Present State Examination; RDC = Research Diagnostic Criteria; SADS = Schedule for Affective Disorders and Schizophrenia; SCL = Symptom Check List.

which mediate 'reward' (Wise 1982; Harrow *et al.* 1994). The reasoning is that, if a neuroleptic interfered with the experience of reward or pleasure, the resultant experience of relative anhedonia could become a phenocopy of a depressed state. Interestingly, a large prospective study found that patients who were maintained on neuroleptic medication manifest more depression than those who were randomized to receive neuroleptic medication only on an 'early intervention' or 'crisis intervention' basis, and patients in that study were found to have lower depression ratings after being taken off neuroleptic medication (Bandelow *et al.* 1992). Another well-designed study specifically comparing anhedonia in schizophrenic patients on vs. off neuroleptics found significantly more anhedonia as well as more depression in those patients who were being treated with neuroleptics (Harrow *et al.* 1994). Notably, several much earlier reports had also implicated neuroleptics as an aetiological agent for depression among schizophrenic patients (DeAlarcon & Carney 1969; Floru *et al.* 1975; Galdi *et al.* 1981; Johnson 1981b; Galdi 1983).

The majority of evidence, however, has tended to refute the notion that appropriately administered neuroleptic medication causes a full depressive state to emerge in schizophrenic patients (Knights & Hirsch 1981; Moller & Von Zerssen 1986; Siris 1991, 2000). This negative evidence comes from three perspectives. First, evaluating psychotic schizophrenic patients throughout the course of treatment for their acute episodes has revealed that the greatest levels of depressive symptomatology exist at the height of the psychosis, and tend to resolve, although often at a slower rate than the psychosis, when the psychosis is treated with a neuroleptic agent (Knights & Hirsch 1981; Möller & von Zerssen 1982; Strian *et al.* 1982; Szymanski *et al.* 1983; Leff *et al.* 1988; Hirsch *et al.* 1989; Green *et al.* 1990; Nakaya *et al.* 1997). These observations oppose the notion that depression is caused by neuroleptics by demonstrating that depressive symptomatology was present before the neuroleptic was administered, and that levels of depression actually decrease as the patient comes under treatment with these compounds. Secondly, a number of studies have found that, when patients being treated with neuroleptics were compared with patients not being treated with neuroleptics, the patients treated with neuroleptics were not observed to be more depressed (Hirsch *et al.* 1973, 1989; Wistedt & Palmstierna 1983; Hogarty & Munetz 1984). Thirdly, when schizophrenic patients with and without depression were compared with each other, in most studies the depressed group was not found to be receiving higher doses of neuroleptic drugs or to have higher neuroleptic blood levels (Roy *et al.* 1983; Roy 1984; Berrios & Bulbena 1987; Siris *et al.* 1988a; Barnes *et al.* 1989; Bandelow *et al.* 1990, 1992; Tugg *et al.* 1997; Peralta & Cuesta 1999; Zisook *et al.* 1999). On the other hand, at least one study did find a positive relationship between haloperidol plasma levels and depressive symptoms in the context of a positive association between extrapyramidal and depressive symptoms (Krakowski *et al.* 1997), and another study found a trend level association

between degree of depression and neuroleptic dose (Perenyi *et al.* 1998). Thus, this 'preponderance of the evidence' refutation of the hypothesis that neuroleptic drugs can cause depression is not entirely conclusive, especially in the presence of one well-designed prospective positive study (Harrow *et al.* 1994), and we certainly cannot rule out the possibility that neuroleptics might not be an important contributing factor to depression in certain individual cases.

Akinesia and akathisia

Antipsychotic drugs may clearly be a factor in generating depression-like states when depressive-like features occur in association with the extrapyramidal neuroleptic side-effects of akinesia and akathisia. Neuroleptic-induced akinesia, a syndrome of reduced spontaneity as well as reduced generalized motor activity, at times can produce a rather exact phenocopy of depression, even when muscle stiffness or cogwheeling is not present (Rifkin *et al.* 1975, 1978; Van Putten & May 1978; Martin *et al.* 1985; Bermanzohn & Siris 1992). This phenocopy includes blue mood as well as reduced energy, pessimism and anhedonia, and is principally differentiated from depression by its responsiveness to antiparkinsonian medication, which is usually not thought to be a treatment for other forms of 'depression'. Akinesia may be particularly problematic in terms of its diagnosis when it occurs in an insidious or subtle form, or when it occurs in the absence of large muscle extrapyramidal signs such as shuffling gait or reduced arm swing. Unfortunately, most of the studies of depression in the course of schizophrenia have made little effort to evaluate the potential presence of neuroleptic-induced akinesia or to rule it out as a confounding factor.

Neuroleptic-induced akathisia is another extrapyramidal side-effect which can easily be confused with depression. It is easy to diagnose in its blatant form, because of prominent motor restlessness, but equally easy to misdiagnose in its subtle form where the patient may be more dysphoric than outwardly restless (Van Putten 1975; Siris 1985; Halstead *et al.* 1994). Patients with less blatant akathisia may still be prone, however, to subtle behavioural excesses such as overtalkativeness or wandering into other people's territory. Dysphoria is often associated with akathisia, and dysphoric akathisia can be easily mistaken for agitated depression. Indeed, the dysphoria of akathisia may be intense, and both suicidal ideation and suicidal behaviour have been associated with this state (Shear *et al.* 1983; Drake & Ehrlich 1985).

Negative symptoms

The negative symptom syndrome of schizophrenia can also present in a way which resembles depression in a number of crucial respects (Crow 1980; Andreasen & Olsen 1982; Carpenter *et al.* 1985; Siris *et al.* 1988b; Kulhara *et al.* 1989; Bermanzohn & Siris 1992; Siris 2000), although clear distinctions may also be evident (Barnes *et al.* 1989; Lindenmayer *et al.* 1991;

Norman & Malla 1991; Kuck *et al.* 1992; Kibel *et al.* 1993). Clinical features such as anhedonia, anergia, social withdrawal and poor motivation may be common between these two states (Bermanzohn & Siris 1992; Sax *et al.* 1996). However, Barnes *et al.* (1989) and Baynes *et al.* (2000) found very little overlap between the diagnosis of the negative symptoms of schizophrenia and diagnosis of depression in chronic inpatients, and some investigators (Norman & Malla 1991, 1994; Sax *et al.* 1996; Nakaya *et al.* 1997; Zisook *et al.* 1999), but not others (Dollfus *et al.* 1993), have found correlations between depression and positive symptoms, perhaps particularly suspiciousness (Kirkpatrick *et al.* 1996; Baynes *et al.* 2000), in schizophrenia.

With careful attention, depression and negative symptoms in schizophrenia need not ordinarily be confused. The symptom which is most likely to set these two conditions apart is blue mood, a clinical feature which is generally present in depression. The negative symptom syndrome, on the other hand, is usually marked by blunted affect.

As one prominent hypothesis concerning the pathogenesis of negative symptoms involves it representing a hypodopaminergic state (Davis *et al.* 1991), it is conceivable that neuroleptic medications, at more than the required dosage, may exacerbate this condition, thereby contributing to the reputation of neuroleptic agents as being 'depressogenic'.

Disappointment reactions

Schizophrenic patients often have a considerable amount to feel disappointed about in the ways in which their lives are progressing (or not progressing), and they may certainly manifest this psychological reaction. An acute disappointment reaction may occur in reaction to any event which goes awry in an individual's life. Operationally, this is most easily distinguished from other forms of depression by the presence of an immediate stressful event and the fact that the reaction is transient – seldom lasting more than a week or two. The chronic variety of disappointment reaction, known as the demoralization syndrome (Frank 1973; Klein 1974), can be more difficult to distinguish from depression. In this situation, patients may become chronically discouraged and dispirited on the basis of repeated failures or losses and/or the impression that important life goals have become impossible to achieve. 'Insight' (Peralta & Cuesta 1994; Kemp & Lambert 1995; Smith *et al.* 2000) or self-awareness of symptoms or psychological deficits may have an important role (Liddle *et al.* 1993; Lysaker *et al.* 1995) and a sense of incompetence may also be prominently involved (deFigueiredo 1993). Of interest, in this regard, is the observation that schizophrenic patients who feel less of a sense of control concerning their illness have been noted to be more prone to experience depression (Birchwood *et al.* 1993; Hoffmann *et al.* 2000). From a clinical perspective, demoralization reactions may be particularly worth diagnosing, because they may represent a condition particularly amenable to psychosocial treatments and supports.

Prodrome of psychotic relapse

Depression has been described as a common symptom which may be manifest by schizophrenic patients during the process of decompensation into a new psychotic episode (Docherty *et al.* 1978; Herz & Melville 1980; Herz 1985; Johnson 1988; Subotnik & Nuechterlein 1988; Hirsch & Jolley 1989; Green *et al.* 1990; Malla & Norman 1994; Tollefson *et al.* 1999). In these cases, the dysphoric state is often accompanied by social withdrawal, anxiety and/or other stigmata such as hypervigilance suggestive of early manifestations of psychosis, but the differential diagnosis may be difficult. Because of this possibility, the lowering of neuroleptic dosage is not necessarily advisable for schizophrenic patients with newly emergent depressive-like symptomatology. Rather, increased monitoring and non-specific support may be the indicated intervention. Initiation of antidepressant medications for patients already in the process of undergoing a psychotic decompensation may have contributed to the early impression, not subsequently validated, that antidepressant medications may be psychotogenic in schizophrenic patients even if neuroleptic medication treatment is maintained (Siris *et al.* 1978).

Schizoaffective disorder

Another condition involving the syndrome of depression and the phenotypic psychosis of schizophrenia, which belongs in the differential diagnosis of secondary depression in schizophrenia, occurs in schizoaffective disorder. In this instance, the full depressive syndrome coincides with the florid psychotic syndrome in ways which have been variously defined over the years and according to different diagnostic schemes (Levitt & Tsuang 1988; Coryell *et al.* 1990; Taylor 1992). Because the definition of the requisite level of psychotic symptomatology coexisting with depression has differed according to the diagnostic system employed, the technical boundary between schizoaffective disorder and secondary depression in residually psychotic schizophrenic patients has also varied. Conceptually though, the pertinent issue is that a full depression syndrome coincides with the appropriate manifestations of psychosis during at least a part of an episode of schizoaffective depression (Siris & Lavin 1995; Siris 1996). Schizoaffective disorder additionally enters into the differential diagnosis of postpsychotic depression in schizophrenia in that episodes of secondary depression can also occur in the course of schizoaffective disorder.

Independent diathesis for depression

Separate from schizoaffective disorder, although perhaps related to it, is the concept that some patients with the diathesis for schizophrenia may also, independently, have the biological diathesis for depression. On purely statistical grounds, the chance occurrence of depression in schizophrenia would be expected to happen at the same rate as in the general population, an interaction which could account for occasional cases. But the construct has also been put forward, based on the stress–vulnerability model of schizophrenia (Zubin & Spring 1977; Nuechterlein & Dawson 1984), that interaction between the two diatheses could account for more cases presenting with both depression and schizophrenia than would be expected by chance alone (Siris 2000, 2001b). This possibility results from the observation that the vulnerability to psychosis appears to occur on a continuum in the population, with a tiny fraction having extreme vulnerability and the vast majority having very low vulnerability. In between, there is a limited, but meaningful, portion of the population with a more moderate, but real, level of psychotic vulnerability. Whereas, in the absence of some other major stressor, only those individuals with extreme vulnerability would become psychotic, in the presence of a major stressor the more moderately vulnerable could also be recruited into the phenotypically psychotic group. The occurrence of major depression, in essence, could represent one such major stressor on both a biological and psychosocial level. As a result, more than the expected by chance number of phenotypically schizophrenic patients would be predicted to manifest depressive syndromes as well. Such a hypothesis would be consistent with the common finding of depressive symptoms occurring during the prodrome of psychotic episodes. It also would be consistent with the findings that dysphoria is more associated with positive than with negative symptoms in schizophrenia (Norman & Malla 1994; Sax et al. 1996) and that adjunctive antidepressant maintenance treatment, designed to prevent the recurrence of depression in schizophrenic individuals with histories of postpsychotic depression, apparently may be protective in reducing the rate of psychotic exacerbations (Siris et al. 1994).

Clinical validation of depression in schizophrenia

Prognosis

The literature concerning the prognostic implications of depressive symptomatology in schizophrenia is complicated by a timing issue: do the depressive symptoms coincide with the psychosis or occur apart from it (Siris 1991, 2000). Although depressive symptoms coinciding with the psychosis carry favourable prognostic implications (McGlashan & Carpenter 1976a; Emsley et al. 1999), such symptoms presenting in intervals during which the patient is not psychotic have been found to predict oppositely (Bartels & Drake 1988; Becker 1988). Specifically, those patients who manifest secondary depressions in schizophrenia have been noted to be more likely to experience psychotic relapse, even when 'prodromal' depressive symptomatology has been accounted for (Falloon et al. 1978; Mandel et al. 1982), and 'major depression' in schizophrenia has also been independently associated with early hospital readmission (Olfson et al. 1999). Consistent with this unfavourable impli-

cation is the observation that postpsychotic depression in schizophrenia is also associated with other negative predictors of outcome, such as poor premorbid adjustment and insidious onset of the first or index psychotic episodes (Moller & von Zerssen 1986).

Suicide

The most blatantly disastrous outcome in schizophrenia is suicide, an event which tragically is not rare and which has been estimated to be the way in which between 2% and 13% of schizophrenic lives end (Tsuang 1978; Black et al. 1985; Drake et al. 1985; Nyman & Jonsson 1986; Roy 1986; Black & Fisher 1992; Krausz et al. 1995; Meltzer & Okayli 1995; Fenton et al. 1997; Stephens et al. 1997, 1999; Inskip et al. 1998; Wiersma et al. 1998; Siris 2001a). This figure has often been interpreted as being approximately 10% (Miles 1977; Caldwell & Gottesman 1990). The rates of suicide attempts in schizophrenia are even higher, with estimates ranging from 18% to 55% (Roy 1986; Breier et al. 1991; Asnis et al. 1993; Cohen et al. 1994; Gupta et al. 1998). A greater number of schizophrenic suicides (Roy 1982, 1986; Drake et al. 1985; Drake & Cotton 1986; Dassori et al. 1990; Heilä et al. 1997; Saarinen et al. 1999; Stephens et al. 1999) and suicide attempters (Roy 1986; Prasad & Kumar 1988; Addington & Addington 1992; Bartels et al. 1992; Cohen et al. 1994; Jones et al. 1994) have been found to have past or recent histories of depressive symptomatology, especially psychological aspects such as hopelessness (Drake et al. 1984; Drake & Cotton 1986; Caldwell & Gottesman 1990; Addington & Addington 1992; Meltzer & Okayli 1995; Saarinen et al. 1999) and loss (Caldwell & Gottesman 1990; Heilä et al. 1999; Saarinen et al. 1999). Suicidal ideation has also been found to be associated with depression in schizophrenia (Barnes et al. 1989; Bartels et al. 1992).

Life events

More undesirable events, more exit events, and more life events altogether have been observed in those schizophrenic patients who manifest secondary depressions (Roy 1981). Additionally, schizophrenic patients with secondary depressions have been found to have had histories of more early parental loss (Roy 1980, 1981; Roy et al. 1983).

Biological validation of depression in schizophrenia

A relatively small number of studies have investigated biological correlates of depression within schizophrenia, either at the symptom or diagnosis level. Even fewer have set out a priori to identify patients on the basis of their comorbidity with depression; rather the vast majority have investigated post hoc the relationship of the measures made with depression subscale scores.

Brain structure and function

Structural imaging

Computerized tomography (CT) and magnetic resonance imaging (MRI) in schizophrenia have produced convincing evidence of increased ventricular volume and decreased cortical volume, with greatest reductions in temporal lobe volume. That regional changes are related to characteristic clinical features of the disorder is an attractive hypothesis. To date, the most consistent relationship found has been between ventricular enlargement and negative symptoms. Far fewer studies have shown significant correlations between regional cerebral *volume* and negative symptoms. A single study (Kohler *et al.* 1998b) examined a priori the effect of depressive symptoms in 64 patients with schizophrenia categorized according to their HAM-D scores into HAM-Hi (>18) or HAM-Lo (<18) groups. The more depressed schizophrenic patients had significantly higher temporal lobe volume, although the effect size was small. Gur *et al.* (2000) found that women but not men with schizophrenia had reduced orbitofrontal cortex volume and that lower volume in this region was associated with higher depression ratings on the HAM-D. On the basis of the studies performed to date, it is fair to conclude that there are no consistently demonstrated structural anatomic correlates of depression in schizophrenia. Data-leads methods of image analysis similar to those used in functional imaging will offer greater opportunities for the identification of clinical correlates of structural changes (Wright *et al.* 1999). Chapter 22 contains a wider discussion of the application of brain imaging to schizophrenia research.

Functional neuroimaging

Functional neuroimaging can be broadly divided into two techniques:
1 'brain mapping', which measures regional cerebral blood flow (rCBF) or metabolism as an index of local neural activity; and
2 neurochemical imaging, in which the specific uptake and binding of radiolabelled tracer compounds is measured.

Brain mapping studies

In primary depression, there is reasonable consistency in the finding of functional abnormalities in key regions of prefrontal and limbic cortex and connected subcortical structures (Drevets 1998). In schizophrenia, it has been demonstrated that functional abnormalities may relate to specific symptoms such as hallucinations (McGuire *et al.* 1993) or syndromes (Liddle *et al.* 1992). Furthermore, observed patterns of functional abnormality may be specific to symptoms across diagnoses (Dolan *et al.* 1993). However, as with structural imaging, very few functional imaging studies in schizophrenia have specifically looked for correlates of depression. No activation studies have addressed this issue. Kohler *et al.* (1998b) used fluo-rodeoxyglucose positron emission tomography (FDG-PET) to examine 29 schizophrenic patients categorized according to HAM-D scores into HAM-Hi (>18) or HAM-Lo (<18) groups. These data showed no main effect attributable to depression, but the HAM-Hi group had a relatively lower left–right anterior cingulate metabolic ratio. This result is consistent with the left lateralized decrease in dorsal cingulate function seen in some studies of primary depression (Bench *et al.* 1992). Further studies are required before conclusions can be drawn as to whether depression in schizophrenia has well-defined neural correlates and how the pattern of function compares with that seen in primary depression and with other syndromes of schizophrenia.

Neurochemical imaging

Neurochemical imaging relies on the availability of suitable radioligands to measure physiological processes, biochemical pathways and receptor systems of interest. Hypothesis-led attempts to relate neurochemical imaging to depressive symptoms in schizophrenia have been very limited.

Dopamine synthesis

Striatal uptake of the PET tracer [^{18}F]fluorodopa reflects the synthesis rate of dopamine in the terminals of nigrostriatal fibres. Studies using this method generally agree that acute schizophrenia is associated with increased fluorodopa uptake. In 10 neuroleptic-naive patients, Hietala *et al.* (1999) found that positive symptoms correlated positively with basal ganglia fluorodopa uptake, whereas there was a highly *negative* correlation between core depressive symptoms (guilt and depression subscales of the Positive and Negative Symptom Scale, PANSS) and left striatal fluorodopa uptake. This correlation remained high even after exclusion of three schizoaffective patients.

Dopamine receptors

Two recent meta-analyses of studies of dopamine D_2-receptors suggest that a small increase in striatal D_2 density is found in some patients with schizophrenia (Laruelle 1998; Zakzanis & Hansen 1998). In primary depression, increased D_2 density has also been described (D'haenen & Bossuyt 1994) with a positive association with psychomotor retardation (Ebert *et al.* 1996; Shah *et al.* 1997). The relationship between D_2 binding and depression in schizophrenia is less clear. Two studies in drug-free patients both suggest that decreased dopaminergic function may mediate negative symptoms, with no data presented for depressive symptoms (Martinot *et al.* 1994; Knable *et al.* 1997). In patients treated with olanzapine or risperidone, de Haan *et al.* (2000) found that negative symptom ratings (from the PANSS) and Montgomery–Åsberg depression rating scale scores both correlated with D_2-receptor occupancy. These authors suggested that the relationship between higher D_2-receptor occupancy, psychopathology and subjective experience may have important implications for dosing strategies and compliance with antipsychotic medication.

Dopamine release

Dopamine receptor imaging techniques may be adapted to provide a measure of stimulant-induced dopamine release. Studies by two independent groups have demonstrated that medication-free patients with acute schizophrenia have exaggerated amphetamine-induced dopamine release (Breier *et al.* 1997; Abi-Dargham *et al.* 1998; Laruelle *et al.* 1999). Furthermore, these changes correlate with an increase in positive symptoms and a smaller decrease in negative symptoms. As yet no analysis of the change in depressive symptoms has been reported, but this requires further investigation.

Serotonergic system

The hypothesis of a serotonin dysfunction in schizophrenia has been examined in several PET studies. Of the four published studies to examine cortical 5-HT$_{2A}$-receptors (Trichard *et al.* 1998; Lewis *et al.* 1999; Ngan *et al.* 2000; Verhoeff *et al.* 2000) only Ngan *et al.* found the decrease in prefrontal cortical receptor density predicted by previous postmortem studies. The study by Lewis *et al.* explicitly rated depressive symptoms but no relationship was found with 5-HT$_{2A}$ binding. Laruelle *et al.* (2000) found that the density of brainstem serotonin transporters was unaltered in 24 patients with schizophrenia and not related to symptomatology; depression was not explicitly examined.

Neuropsychology

A single study has been found which examines a priori the effect of depression in schizophrenia on neuropsychological performance. Kohler *et al.* (1998a) examined 128 patients with schizophrenia, categorized according to HAM-D scores into HAM-Hi (>18) or HAM-Lo (<18) groups, on a battery of neuropsychological tests. HAM-Hi patients had a higher score for delusions but the groups were otherwise well matched. The neuropsychological battery revealed that women in the HAM-Hi group were impaired on the vigilance component of the Continuous Performance Task (CPT). While it is tempting to suggest that this deficit is linked to the anatomical changes in the prefrontal cortex in women with schizophrenia previously described, it is impossible to draw any firm conclusions from this single study.

Endocrine and biochemical measures

Inconsistent results have been reported in the several studies which have examined the results of the dexamethasone suppression test (DST) in schizophrenic patients with secondary depressions (Siris *et al.* 1984; Siris 1991). One confounding variable in these investigations may have been the failure to control for the effects of antiparkinsonian or other anticholinergic medications on dexamethasone suppression. Recently, Ismail *et al.* (1998) found very low rates of non-suppression in a group of 64 schizophrenic patients, 36% of whom fulfilled criteria for major depression. Only one study has been reported concerning the thyrotropin-releasing hormone (TRH) test in postpsychotic depressed schizophrenic patients (Siris *et al.* 1991b). Although

that study showed rates of blunted response comparable with that of patients with primary depression, it contained no control group of non-depressed schizophrenic patients. The finding of higher levels of platelet monoamine oxidase (MAO) activity in patients with schizophrenia-related depression (Schildkraut *et al.* 1980) has not been replicated.

Genetic studies

Family studies

Several family studies have examined the relationships between schizophrenia and affective disorder. Kendler *et al.* (1993) reported a familial association between schizophrenia and psychotic affective illness, but not with affective illness in general, and Maier *et al.* (1993) found a familial relationship between schizophrenia and unipolar depressive disorder. Kendler *et al.* (1996) also found a relationship with psychotic affective illness in the parents of offspring with schizophrenia. However, most family studies of schizophrenia do not look specifically for an association between comorbid depression in schizophrenia, either at the symptoms or diagnosis level, with depression in other family members. Kendler and Hays (1983) found that schizophrenic patients who have first-degree relatives with unipolar depression have a significantly higher likelihood of developing a depression syndrome following the resolution of a psychotic episode. On the other hand, two relatively small studies ($n = 44$ and $n = 70$) failed to find significant differences in rates of primary affectively disordered relatives between schizophrenic patients with and without depression (Guze *et al.* 1983; Berrios & Bulbena 1987). One unique study found a relationship between neuroleptic-induced depressive symptomatology and those schizophrenic patients who had depressed relatives (Galdi *et al.* 1981).

Sibling pair studies

DeLisi *et al.* (1987) found a significant intrapair association for the occurrence of RDC major depression in 53 sibling pairs with RDC schizophrenia or schizoaffective disorder, and Kendler *et al.* (1997) found significant associations for the severity of depressive symptoms in 256 sibling pairs with DSM-IIIR schizophrenia. In contrast, Cardno *et al.* (1998) found no familial aggregation of presence/absence of depressive episodes in their sample of 109 sibling pairs with DSM-IV schizophrenia or schizoaffective disorder.

Molecular genetic studies

In linkage studies, large families with several affected members are studied to try to find a genetic marker that cosegregates with the disease. The power of linkage studies may be increased by using phenotypes that include key dimensions of gene expression which may act as quantitative traits (Brzustowicz *et al.* 1997). Asherson *et al.* (1998) have implicated markers on chromosome 4p in the expression of schizophrenia with significant affective symptoms, while Kendler *et al.* (2000) reported that patients from families with evidence for linkage to chromosome 8p displayed fewer depressive symptoms.

In association studies, the frequency of various alleles of a gene that is suspected of involvement in the pathogenesis of the disorder is examined in a series of subjects with schizophrenia as compared with a control group. As in linkage studies, interest has been growing in utilizing phenotypes other than diagnosis, such as neurocognitive measures, brain imaging abnormalities and symptom domains including depression (Malhotra 2001). For example, Serretti *et al.* (1996) developed a phenotype definition based on symptomatological factors within the major psychoses of excitement, depression, delusions and disorganization. This group and others have examined a number of genes for their relationship with symptomatology including depression within major psychoses. Although this is a promising approach, to date only negative studies have been published for the serotonin transporter gene (Serretti *et al.* 1999a) and dopamine D$_3$ and D$_4$ receptors (Serretti *et al.* 1999b,c).

Treatment implications

The existence of a syndrome of depression in schizophrenia raises several important implications for treatment. A newly emergent syndrome of depression in a patient with schizophrenia is certainly cause for an increased level of observation, attention and support. Increased frequency of outpatient appointments and contact with families or residential providers is indicated, and interventions which solve problems, increase structure and decrease both biological and psychosocial stresses are useful. If the appearance of depressive symptomatology was a product of a transient disappointment reaction, such interventions may prove to be adequate.

Antipsychotic medications

As noted in the differential diagnosis above, a manifestation of 'depression' in schizophrenia may represent an early stage in the process of decompensation into a new episode of psychosis. In a closely followed patient, a new psychotic episode will soon declare itself with an increase in psychotic symptoms such as hallucinations, delusions, overinterpretation of perceptions or events, derailment of thought processes, or illogical or magical thinking. If such proves to be the case, augmentation or change of antipsychotic medication may be called for. Intercepting and treating new episodes of psychosis quickly may substantially curtail both psychiatric and social morbidity and it is a crucial objective in the longitudinal treatment of individuals with schizophrenia. Whether to increase dosage or to change antipsychotic medication will need to be decided on an individual basis, with consideration given to past treatment response to particular antipsychotic agents at particular dosage, current pattern and severity of side-effects and level of patient acceptability for these, and plasma levels of medications for those which have available meaningful levels. Assessment of proper medication compliance is always an important issue in such a situation.

When a new state of depression in schizophrenia persists or becomes chronic in a patient who is not manifesting florid psychotic symptomatology, reduction of the dosage of neuroleptic medication should be considered if the patient is being treated with a conventional neuroleptic agent (i.e. a 'typical' antipsychotic agent). Although evidence remains divided with regard to whether standard neuroleptic agents can cause an otherwise characteristic depressed illness in schizophrenic patients, standard neuroleptic drugs certainly may at least have a role in generating syndromes which mimic depression. These include akinesia, akathisia and, perhaps, even the 'negative symptoms' state. Therefore, when treating non-acute episodes of depression in schizophrenia, an effort should be made to decrease the neuroleptic dosage to the lowest level consistent with maintaining remission from flagrant psychotic symptomatology. Indeed, the minimizing of neuroleptic dosage in this manner is generally advocated for the long-term maintenance of patients with schizophrenia as a means of reducing side-effects and optimizing psychosocial functioning (Kane *et al.* 1983; Marder *et al.* 1987).

The obvious alternative to continuing treatment with a standard neuroleptic agent when an enduring pattern of depression has emerged in a patient with schizophrenia is to switch the patient to a so-called 'atypical' antipsychotic agent (Siris 2000). First, atypical antipsychotics have been shown to demonstrate a much more favourable extrapyramidal side-effect profile than standard neuroleptics (Chouinard *et al.* 1993; Marder & Meibach 1994; Peuskens 1995; Borison *et al.* 1996; Tandon *et al.* 1997). Because akinesia and akathisia figure quite prominently in the manifestation of depression-like symptomatology in schizophrenia, this atypical antipsychotic benefit alone could account for much of the more favoured 'depression' findings which have been observed following the use of these agents (Siris 2000). Secondly, in light of atypical antipsychotic agents relying much less on dopaminergic blockade for their therapeutic effect (Meltzer *et al.* 1989; Deutch *et al.* 1991; Seeger *et al.* 1995; Jones 1997; Tandon *et al.* 1997), they would be much less likely to be responsible for a dopamine-blockade-induced anhedonia, which could then either directly or indirectly contribute to depressive symptomatology. Thirdly, atypical antipsychotics have been widely reported to be superior in the treatment of negative symptoms of schizophrenia (Kane *et al.* 1988; Chouinard *et al.* 1993; Marder & Meibach 1994; Buchanan 1995; Möller *et al.* 1995; Beasley *et al.* 1996; Borison *et al.* 1996; Tandon *et al.* 1997; Tollefson & Sanger 1997; Tollefson *et al.* 1997). Again, this could generate a more favourable depression profile in patients either directly, in the case where negative symptoms present a phenocopy of depression, or indirectly, where patients are discouraged by their negative symptoms and manifest depression secondarily.

The above factors (and possibly other factors as well) are likely to be contributors to the observation that atypical antipsychotic agents may be associated with superior outcomes in schizophrenia, as suggested by quality of life measures (Franz *et al.* 1997; Tollefson & Andersen 1999; Voruganti *et al.* 2000). If this is the case, it is logical that both acute and chronic disappointment reactions would be reduced when atypical antipsychotic medications are employed. Beyond this, there is the possibility that atypical antipsychotics may have some direct antidepressant activity on their own. This has been suggested by the results of a number of controlled studies (Azorin 1995; Meltzer & Okayli 1995; Beasley *et al.* 1996; Tandon *et al.* 1997; Tollefson *et al.* 1997, 1998a,b; Keck *et al.* 1998; Walker *et al.* 1998; Daniel *et al.* 1999) but, in light of all the above-mentioned confounding issues, it still remains to be definitively determined (Siris 2000).

Antidepressant medications

After the possibilities of impending psychotic relapse and transient disappointment reaction have been accounted for, and an effort has been made to rule out neuroleptic-induced akinesia or akathisia through appropriate adjustments of medication, the efficacy of treatment with antidepressant medication must be considered. Studies addressing this question have had mixed results, but are generally regarded as being favourable (Plasky 1991; Siris 1991, 2000; Levinson *et al.* 1999). Table 9.2 reviews the double-blind, placebo-controlled studies which have been reported concerning the addition of an adjunctive antidepressant medication in cases of secondary depression in schizophrenia.

Most of the negative reports in Table 9.2 have design issues which make their interpretation difficult. These include brief duration of treatment (4 weeks), low antidepressant dosage (maprotiline as low as 50 mg/day), antidepressant dosage which may be too high for some patients (nortriptyline 150 mg/day, especially in the presence of a concomitant neuroleptic which could reduce metabolism), antidepressant medication being given to patients on one antipsychotic agent while placebo is given to patients receiving a different antipsychotic, or a small *n* limiting the power of the comparison. The studies in Table 9.2 which are positive have fewer limitations of design, although even the most favourable-appearing study (Siris *et al.* 1987) demonstrated 'much improved' responses in fewer than half (42%) of the patients treated with adjunctive antidepressant. Additionally, the large majority of studies in Table 9.2 did not make an attempt to rule out the syndrome of akinesia in their design, so their results have to be interpreted in that light. Finally, the study by Kramer *et al.* (1989) differs from most of the others in that it involved patients who were floridly psychotic at the time of the treatment trial (acutely admitted patients with schizoaffective depressions). The fact that these patients did not benefit from the addition of an antidepressant to their neuroleptic regimen may relate to their being flagrantly psychotic at the time of the trial (Siris 1991).

In general, outpatients in the studies in Table 9.2 did better with an adjunct antidepressant than inpatients did (Fisher Exact Test for this question, $P = 0.015$, for those studies in Table 9.2 which specified whether inpatients or outpatients were involved). However, it is unclear why that is the case. It might be a result of outpatients being likely to have less florid psychotic symptoms, or it might be because of other factors such as more constructive and/or less problematic outlets being available in the outpatient setting for the expression of restored energy.

It is more difficult to assess the impact of adjunctive antidepressant medications in double-blind studies that involved more unselected populations of schizophrenic patients, because absence of depression may have left little or no room for improvement in this dimension, but even in this case there have been some reported improvements (Taiminen *et al.* 1997).

MAO inhibitor antidepressants have not been adequately studied in schizophrenic patients with depressions. Of possible relevance, however, is a double-blind adjunctive tranylcypromine study which found this MAO inhibitor to be of benefit for schizophrenic patients with negative symptoms (Bucci 1987). Preliminary results have suggested that selegiline, an MAO-B inhibitor, may have value as an adjunctive treatment for negative symptoms (Perenyi *et al.* 1992; Bodkin *et al.* 1996), but interpretation of these results is complicated by the fact that selegiline has antiparkinsonian properties (Parkinson Study Group 1993) and the effects being observed may therefore represent treatment of akinesia. One double-blind study which did not show a favourable impact of selegiline on negative symptoms (Goff *et al.* 1993) was fundamentally a study of tardive dyskinesia and had the weakness, for these purposes, of not having originally selected the patients for the presence of negative symptoms, but another negative double-blind study, while small and therefore lacking in statistical power ($n = 16$), did not suffer from this limitation (Jungerman *et al.* 1999). The reversible MAO-A inhibitor meclobemide also appeared to be beneficial in one small open study of adjunctive treatment for negative symptoms (Silver *et al.* 1999).

Several double-blind studies have indicated that an adjunctive serotonin reuptake-inhibitor (SSRI) (Silver & Nassar 1992; Spina *et al.* 1994; Goff *et al.* 1995; Silver & Shmugliakov 1998) or possibly a tricyclic (Collins & Dundas 1967; Siris *et al.* 1991a) or similar (Yamagami & Soejima 1989; Decina *et al.* 1994) antidepressant may be of use in ameliorating negative symptoms in some schizophrenic patients (Evins & Goff 1996), although other double-blind studies have not found such an effect (Buchanan *et al.* 1996; Salokangas *et al.* 1996; Taiminen *et al.* 1997; Lee *et al.* 1998; Arango *et al.* 2000). Careful distinctions would have to be made to differentiate improvements in negative symptoms from improvements in depression among such individuals (Goff & Evins 1998), and the use of instruments which are specifically targeted to depression in schizophrenia may be helpful in targeting these changes (Addington *et al.* 1996b; Collins *et al.* 1996). Otherwise, while the use of antidepressant agents in the absence of antipsychotic drugs is certainly not recommended in patients with schizophrenia (Siris *et al.* 1978), there have not been direct studies of the impact of antidepressant agents on chronic symptoms of schizophrenia

Table 9.2 Double-blind studies of antidepressants in 'depressed' schizophrenic patients. (Modified and supplemented after Siris 1991.)

Study (n)	Patients	Antipsychotic	Antidepressant	Duration	Result
Singh et al. (1978) n = 60	Schizophrenia by Feighner criteria Chronic patients with symptoms of depression HAM-D score >18 Inpatients	Previous phenothiazine continued	Trazodone 300 mg/day or placebo	6 weeks	Trazadone favoured by HAM-D and CGI scale changes No significant differences in BPRS
Prusoff et al. (1979) n = 35	Schizophrenia by New Haven Index criteria A score of at least 7 on the Raskin Depression Rating Scale Outpatients	Perphenazine 16–48 mg/day	Amitriptyline 100–200 mg/day or placebo	1, 2, 4 or 6 months	With amitriptyline: some decrease in depression ratings some increase in thought disorder and agitation ratings improvement in social well-being overall impression: mildly positive
Waehrens & Gerlach (1980) n = 17	'Schizophrenia' (no criteria given) Chronic and 'emotionally withdrawn 'Long-term' inpatients (cross-over design)	Continuation of previous neuroleptics	Maprotiline 50–200 mg/day or placebo	8 weeks	No benefit found from addition of maprotiline
Johnson (1981a) n = 50	Schizophrenia by Feighner or Schneiderian symptoms BDI score 15 or more for episode of 'acute' depression All 'chronic' patients (unstated if inpatients or outpatients)	Fluphenazine decanoate or flupenthixol decanoate (doses not specified)	Nortriptyline 150 mg/day or placebo	5 weeks	No statistically significant benefit to depression from adding nortriptyline, though 40% placebo response rate would make such a finding difficult to detect Increased side-effects with nortriptyline
Kurland & Nagaraju (1981) n = 22	Schizophrenia (no criteria given) HAM-D score of 18 or more Patients treated with antiparkinsonian medications were specifically excluded Inpatients	Chlorpromazine 75–300 mg/day or haloperidol 6–15 mg/day	Viloxazine to 300 mg/day maximum in final week only or placebo	4 weeks	No differences between groups Majority of patients in both groups improved
Becker (1983) n = 52	Schizophrenia by RDC RDC for major depressive syndrome (superimposed on schizophrenia) Inpatients	Chlorpromazine 100–1200 mg/day or thiothixene 5–60 mg/day	Imipramine 150–250 mg/day for patients on chlorpromazine, or placebo for patients on thiothixene	4 weeks (after 2 weeks drug free)	Both treatments effective compared with baseline on BPRS and HAM-D but neither treatment statistically superior to the other More sedative and autonomic side-effects with chlorpromazine–imipramine combination

Table 9.2 (cont.)

Study (n)	Patients	Antipsychotic	Antidepressant	Duration	Result
Siris et al. (1987a) n = 33	Schizophrenia or schizoaffective disorder by RDC (non-psychotic or residually psychotic) RDC for major or minor depression Depression unresponsive to benztropine 2 mg p.o. t.i.d. Outpatients	Fluphenazine decanoate – clinically adjusted stable weekly dose	Imipramine 150–200 mg/day or placebo	6 weeks	Imipramine group superior on global measure (CGI) and depression scales No difference between groups in psychosis or side-effects
Dufresne et al. (1988) n = 38	Schizophrenia by DSM-III Superimposed atypical affective disorder (equivalent to DSM-III major depression) Inpatients	Thiothixene – clinically adjusted stable dose	Bupropion 150–750 mg/day flexible dose or placebo	4 weeks	Both groups improved, but placebo group improved more Majority of bupropion-treated patients dropped out
Siris et al. (1989, 1994) n = 24	Schizophrenia or schizoaffective disorder by RDC (non-psychotic or residually psychotic) RDC for major depression History of favourable response to adjunctive imipramine (150–300 mg/day) Outpatients	Fluphenazine decanoate – clinically adjusted stable dose	Six months open continuation treatment with imipramine 100–300 mg/day, then either maintained on imipramine or tapered to placebo double-blind for 1 year	18 months	Significantly more relapses into depression in group tapered to adjunctive placebo than in those maintained on adjunctive imipramine ($P < 0.001$) No exacerbation of psychosis while on adjunctive imipramine Significantly fewer episodes of psychotic exacerbation in group maintained on adjunctive imipramine ($P < 0.02$)
Kramer et al. (1989) n = 58	Initial DSM-III diagnosis of schizophrenia RDC for schizophrenia disorder (mainly schizophrenic), depressive subtype HAM-D score >17 Treated with benztropine 2–8 mg/day Inpatients, actively psychotic	Haloperidol 0.4 mg/kg/day p.o.	Amitriptyline 3.5 mg/kg/day, Desipramine 3.5 mg/kg/day, or placebo	4 weeks	Neither addition of amitriptyline nor desipramine showed significant therapeutic advantage. Patients treated with antidepressant tended to score worse at the end on BPRS hallucinatory behaviour and thinking disturbance

Table 9.2 (cont.)

Study (n)	Patients	Antipsychotic	Antidepressant	Duration	Result
Müller-Siecheneder et al. (1998) n = 19	Inpatient admissions with schizophrenia or schizophreniform disorder by DSM-IIIR, who had scores of at least 15 on the BRMES and a score of at least 3 on the BRMES depression item	Risperidone 2–12 mg/day (mean = 6.9) vs. haloperidol 2.5–15 mg/day (mean = 9.0)	Amitriptyline 50–300 mg/day for the haloperidol group only	6 weeks	Decreases in the BRMES and BPRS scores were greater in the haloperidol/amitriptyline group, but this finding did not achieve statistical significance (P = 0.11 and 0.17, respectively). (Small n limits the power of this comparison, which was part of a much larger study involving patients with combined psychotic and depressive syndromes, the results of which were statistically significant)
Kirli & Çaliskan (1998) n = 40	Schizophrenia with postpsychotic depressive disorder according to DSM-IV HAM-D score of 14 or more No mention if inpatient or outpatient	Continuation of previous antipsychotic regimen (mean equivalent haloperidol dose = 6 mg/day)	Sertraline 50 mg/day vs. imipramine 150 mg/day	5 weeks	Significant reduction in HAM-D score in both groups (P < 0.01) in both groups after 5 weeks Significant reduction after 2 weeks in sertraline group only (P < 0.05). CGI improvement (P < 0.01) for sertraline beginning after first week and for imipramine after 2 weeks No placebo control group
Cooper et al. (2000) n = 24	Stable outpatients diagnosed with schizophrenia by DSM-IIIR criteria BPRS Depression item > 3 and BDI > 14	On stable antipsychotic medication (otherwise unstated)	Sertraline 'up to 100 mg daily' vs. placebo	Unstated	BDI score fell 15.8% in the sertraline group vs. 6.0% in the placebo group (P < 0.05). On CGI Change Scale 10/12 on sertraline improved vs. 4/12 on placebo (P < 0.01)
Vlokh et al. (2000) n = 40	Clinic patients with schizophrenia (criteria not stated), who also had 'depressions' (criteria not stated)	Unstated	Sertraline (doses not stated) vs. placebo	Mean course of treatment = 6 weeks	'Positive dynamics' on basis of HAM-D evaluation in 56.7% of sertraline-treated patients vs. 10.5% of placebo patients (no statistics reported)

BDI = Beck Depression Inventory; BMRES = Bech-Rafaelsen Melancholia Scale; BPRS = Brief Psychiatric Rating Scale; CGI = Clinical Global Impression; DSM = Diagnostic and Statistical Manual; HAM-D = Hamilton Depression Rating Scale; n = number of subjects; RDC = Research Diagnostic Criteria.

other than depression or negative symptoms among patients undergoing maintenance treatment with antipsychotic medication. The assessments of schizophrenic patients with depression or negative symptoms who have received antidepressant medication as an adjunct to an antipsychotic compound, however, have not suggested that ill effects have resulted. The reader is referred to Chapter 25 on the maintenance treatment of schizophrenia for additional discussion of negative and other chronic symptoms of schizophrenia and their treatments.

When adding adjunctive antidepressant medication to antipsychotic medication, the prescriber needs to be cognizant of the possibility that each of these drugs can potentially influence the metabolism of the other. The combination of neuroleptics plus tricyclic antidepressants has been described as raising blood levels in the past (Vandel *et al.* 1979; Nelson & Jatlow 1980; Siris *et al.* 1988c,d), and combinations involving more recently introduced compounds may do the same (Centorrino *et al.* 1996; Ereshefsky 1996). Appropriate cautions include conservatism in terms of rapidity of dosage increase, alertness to side-effects and adverse reactions, awareness of the potential for prolonged medication half-lives, sensitivity to pre-existing conditions which could be problematic (such as heart or liver disease), and monitoring of plasma concentrations where appropriate and available.

Large prospective controlled studies involving the combination of an antidepressant medication with an atypical antipsychotic medication have not as yet been published. It is tempting to extrapolate from the literature regarding standard neuroleptic agents that there might be a useful role for this combination, and clinicians in the field seem to be utilizing such combinations already (Siris *et al.* 2001), but a conclusive assessment is not yet available.

Lithium

Most of the studies involving the use of lithium in schizophrenia have involved the acute treatment of psychotic exacerbations, rather than its use in the maintenance phase of treatment (Christison *et al.* 1991; Plasky 1991), and the most frequently cited predictors of favourable response are excitement, overactivity and euphoria. Little evidence has been gathered concerning the use of lithium when depressive symptoms appear in schizophrenia (Levinson *et al.* 1999). Nevertheless, one small study has identified depressive symptomatology as a positive prognosticator of adjunctive lithium response in schizophrenia (Lerner *et al.* 1988). Previous affective episodes, family history of affective disorder and an overall episodic course may also be favourable indicators (Atre-Vaidya & Taylor 1989). It is therefore reasonable to attempt a trial of adjunctive lithium in patients with postpsychotic depression who have been otherwise non-responsive, especially if there are any other features of bipolar disorder involved in the clinical picture or if there is a family history suggestive of bipolar disorder. Similarly, it is rational to try lithium in addition to an adjunctive antidepressant for schizophrenic patients whose depression does not respond, although, again, specific documentation for this approach does not exist in the literature. Support for the use and safety of lithium, in patients who have both affective and psychotic characteristics, derives from the fact that it may be useful in patients with the closely related symptomatology of schizoaffective disorder (Siris 1996).

Psychosocial interventions

Although psychosocial interventions have not specifically been studied in a controlled fashion in schizophrenic patients with depression, it is clear that appropriate psychosocial approaches can be valuable in the long-term management of schizophrenia (Hogarty *et al.* 1986), and these benefits would logically be expected to be extended to schizophrenic patients with depressions. Such interventions include skill building, psychoeducation, stress reduction, problem-solving and family work aimed at reducing expressed emotion. Appropriate structure and support, along with treatments aimed at building self-esteem and realistic components of hope and confidence, may also be quite useful. Schizophrenic patients with depressions would appear to be particularly likely to benefit from such interventions because of their otherwise compromised status and fragility.

Conclusions

Depressive syndromes occur frequently during the longitudinal course of schizophrenia. These states are associated with considerable morbidity and even the risk of mortality. They carry important prognostic implications, and a number of differential diagnostic alternatives must be considered to undertake their treatment most usefully. Their proper understanding may also have heuristic relevance.

References

Abi-Dargham, A., Gil, R., Krystal, J. *et al.* (1998) Increased striatal dopamine transmission in schizophrenia: confirmation in a second cohort. *American Journal of Psychiatry* **155**, 761–767.

Addington, D. & Addington, J. (1990) Depression dexamethasone nonsuppression and negative symptoms in schizophrenia. *Canadian Journal of Psychiatry* **35**, 430–433.

Addington, D.E. & Addington, J.M. (1992) Attempted suicide and depression in schizophrenia. *Acta Psychiatrica Scandinavica* **85**, 288–291.

Addington, D., Addington, J. & Patten, S. (1996a) Gender and affect in schizophrenia. *Canadian Journal of Psychiatry* **41**, 265–268.

Addington, D., Addington, J. & Atkinson, M. (1996b) A psychometric comparison of the Calgary Depression Scale for Schizophrenia and the Hamilton Depression Rating Scale. *Schizophrenia Research* **19**, 205–212.

Andreasen, N.C. & Olsen, S. (1982) Negative symptoms in schizophrenia: definition and reliability. *Archives of General Psychiatry* **39**, 789–794.

Andreasen, N.C., Arndt, S., Alliger, R., Miller, D. & Flaum, M. (1995) Symptoms of schizophrenia: methods, meanings, and mechanisms. *Archives of General Psychiatry* **52**, 341–351.

Arango, C., Kirkpatrick, B. & Buchanan, R.W. (2000) Fluoxetine as an adjunct to conventional antipsychotic treatment of schizophrenia patients with residual symptoms. *Journal of Nervous and Mental Disease* **188**, 50–53.

Asherson, P., Mant, R., Williams, N. *et al.* (1998) A study of chromosome 4p markers and dopamine D5 receptor gene in schizophrenia and bipolar disorder. *Molecular Psychiatry* **3**, 310–320.

Asnis, G.M., Friedman, T.A., Sanderson, W.C. *et al.* (1993) Suicidal behaviors in adult psychiatric outpatients. I. Description and prevalance. *American Journal of Psychiatry* **150**, 108–112.

Atre-Vaidya, N. & Taylor, M.A. (1989) Effectiveness of lithium and schizophrenia: do we really have an answer? *Journal of Clinical Psychiatry* **50**, 170–173.

Awad, A.G. (1993) Subjective response to neuroleptics in schizophrenia. *Schizophrenia Bulletin* **19**, 609–618.

Azorin, J.M. (1995) Long-term treatment of mood disorders in schizophrenia. *Acta Psychiatrica Scandanavica* **91** (Suppl.), 20–23.

Bandelow, B., Müller, P., Gaebel, W. *et al.* (1990) Depressive syndromes in schizophrenic patients after discharge from hospital. *European Archives of Psychiatry and Clinical Neuroscience* **240**, 113–120.

Bandelow, B., Müller, P., Frick, U. *et al.* (1992) Depressive syndromes in schizophrenic patients under neuroleptic therapy. *European Archive of Psychiatry and Clinical Neuroscience* **241**, 291–295.

Barnes, T.R.E., Curson, D.A., Liddle, P.F. & Patel, M. (1989) The nature and prevalence of depression in chronic schizophrenic in-patients. *British Journal of Psychiatry* **154**, 486–491.

Bartels, S.J. & Drake, R.E. (1988) Depressive symptoms in schizophrenia: comprehensive differential diagnosis. *Comprehensive Psychiatry* **29**, 467–483.

Bartels, S.J. & Drake, R.E. (1989) Depression in schizophrenia: current guidelines to treatment. *Psychiatric Quarterly* **60**, 337–357.

Bartels, S.J., Drake, R.E. & McHugo, G.J. (1992) Alcohol abuse, depression, and suicidal behavior in schizophrenia. *American Journal of Psychiatry* **149**, 394–395.

Baynes, D., Mulholland, C., Cooper, S.J. *et al.* (2000) Depressive symptoms in stable chronic schizophrenia: prevalence and relationship to psychopathology and treatment. *Schizophrenia Research* **45**, 47–56.

Beasley, C.M., Tollefson, G., Tran, P. *et al.* (1996) Olanzapine versus placebo and haloperidol: acute phase results of the North American double-blind olanzapine trial. *Neuropsychopharmacology* **14**, 111–123.

Becker, R.E. (1983) Implications of the efficacy of thiothixene and a chlorpromazine–imipramine combination for depression in schizophrenia. *American Journal of Psychiatry* **140**, 208–211.

Becker, R.E. (1988) Depression in schizophrenia. *Hospital and Community Psychiatry* **39**, 1269–1275.

Bench, C.J., Friston, K.J., Brown, R.G. *et al.* (1992) The anatomy of melancholia: focal abnormalities of cerebral blood flow in major depression. *Psychological Medicine* **22**, 607–615.

Bermanzohn, P.C. & Siris, S.G. (1992) Akinesia: a syndrome common to parkinsonism, retarded depression, and negative symptoms. *Comprehensive Psychiatry* **33**, 221–232.

Berrios, G.E. & Bulbena, A. (1987) Post psychotic depression: the Fulbourn cohort. *Acta Psychiatrica Scandinavica* **76**, 89–93.

Birchwood, M., Mason, R., Macmillan, F. & Healy, J. (1993) Depression, demoralization and control over psychotic illness: a comparison of depressed and non-depressed patients with a chronic psychosis. *Psychological Medicine* **23**, 387–395.

Black, D.W. & Fisher, R. (1992) Mortality in DSM-IIIR schizophrenia. *Schizophrenia Research* **7**, 109–116.

Black, D.W., Winokur, G. & Warrack, G. (1985) Suicide in schizophrenia: the Iowa record linkage study. *Journal of Clinical Psychiatry* **46**, 14–17.

Bleuler, E. (1950) *Dementia Praecox or the Group of Schizophrenias*, p. 208. International Universities Press, New York.

Bodkin, A., Cohen, B.M., Salomon, M.S. *et al.* (1996) Treatment of negative symptoms in schizophrenia and schizoaffective disorder by selegiline augmentation of antipsychotic medication: a pilot study examining the role of dopamine. *Journal of Nervous and Mental Disease* **184**, 295–301.

Borison, R.L., Arvanitis, L.A. & Miller, B.G. (1996) ICI 204,636, an atypical antipsychotic: efficacy and safety in a multicenter, placebo-controlled trial in patients with schizophrenia. *Journal of Clinical Psychopharmacology* **16**, 158–169.

Bowers, M.D. & Astrachan, B.M. (1967) Depression in acute schizophrenic psychosis. *American Journal of Psychiatry* **123**, 976–979.

Breier, A., Schreiber, J.L., Dyer, J. & Pickar, D. (1991) National Institute of Mental Health longitudinal study of chronic schizophrenia: prognosis and predictors of outcome. *Archives of General Psychiatry* **48**, 239–246.

Breier, A., Su, T.-P., Saunders, R. *et al.* (1997) Schizophrenia is associated with elevated amphetamine-induced synaptic dopamine concentrations: evidence from a novel positron emission tomography method. *Proceedings of the National Academy of Science USA* **94**, 2569–2574.

Browne, S., Garavan, J., Gervin, M. *et al.* (1998) Quality of life in schizophrenia: insight and subjective response to neuroleptics. *Journal of Nervous and Mental Disease* **186**, 74–78.

Brzustowicz, L.M., Honer, W.G., Chow, E.W. *et al.* (1997) Use of a quantitative trait to map a locus associated with severity of positive symptoms in familial schizophrenia to chromosome 6p. *American Journal of Human Genetics* **61**, 1388–1396.

Bucci, L. (1987) The negative symptoms of schizophrenia and monamine oxidase inhibitors. *Psychopharmacology* **91**, 104–108.

Buchanan, R.W. (1995) Clozapine: efficacy and safety. *Schizophrenia Bulletin* **21**, 579–591.

Buchanan, R.W., Kirkpatrick, B., Bryant, N., Ball, P. & Brier, A. (1996) Fluoxetine augmentation of clozapine treatment in patients with schizophrenia. *American Journal of Psychiatry* **153**, 1625–1627.

Caldwell, C.B. & Gottesman, I.I. (1990) Schizophrenics kill themselves too: a review of risk factors for suicide. *Schizophrenia Bulletin* **16**, 571–589.

Cardno, A.G., Jones, L.A., Murphy, K.C. *et al.* (1998) Sibling pairs with schizophrenia or schizoaffective disorder: associations of subtypes, symptoms and demographic variables. *Psychological Medicine* **28**, 815–823.

Carpenter, W.T. Jr, Heinrichs, D.W. & Alphs, L.D. (1985) Treatment of negative symptoms. *Schizophrenia Bulletin* **11**, 440–452.

Centorrino, F., Baldessarini, R.J., Frankenburg, F.R. *et al.* (1996) Serum levels of clozapine and norclozapine in patients treated with selective serotonin reuptake inhibitors. *American Journal of Psychiatry* **153**, 820–822.

Chouinard, G., Jones, B., Remington, G. *et al.* (1993) A Canadian multicenter placebo-controlled study of fixed doses of risperidone and haloperidol in the treatment of chronic schizophrenic patients. *Journal of Clinical Psychopharmacology* **13**, 25–40.

Christison, G.W., Kirch, D.G. & Wyatt, R.J. (1991) When symptoms persist: choosing among alternative somatic treatments for schizophrenia. *Schizophrenia Bulletin* **17**, 217–240.

Cohen, S., Lavelle, J., Rich, C.L. & Bromet, E. (1994) Rates and correlates of suicide attempts in first-admission psychotic patients. *Acta Psychiatrica Scandinavica* **90**, 167–171.

Collins, A.A., Remington, G., Coulter, K. & Birkett, K. (1996) Depression in schizophrenia: a comparison of three measures. *Schizophrenia Research* **20**, 205–209.

Collins, A.D. & Dundas, J. (1967) A double-blind trial of amitriptyline/perphenazine, perphenazine, and placebo in chronic withdrawn inert schizophrenics. *British Journal of Psychiatry* **113**, 1425–1429.

Cooper, S.J., Mulholland, C., Lynch, G., Baynes, D. & King, D.J. (2000) Sertraline in the treatment of depressive symptoms in stable, chronic schizophrenia: a placebo controlled trial [Abstract]. *Schizophrenia Research* **41**, 209.

Coryell, W., Keller, M., Lavori, P. & Endicott, J. (1990) Affective syndromes, psychotic features, and prognosis. I. Depression. *Archives of General Psychiatry* **47**, 651–657.

Crow, T.J. (1980) Molecular pathology of schizophrenia: more than one disease process? *British Medical Journal* **280**, 66–68.

Dalack, G.W., Healy, D.J. & Meador-Woodruff, J.H. (1998) Nicotine dependence in schizophrenia: clinical phenomena and laboratory findings. *American Journal of Psychiatry* **155**, 1490–1501.

Daniel, D.G., Zimbroff, D.L., Potkin, S.G. *et al.* & the Ziprasidone Study Group (1999) Ziprasidone 80 mg/day and 160 mg/day in the acute exacerbation of schizophrenia and schizoaffective disorder: a 6-week placebo-controlled trial. *Neuropsychopharmacology* **20**, 491–505.

Dassori, A.M., Mezzich, J.E. & Keshavan, M. (1990) Suicidal indicators in schizophrenia. *Acta Psychiatrica Scandanavica* **81**, 409–413.

Davis, K.L., Kahn, R.S., Ko, G. & Davidson, M. (1991) Dopamine in schizophrenia: a review and reconceptualization. *American Journal of Psychiatry* **148**, 1474–1486.

DeAlarcon, R. & Carney, M.W.P. (1969) Severe depressive mood changes following slow-release intramuscular fluphenazine injection. *British Medical Journal* **3**, 564–567.

Decina, P., Mukherjee, S., Bocola, V. *et al.* (1994) Adjunctive trazodone in the treatment of negative symptoms of schizophrenia. *Hospital and Community Psychiatry* **45**, 1220–1223.

DeLisi, L.E., Goldin, L.R., Maxwell, E., Kazuba, D.M. & Gershon, E.S. (1987) Clinical features of illness in siblings with schizophrenia or schizoaffective disorder. *Archives of General Psychiatry* **44**, 891–896.

Deutch, A.Y., Moghaddam, B., Innes, R.B. *et al.* (1991) Mechanisms of actions of atypical antipsychotic drugs: implications for novel therapeutic strategies for schizophrenia. *Schizophrenia Research* **4**, 121–156.

D'haenen, H.A. & Bossuyt, A. (1994) Dopamine D$_2$ receptors in depression measured with single photon emission tomography. *Biological Psychiatry* **35**, 128–132.

Docherty, J.P., van Kammen, D.P., Siris, S.G. & Marder, S.R. (1978) Stages of onset of schizophrenic psychosis. *American Journal of Psychiatry* **135**, 420–426.

Dolan, R.J., Bench, C.J., Liddle, P.F. *et al.* (1993) Dorsolateral prefrontal cortex dysfunction in the major psychoses; symptom or disease specificity? *Journal of Neurology, Neurosurgery and Psychiatry* **56**, 1290–1294.

Dollfus, S., Petit, M. & Menard, J.F. (1993) Relationship between depressive and positive symptoms in schizophrenia. *Journal of Affective Disorders* **28**, 61–69.

Drake, R.E. & Cotton, P.G. (1986) Depression, hopelessness and suicide in chronic schizophrenia. *British Journal of Psychiatry* **148**, 554–559.

Drake, R.E. & Ehrlich, J. (1985) Suicide attempts associated with akathisia. *American Journal of Psychiatry* **142**, 499–501.

Drake, R.E., Gates, C., Cotton, P.G. & Whitaker, A. (1984) Suicide among schizophrenics: who is at risk? *Journal of Nervous and Mental Disease* **172**, 613–617.

Drake, R.E., Gates, C., Whitaker, A. & Cotton, P.G. (1985) Suicide among schizophrenics: a review. *Comprehensive Psychiatry* **26**, 90–100.

Drevets, W.C. (1998) Functional neuroimaging studies of depression: the anatomy of melancholic. *Annual Reviews of Medicine* **49**, 341–361.

Dufresne, R.L., Kass, D.J. & Becker, R.E. (1988) Bupropion and thiothixene versus placebo and thiothixene in the treatment of depression in schizophrenia. *Drug Development Research* **12**, 259–266.

Ebert, D., Feistel, H., Loew, T. & Pirner, A. (1996) Dopamine and depression: striatal dopamine D$_2$ receptor SPECT before and after antidepressant therapy. *Psychopharmacology* **126**, 91–94.

Eissler, K.R. (1951) Remarks on the psycho-analysis of schizophrenia. *International Journal of Psychoanalysis* **32**, 139–156.

Emsley, R.A., Oosthuizen, P.P., Joubert, A.F., Roberts, M.C. & Stein, D.J. (1999) Depressive and anxiety symptoms in patients with schizophrenia and schizophreniform disorder. *Journal of Clinical Psychiatry* **60**, 747–751.

Ereshefsky, L. (1996) Pharmacokinetics and drug interactions: update for new antipsychotics. *Journal of Clinical Psychiatry* **57** (Suppl. 11), 12–25.

Evins, A.E. & Goff, D.C. (1996) Adjunctive antidepressant drug therapies in the treatment of negative symptoms of schizophrenia. *CNS Drugs* **6**, 130–147.

Falloon, I., Watt, D.C. & Shepherd, M. (1978) A comparative controlled trial of pimozide and fluphenazine decanoate in the continuation therapy of schizophrenia. *Psychological Medicine* **8**, 59–70.

Fenton, W.S., McGlashan, T.H., Victor, B.J. & Blyler, C.R. (1997) Symptoms, subtype, and suicidality in patients with schizophrenia spectrum disorders. *American Journal of Psychiatry* **154**, 199–204.

deFigueiredo, J.M. (1993) Depression and demoralization: phenomenologic differences and research perspectives. *Comprehensive Psychiatry* **34**, 308–311.

Floru, L., Heinrich, K. & Wittek, F. (1975) The problem of post-psychotic schizophrenic depressions and their pharmacological induction. *International Pharmacopsychiatry* **10**, 230–239.

Frank, J.D. (1973) *Persuasion and Healing.* Johns Hopkins University Press, Baltimore.

Franz, M., Lis, S., Pluddemann, K. & Gallhofer, B. (1997) Conventional versus atypical neuroleptics: subjective quality of life in schizophrenic patients. *British Journal of Psychiatry* **170**, 422–425.

Galdi, J. (1983) The causality of depression in schizophrenia. *British Journal of Psychiatry* **142**, 621–625.

Galdi, J., Rieder, R.O., Silber, D. & Bonato, R.R. (1981) Genetic factors in the response to neuroleptics in schizophrenia: a pharmacogenetic study. *Psychological Medicine* **11**, 713–728.

Goff, D.C. & Evins, A.E. (1998) Negative symptoms in schizophrenia: neurobiological models and treatment response. *Harvard Review of Psychiatry* **6**, 59–77.

Goff, D.C., Renshaw, P.F., Sarid-Segal, O. *et al.* (1993) A placebo-controlled trial of selegiline (L-depreyl) in the treatment of tardive dyskinesia. *Biological Psychiatry* **33**, 700–706.

Goff, D.C., Midha, K.K., Sarid-Segal, O., Hubbard, J.W. & Amico, E. (1995) A placebo-controlled trial of fluoxetine added to neuroleptic in patients with schizophrenia. *Psychopharmacology* **117**, 417–423.

Goldstein, J.M. & Link, B.G. (1988) Gender and the expression of schizophrenia. *Journal of Psychiatric Research* **22**, 141–155.

Goldstein, J.M., Santangelo, S.L., Simpson, J.C. & Tsuang, M.T. (1990) The role of gender in identifying subtypes of schizophrenia: a latent class analytic approach. *Schizophrenia Bulletin* **16**, 263–275.

Green, M.F., Nuechterlein, K.H., Ventura, J. & Mintz, J. (1990) The temporal relationship between depressive and psychotic symptoms in recent-onset schizophrenia. *American Journal of Psychiatry* **147**, 179–182.

Griffiths, R.R. & Mumford, G.K. (1995) Caffeine: a drug of abuse? In: *Psychopharmacology: the Fourth Generation of Progress* (eds F.E. Bloom & D.J. Kupfer), pp. 1699–1713. Raven Press, New York.

Gupta, S., Black, D.W., Arndt, S., Hubbard, W.C. & Andreasen, N.C. (1998) Factors associated with suicide attempts among patients with schizophrenia. *Psychiatric Services* **49**, 1353–1355.

Gur, R.E., Cowell, P.E., Latshaw, A. *et al.* (2000) Reduced dorsal and orbital prefrontal gray matter volumes in schizophrenia. *Archives of General Psychiatry* **57**, 76–768.

Guze, S.B., Cloninger, C.R., Martin, R.L. & Clayton, P.J. (1983) A follow-up and family study of schizophrenia. *Archives of General Psychiatry* **40**, 1273–1276.

de Haan, L., Lavalaye, J., Linszen, D., Dingemans, P.M.A.J. & Booij, J. (2000) Subjective experience and striatal dopamine D₂ receptor occupancy in patients with schizophrenia stabilized with olanzapine or risperidone. *American Journal of Psychiatry* **157**, 1019–1020.

Haas, G.L., Glick, I.D., Clarkin, J.F., Spencer, J.H. & Lewis, A.B. (1990) Gender and schizophrenia outcome: a clinical trial of an inpatient family intervention. *Schizophrenia Bulletin* **16**, 277–292.

Häfner, H., Maurer, K., Löffler, W. *et al.* (1994) The epidemiology of early schizophrenia: influence of age and gender on onset and early course. *British Journal of Psychiatry* **164** (Suppl. 23), 29–38.

Halstead, S.M., Barnes, T.R.E. & Speller, J.C. (1994) Akathisia: pre-valence and associated dysphoria in an in-patient population with chronic schizophrenia. *British Journal of Psychiatry* **164**, 177–183.

Harrow, M., Yonan, C.A., Sands, J.F. & Marengo, J. (1994) Depression in schizophrenia: are neuroleptics, akinesia, or anhedonia involved? *Schizophrenia Bulletin* **20**, 327–338.

Heilä, H., Isometsä, E.T., Henriksson, M.M. *et al.* (1997) A nationwide psychological autopsy study on age- and sex-specific clinical characteristics of 92 suicide victims with schizophrenia. *American Journal of Psychiatry* **154**, 1235–1242.

Heilä, H., Heikkinen, M.E., Isometsä, E.T. *et al.* (1999) Life events and completed suicide in schizophrenia: a comparison of suicide victims with and without schizophrenia. *Schizophrenia Bulletin* **25**, 519–531.

Herz, M. (1985) Prodromal symptoms and prevention of relapse in schizophrenia. *Journal of Clinical Psychiatry* **46** (11), 22–25.

Herz, M. & Melville, C. (1980) Relapse in schizophrenia. *American Journal of Psychiatry* **137**, 801–805.

Hietala, J., Syvälahti, E., Vilkman, H. *et al.* (1999) Depressive symptoms and presynaptic dopamine function in neuroleptic-naive schizophrenia. *Schizophrenia Research* **35**, 41–50.

Hirsch, S.R. & Jolley, A.G. (1989) The dysphoric syndrome in schizophrenia and its implications for relapse. *British Journal of Psychiatry* **155** (Suppl. 5), 46–50.

Hirsch, S.R., Gaind, R., Rohde, P.D., Stevens, B.C. & Wing, J.T. (1973) Outpatient maintenance of chronic schizophrenic patients with long-acting fluphenazine: double-blind placebo trial. *British Medical Journal* **1**, 633–637.

Hirsch, S.R., Jolley, A.G., Barnes, T.R.E. *et al.* (1989) Dysphoric and depressive symptoms in chronic schizophrenia. *Schizophrenia Research* **2**, 259–264.

Hoffmann, H., Kupper, Z. & Kunz, B. (2000) Hopelessness and its impact on rehabilitation outcome in schizophrenia: an exploratory study. *Schizophrenia Research* **43**, 147–158.

Hogarty, G.E. & Munetz, M.R. (1984) Pharmacogenic depression among outpatient schizophrenic patients: a failure to substantiate. *Journal of Clinical Psychopharmacology* **4**, 17–24.

Hogarty, G.E., Anderson, C.M., Reiss, D.J. *et al.* (1986) Family psychoeducational, social skills training, and maintenance chemotherapy in the aftercare treatment of schizophrenia. I. One-year effects of a controlled study on relapse and expressed emotion. *Archives of General Psychiatry* **43**, 633–642.

Inskip, H.M., Harris, E.C. & Barraclough, B. (1998) Lifetime risk of suicide for affective disorder, alcoholism and schizophrenia. *British Journal of Psychiatry* **172**, 35–37.

Ismail, K., Murray, R.M., Wheeler, M.J. & O'Keane, V. (1998) The dexamethasone suppression test in schizophrenia. *Psychological Medicine* **28**, 311–317.

Johnson, D.A.W. (1981a) Studies of depressive symptoms in schizophrenia. *British Journal of Psychiatry* **139**, 89–101.

Johnson, D.A.W. (1981b) Depressions in schizophrenia: some observations on prevalence, etiology, and treatment. *Acta Psychiatrica Scandinavica* **63** (Suppl. 291), 137–144.

Johnson, D.A.W. (1988) The significance of depression in the prediction of relapse in chronic schizophrenia. *British Journal of Psychiatry* **152**, 320–323.

Jones, H. (1997) Risperidone: a review of its pharmacology and use in the treatment of schizophrenia. *Journal of Serotonin Research* **4**, 17–28.

Jones, J.S., Stein, D.J., Stanley, B. *et al.* (1994) Negative and depressive symptoms in suicidal schizophrenics. *Acta Psychiatrica Scandinavica* **89**, 81–87.

Jungerman, T., Rabinowitz, D. & Klein, E. (1999) Depreyl augmentation for treating negative symptoms of schizophrenia: a double-blind, controlled study. *Journal of Clinical Psychopharmacology* **19**, 522–525.

Kane, J.M., Rifkin, A., Woerner, M. *et al.* (1983) Low dose neuroleptic treatment of outpatient schizophrenics. I. Preliminary results for relapse rates. *Archives of General Psychiatry* **40**, 893–896.

Kane, J., Honigfeld, G., Singer, J. & Meltzer, H. (1988) Clozapine for the treatment-resistant schizophrenic: a double-blind comparison with chlorpromazine. *Archives of General Psychiatry* **45**, 789–796.

Keck, P., Buffenstein, A., Ferguson, J. *et al.* (1998) Ziprasidone 40 and 120 mg/day in the acute exacerbation of schizophrenia and schizoaffective disorder: a 4-week placebo-controlled trial. *Psychopharmacology (Berl)* **140**, 173–184.

Kemp, R.A. & Lambert, T.J.R. (1995) Insight in schizophrenia and its relationship to psychopathology. *Schizophrenia Research* **18**, 21–28.

Kendler, K.S. & Hays, P. (1983) Schizophrenia subdivided by the family history of affective disorder: a comparison of symptomatology and cause of illness. *Archives of General Psychiatry* **40**, 951–955.

Kendler, K.S., McGuire, M., Gruenberg, A.M. *et al.* (1993) The Roscommon family study. I. methods, diagnosis of probands, and risk of schizophrenia in relatives. *Archives of General Psychiatry* **50**, 527–540.

Kendler, K.S., Karkowski-Shuman, L. & Walsh, D. (1996) The risk for psychiatric illness in siblings of schizophrenics: the impact of psychotic and non-psychotic affective illness and alcoholism in parents. *Acta Psychiatrica Scandinavica* **94**, 49–55.

Kendler, K.S., Karkowski-Shuman, L., O'Neill, A. *et al.* (1997) Resemblance of psychotic symptoms and syndromes in affected sibling pairs from the Irish study of high-density schizophrenia families: evidence for possible etiologic heterogeneity. *American Journal of Psychiatry* **154**, 191–198.

Kendler, K.S., Myers, J.M., O'Neill, F.A. *et al.* (2000) Clinical features of schizophrenia and linkage to chromosomes 5q, 6p, 8p, and 10p in the Irish study of high-density schizophrenia families. *American Journal of Psychiatry* **157**, 402–408.

Kibel, D.A., Laffont, I. & Liddle, P.F. (1993) The composition of the negative syndrome of chronic schizophrenia. *British Journal of Psychiatry* **162**, 744–750.

Kirkpatrick, B., Amador, X.F., Yale, S.A. *et al.* (1996) The deficit syndrome in the DSM-IV field trial. II. Depressive episodes and persecutory beliefs. *Schizophrenia Research* **20**, 79–90.

Kirli, S. & Çaliskan, M. (1998) A comparative study of sertraline versus imipramine in postpsychotic depressive disorder of schizophrenia. *Schizophrenia Research* **33**, 103–111.

Klein, D.F. (1974) Endomorphic depression: a conceptual and terminological revision. *Archives of General Psychiatry* **31**, 447–454.

Knable, M.B., Egan, M.F., Heinz, A. *et al.* (1997) Altered dopaminergic function and negative symptoms in drug-free patients with schizophrenia: [^{123}I]-iodobenzamine SPECT study. *British Journal of Psychiatry* **171**, 574–577.

Knights, A. & Hirsch, S.R. (1981) 'Revealed' depression and drug treatment for schizophrenia. *Archives of General Psychiatry* **38**, 806–811.

Knights, A., Okasha, M.S., Salih, M.A. & Hirsch, S.R. (1979) Depressive and extrapyramidal symptoms and clinical effects: a trial of fluphenazine versus flupenthixol in maintenance of schizophrenic out-patients. *British Journal of Psychiatry* **135**, 515–523.

Kohler, C., Gur, R.C., Swanson, C.L., Petty, R. & Gur, R.E. (1998a) Depression in schizophrenia. I. Association with neuroopsychological deficits. *Biological Psychiatry* **43**, 165–172.

Kohler, C., Swanson, C.L., Gur, R.C., Mozley, L.H. & Gur, R.E. (1998b) Depression in schizophrenia. II. MRI and PET findings. *Biological Psychiatry* **43**, 173–180.

Koreen, A.R., Siris, S.G., Chakos, M. *et al.* (1993) Depression in first-episode schizophrenia. *American Journal of Psychiatry* **150**, 1643–1648.

Krakowski, M., Czobor, P. & Volavka, J. (1997) Effect of neuroleptic treatment on depressive symptoms in acute schizophrenic episodes. *Psychiatric Research* **71**, 19–26.

Kramer, M.S., Vogel, W.H., DiJohnson, C. *et al.* (1989) Antidepressants in 'depressed' schizophrenic inpatients: a controlled trial. *Archives of General Psychiatry* **46**, 922–928.

Krausz, M., Müller-Thomsen, T. & Hassen, C. (1995) Suicide among schizophrenic adolescents in the long-term course of illness. *Psychopathology* **28**, 95–103.

Kuck, J., Zisook, S., Moranville, J.T., Heaton, R.K. & Braff, D.L. (1992) Negative symptomatology in schizophrenic outpatients. *Journal of Nervous and Mental Disease* **180**, 510–515.

Kulhara, P., Avasthi, A., Chadda, R. *et al.* (1989) Negative and depressive symptoms in schizophrenia. *British Journal of Psychiatry* **154**, 207–211.

Kurland, A.A. & Nagaraju, A. (1981) Viloxazine and the depressed schizophrenic: methodological issues. *Journal of Clinical Pharmacology* **21**, 37–41.

Laruelle, M. (1998) Imaging dopamine neurotransmission in schizophrenia: a review and meta-analysis. *Quarterly Journal of Nuclear Medicine* **42**, 211–221.

Laruelle, M., Abi-Dargham, A., Gil, R., Kegeles, L. & Innis, R. (1999) Increased dopamine transmission in schizophrenia: relationship to illness phases. *Biological Psychiatry* **46**, 56–72.

Laruelle, M., Abi-Dargham, A., van Dyck, C. *et al.* (2000) Dopamine and serotonin transporters in patients with schizophrenia: an imaging study with [^{123}]-CIT. *Biological Psychiatry* **47**, 371–379.

Lee, M.S., Kim, Y.K., Lee, S.K. & Suh, K.Y. (1998) A double-blind study of adjunctive sertraline in haloperidol-stabilized patients with chronic schizophrenia. *Journal of Clinical Psychopharmacology* **18**, 399–403.

Leff, J., Tress, K. & Edwards, B. (1988) The clinical course of depressive symptoms in schizophrenia. *Schizophrenia Research* **1**, 25–30.

Lerner, Y., Mintzer, Y. & Schestatzky, M. (1988) Lithium combined with haloperidol in schizophrenic patients. *British Journal of Psychiatry* **153**, 359–362.

Levinson, D.F., Umapathy, C. & Musthaq, M. (1999) Treatment of schizoaffective disorder and schizophrenia with mood symptoms. *American Journal of Psychiatry* **156**, 1138–1148.

Levitt, J.J. & Tsuang, M.T. (1988) The heterogeneity of schizoaffective

disorder: implications for treatment. *American Journal of Psychiatry* **145**, 926–936.

Lewis, R., Kapur, S., Jones, C. *et al.* (1999) Serotonin 5-HT$_2$ receptors in schizophrenia: a PET study unsing [^{18}F]setoperone in neuroleptic-naive patients and normal subjects. *American Journal of Psychiatry* **156**, 72–78.

Liddle, P.F., Friston, K.J., Frith, C.D. *et al.* (1992) Patterns of cerebral blood flow in schizophrenia. *British Journal of Psychiatry* **160**, 179–186.

Liddle, P.F., Barnes, T.R.E., Curson, D.A. & Patel, M. (1993) Depression and the experience of psychological deficits in schizophrenia. *Acta Psychiatrica Scandanavica* **88**, 243–247.

Lindenmayer, J.-P., Grochowski, S. & Kay, S.R. (1991) Schizophrenic patients with depression: psychopathological profiles and relationship with negative symptoms. *Comprehensive Psychiatry* **32**, 528–533.

Lindenmayer, J.P., Grochowski, S. & Hyman, R.B. (1995) Five factor model of schizophrenia: replication across samples. *Schizophrenia Research* **14**, 229–234.

Lysaker, P.H., Bell, M.D., Bioty, S.M. & Zito, W.S. (1995) The frequency of associations between positive and negative symptoms and dysphoria in schizophrenia. *Comprehensive Psychiatry* **36**, 113–117.

McGlashan, T.H. & Bardenstein, K.K. (1990) Gender differences is affective, schizoaffective, and schizophrenic disorders. *Schizophrenia Bulletin* **16**, 319–329.

McGlashan, T.H. & Carpenter, W.T. Jr (1976a) Postpsychotic depression in schizophrenia. *Archives of General Psychiatry* **33**, 231–239.

McGlashan, T.H. & Carpenter, W.T. Jr (1976b) An investigation of the post psychotic depressive syndrome. *American Journal of Psychiatry* **133**, 14–19.

McGuire, P.K., Shah, G.M.S. & Murray, R.M. (1993) Increased blood flow in Broca's area during auditory hallucinations in schizophrenia. *Lancet* **342**, 703–706.

Maier, W., Lichtermann, D., Minges, J. *et al.* (1993) Continuity and discontinuity of affective disorders and schizophrenia: results of a controlled family study. *Archives of General Psychiatry* **50**, 871–883.

Malhotra, A. (2001) The genetics of schizophrenia. *Current Opinion in Psychiatry* **14**, 3–7.

Malla, A.K. & Norman, R.M.G. (1994) Prodromal symptoms in schizophrenia. *British Journal of Psychiatry* **164**, 287–293.

Mandel, M.R., Severe, J.B., Schooler, N.R., Gelenberg, A.J. & Mieske, M. (1982) Development and prediction of post-psychotic depression in neuroleptic-treated schizophrenics. *Archives of General Psychiatry* **39**, 197–203.

Marder, S.R. & Meibach, R.C. (1994) Risperidone in the treatment of schizophrenia. *American Journal of Psychiatry* **151**, 825–835.

Marder, S.R., Van Putten, T., Mintz, J. *et al.* (1987) Low- and conventional-dose maintenance therapy with fluphenazine decanoate: two year outcome. *Archives of General Psychiatry* **44**, 518–521.

Markou, P. (1996) Depression in schizophrenia: a descriptive study. *Australian and New Zealand Journal of Psychiatry* **30**, 354–357.

Martin, R.L., Cloninger, R.C., Guze, S.B. & Clayton, P.J. (1985) Frequency and differential diagnosis of depressive syndromes in schizophrenia. *Journal of Clinical Psychiatry* **46** (11), 9–13.

Martinot, J.L., Paillère-Martinot, M.L., Loc'h, C. *et al.* (1994) Central D$_2$ receptors and negative symptoms of schizophrenia. *British Journal of Psychiatry* **164**, 27–34.

Mauri, M.C., Bravin, S., Fabiano, L. *et al.* (1995) Depressive symptoms and schizophrenia: a psychopharmacological approach. *L'Encephale* **21**, 555–558.

Meltzer, H.Y. & Okayli, G. (1995) Reduction of suicidality during clozapine treatment of neuroleptic-resistant schizophrenia: impact on risk-benefit assessment. *American Journal of Psychiatry* **152**, 183–190.

Meltzer, H.Y., Matsubara, S. & Lee, J.C. (1989) Classification of typical and atypical antipsychotic drugs on the basis of dopamine D_1, D_2 and serotonin$_2$ pKi values. *Journal of Pharmacology and Experimental Therapeutics* **25**, 238–246.

Miles, C. (1977) Conditions predisposing to suicide: a review. *Journal of Nervous and Mental Disease* **164**, 221–246.

Miller, J.B. & Sonnenberg, S.M. (1973) Depression following psychotic episodes: a response to the challenge of change? *Journal of the American Academy of Psychoanalysis* **1**, 253–270.

Möller, H.J. & von Zerssen, D. (1982) Depressive states occurring during the neuroleptic treatment of schizophrenia. *Schizophrenia Bulletin* **8**, 109–117.

Möller, H.J. & von Zerssen, D. (1986) Depression in schizophrenia. In: *Handbook of Studies on Schizophrenia, Part 1* (eds G.D. Burrows, T.R. Norman & G. Rubinstein), pp. 183–191. Elsevier, Amsterdam.

Möller, H.J., Muller, H., Borison, R., Schooler, N.R. & Chouinard, G. (1995) A path analytical approach to differentiate between direct and indirect drug effects on negative symptoms in schizophrenic patients: a re-evaluation of the North American risperidone study. *European Archives of Clinical Neuroscience* **245**, 45–49.

Müller, M.J. & Wetzel, H. (1998) Dimensionality of depression in acute schizophrenia: a methodological study using the Bech–Rafaelsen Melancholia Scale (BRMES). *Journal of Psychiatric Research* **32**, 369–378.

Müller-Siecheneder, F., Müller, M.J., Hillert, A. *et al.* (1998) Risperidone versus haloperidol and amitriptyline in the treatment of patients with a combined psychotic and depressive syndrome. *Journal of Clinical Psychopharmacology* **18**, 111–120.

Munro, J.G., Hardiker, T.M. & Leonard, D.P. (1984) The dexamethasone suppression test in residual schizophrenia with depression. *American Journal of Psychiatry* **141**, 250–252.

Nakaya, M., Ohmori, K., Komahashi, T. & Suwa, H. (1997) Depressive symptoms in acute schizophrenic inpatients. *Schizophrenia Research* **25**, 131–139.

Nelson, J.C. & Jatlow, P.I. (1980) Neuroleptic effect on desipramine steady-state plasma concentrations. *American Journal of Psychiatry* **137**, 1232–1234.

Ngan, E.T.C., Yatham, L.N., Ruth, T.J. & Liddle, P.F. (2000) Decreased serotonin 2A receptor densities in neuroleptic-naive patients with schizophenia: a PET study using [^{18}F]setoperone. *American Journal of Psychiatry* **157**, 1016–1018.

Norman, R.M.G. & Malla, A.K. (1991) Dysphoric mood and symptomatology in schizophrenia. *Psychological Medicine* **21**, 897–903.

Norman, R.M.G. & Malla, A.K. (1994) Correlations over time between dysphoric mood and symptomatology in schizophrenia. *Comprehensive Psychiatry* **35**, 34–38.

Norman, R.M.G., Malla, A.K., Cortese, L. & Diaz, F. (1998) Aspects of dysphoria and symptoms of schizophrenia. *Psychological Medicine* **28**, 1433–1441.

Nuechterlein, K.H. & Dawson, M.D. (1984) A heuristic vulnerability/stress model of schizophrenic episodes. *Schizophrenia Bulletin* **10**, 300–312.

Nyman, A.K. & Jonsson, H. (1986) Patterns of self-destructive behaviour in schizophrenia. *Acta Psychiatrica Scandinavica* **73**, 252–262.

Olfson, M., Mechanic, D., Boyer, C.A. *et al.* (1999) Assessing clinical predictions of early rehospitalization in schizophrenia. *Journal of Nervous and Mental Disease* **187**, 721–729.

Parkinson Study Group (1993) Effects of tocopherol and deprenyl on the progression of disability in early Parkinson's disease. *New England Journal of Medicine* **328**, 176–183.

Peralta, V. & Cuesta, M.J. (1994) Lack of insight: its status within schizophrenic psychopathology. *Biological Psychiatry* **36**, 559–561.

Peralta, V. & Cuesta, M.J. (1999) Negative, parkinsonian, depressive and catatonic symptoms in schizophrenia: a conflict of paradigms revisited. *Schizophrenia Research* **40**, 245–253.

Perenyi, A., Goswami, U., Frecska, E. & Arato, M. (1992) L-deprenyl in treating negative symptoms of schizophrenia. *Psychiatry Research* **42**, 189–191.

Perenyi, A., Norman, T., Hopwood, M. & Burrows, G. (1998) Negative symptoms, depression and parkinsonian symptoms in chronic, hospitalised schizophrenic patients. *Journal of Affective Disorders* **48**, 163–169.

Peuskens, J. (1995) Risperidone in the treatment of patients with chronic schizophrenia: a multinational, multi-center, double-blind, parallel group study versus haloperidol. *British Journal of Psychiatry* **166**, 712–726.

Plasky, P. (1991) Antidepressant usage in schizophrenia. *Schizophrenia Bulletin* **17**, 649–657.

Prasad, A.J. & Kumar, N. (1988) Suicidal behavior in hospitalized schizophrenics. *Suicide and Life-Threatening Behavior* **18**, 265–269.

Prusoff, B.A., Williams, D.H., Weissman, M.M. & Astrachan, B.M. (1979) Treatment of secondary depression in schizophrenia. *Archives of General Psychiatry* **36**, 569–575.

Rifkin, A., Quitkin, F. & Klein, D.F. (1975) Akinesia: a poorly recognized drug-induced extrapyramidal behavioral disorder. *Archives of General Psychiatry* **32**, 672–674.

Rifkin, A., Quitkin, F., Kane, J., Struve, F. & Klein, D.F. (1978) Are prophylactic antiparkinsonian drugs necessary? A controlled study of procyclidine withdrawal. *Archives of General Psychiatry* **35**, 483–489.

Roth, S. (1970) The seemingly ubiquitous depression following acute schizophrenic episodes, a neglected area of clinical discussion. *American Journal of Psychiatry* **127**, 51–58.

Roy, A. (1980) Depression in chronic paranoid schizophrenia. *British Journal of Psychiatry* **137**, 138–139.

Roy, A. (1981) Depression in the course of chronic undifferentiated schizophrenia. *Archives of General Psychiatry* **38**, 296–297.

Roy, A. (1982) Suicide in chronic schizophrenia. *British Journal of Psychiatry* **141**, 171–177.

Roy, A. (1984) Do neuroleptics cause depression? *Biological Psychiatry* **19**, 777–781.

Roy, A. (1986) Depression, attempted suicide, and suicide in patients with chronic schizophrenia. *Psychiatric Clinics of North America* **9**, 193–206.

Roy, A., Thompson, R. & Kennedy, S. (1983) Depression in chronic schizophrenia. *British Journal of Psychiatry* **142**, 465–470.

Saarinen, P.I., Lehtonen, J. & Lönnqvist, J. (1999) Suicide risk in schizophrenia: an analysis of 17 consecutive suicides. *Schizophrenia Bulletin* **25**, 533–542.

Salokangas, R.K.R., Saarijärvi, S., Taiminen, T. *et al.* (1996) Citalopram as an adjuvant in chronic schizophrenia: a double-blind placebo-controlled study. *Acta Psychiatrica Scandinavica* **94**, 175–180.

Sands, J.R. & Harrow, M. (1999) Depression during the longitudinal course of schizophrenia. *Schizophrenia Bulletin* **25**, 157–171.

Sax, K.W., Strakowski, S.M., Keck, P.E. *et al.* (1996) Relationships amond negative, positive, and depressive symptoms in schizophrenia and psychotic depression. *British Journal of Psychiatry* **168**, 68–71.

Schildkraut, J.J., Orsulak, P.J., Schatzberg, A.F. & Herzog, J.M. (1980)

Platelet monoamine oxidase activity in subgroups of schizophrenic disorders. *Schizophrenia Bulletin* 6, 220–225.

Seeger, T.F., Seymour, P.A., Schmidt, A.W. *et al.* (1995) Ziprasidone (CP-88,059): a new antipsychotic with combined dopamine and serotonin receptor antagonist activity. *Journal of Pharmacology and Experimental Therapeutics* 275, 101–113.

Semrad, E.V. (1966) Long-term therapy of schizophrenia: formulation of the clinical approach. In: *Psychoneuroses and Schizophrenia* (ed. G. Usdin), pp. 155–173. J.B. Lippincott, Philadelphia.

Serretti, A., Macciardi, F.M. & Smeraldi, E. (1996) Identification of symptomatologic patterns common to major psychoses: proposal for a phenotype definition. *American Journal of Medical Genetics* 67, 393–400.

Serretti, A., Catalano, M. & Smeraldi, E. (1999a) Serotonin transporter gene is not associated with symptomatology of schizophrenia. *Schizophrenia Research* 35, 33–39.

Serretti, A., Lattuada, E., Cusin, C. *et al.* (1999b) Dopamine D_3 receptor gene not associated with symptomatology of major psychoses. *American Journal of Medical Genetics* 88, 476–480.

Serretti, A., Cusin, C., Lattuada, E. *et al.* (1999c) No interaction between serotonin transporter gene and dopamine receptor D_4 gene in symptomatology of major psychoses. *American Journal of Medical Genetics* 88, 481–485.

Shah, P.J., Ogilvie, A.D., Goodwin, G.M. & Ebmeier, K.P. (1997) Clinical and psychometric correlates of dopamine D_2 binding in depression. *Psychological Medicine* 27, 1247–1256.

Shear, K., Frances, A. & Weiden, P. (1983) Suicide associated with akathisia and depot fluphenazine treatment. *Journal of Clinical Psychopharmacology* 3, 235–236.

Shtasel, D.L., Gur, R.E., Gallacher, F., Heimberg, C. & Gur, R.C. (1992) Gender differences in the clinical expression of schizophrenia. *Schizophrenia Research* 7, 225–231.

Silver, H. & Nassar, A. (1992) Fluvoxamine improves negative symptoms in treated chronic schizophrenia: an add-on double-blind, placebo-controlled study. *Biological Psychiatry* 31, 698–704.

Silver, H. & Shmugliakov, N. (1998) Augmentation with fluvoxamine but not maprotiline improves negative symptoms in treated schizophrenia: evidence for a specific serotonergic effect from a double-blind study. *Journal of Clinical Psychopharmacology* 18, 208–211.

Silver, H., Aharon, N., Hausfater, N. & Jhahah, N. (1999) The effect of augmentation with moclobemide on symptoms of schizophrenia. *International Clinical Psychopharmacology* 14, 193–195.

Singh, A.N., Saxena, B. & Nelson, H.L. (1978) A controlled clinical study of trazodone in chronic schizophrenic patients with pronounced depressive symptomatology. *Current Therapeutics Research* 23, 485–501.

Siris, S.G. (1985) Akathisia and 'acting-out. *Journal of Clinical Psychiatry* 46, 395–397.

Siris, S.G. (1991) Diagnosis of secondary depression in schizophrenia: implications for DSM-IV. *Schizophrenia Bulletin* 17, 75–98.

Siris, S.G. (1996) The treatment of schizoaffective disorder. In: *Current Psychiatric Therapy II* (ed. D.L. Dunner), pp. 196–201. W.B. Saunders, Philadelphia.

Siris, S.G. (2000) Depression in schizophrenia: perspective in the era of 'atypical' antipsychotic agents. *American Journal of Psychiatry* 157, 1379–1389.

Siris, S.G. (2001a) Suicide and schizophrenia. *Journal of Psychopharmacology* 15, 129–137.

Siris, S.G. (2001b) Depression in the course of schizophrenia. In: *Schizophrenia and Comorbid Conditions: Diagnosis and Treatment* (eds. M.Y. Hwang & P.C. Bermanzohn), pp. 31–56. American Psychiatric Press, Washington, DC.

Siris, S.G. & Lavin, M.R. (1995) Schizoaffective disorder, schizophreniform disorder, and acute psychotic disorder. In: *Comprehensive Textbook of Psychiatry* Vol. 1, 6th edn (eds H.I. Kaplan & B.J. Sadock), pp. 1019–1031, Williams & Wilkins, Baltimore.

Siris, S.G., van Kammen, D.P. & Docherty, J.P. (1978) The use of antidepressant medication in schizophrenia: a review of the literature. *Archives of General Psychiatry* 35, 1368–1377.

Siris, S.G., Harmon, G.K. & Endicott, J. (1981) Postpsychotic depressive symptoms in hospitalized schizophrenic patients. *Archives of General Psychiatry* 38, 1122–1123.

Siris, S.G., Rifkin, A., Reardon, G.T. *et al.* (1984) The dexamethasone suppression test in patients with post-psychotic depressions. *Biological Psychiatry* 19, 1351–1356.

Siris, S.G., Morgan, V., Fagerstrom, R., Rifkin, A. & Cooper, T.B. (1987) Adjunctive imipramine in the treatment of post-psychotic depression: a controlled trial. *Archives of General Psychiatry* 44, 533–539.

Siris, S.G., Strahan, A., Mandeli, J., Cooper, T.B. & Casey, E. (1988a) Fluphenazine decanoate dose and severity of depression in patients with post-psychotic depression. *Schizophrenia Research* 1, 31–35.

Siris, S.G., Adan, F., Cohen, M. *et al.* (1988b) Post-psychotic depression and negative symptoms: an investigation of syndromal overlap. *American Journal of Psychiatry* 145, 1532–1537.

Siris, S.G., Adan, F., Lee, A. *et al.* (1988c) Patterns of plasma imipramine/desipramine concentrations in patients receiving concomitant fluphenazine decanoate. *Journal of Clinical Psychiatry* 49, 64–65.

Siris, S.G., Sellew, A.P., Frechen, K. *et al.* (1988d) Antidepressants in the treatment of post-psychotic depression in schizophrenia: drug interactions and other considerations. *Journal of Clinical Chemistry* 34, 837–840.

Siris, S.G., Cutler, J., Owen, K. *et al.* (1989) Adjunctive imipramine maintenance in schizophrenic patients with remitted post-psychotic depressions. *American Journal of Psychiatry* 146, 1495–1497.

Siris, S.G., Bermanzohn, P.C., Gonzalez, A. *et al.* (1991a) The use of antidepressants for negative symptoms in a subset of schizophrenic patients. *Psychopharmacology Bulletin* 27, 331–335.

Siris, S.G., Frechen, K., Strahan, A. *et al.* (1991b) Thyroid-releasing hormone test in schizophrenic patients with post-psychotic depression. *Progress in Neuro-Psychopharmacology and Biological Psychiatry* 15, 369–378.

Siris, S.G., Bermanzohn, P.C., Mason, S.E. & Shuwall, M.A. (1994) Maintenance imipramine for secondary depression in schizophrenia: a controlled trial. *Archives of General Psychiatry* 51, 109–115.

Siris, S.G., Addington, D., Azorin, J.-M. *et al.* (2001) Depression in schizophrenia: recognition and management in the USA. *Schizophrenia Research* 47, 185–197.

Smith, T.E., Hull, J.W., Israel, L.M. & Willson, D.F. (2000) Insight, symptoms, and neurocognition in schizophrenia and schizoaffective disorder. *Schizophrenia Bulletin* 26, 193–200.

Spina, E., DeDomenico, P., Ruello, C. *et al.* (1994) Adjunctive fluoxetine in the treatment of negative symptoms in chronic schizophrenic patients. *International Clinical Psychopharmacology* 9, 281–285.

Spitzer, R.L., Endicott, J. & Robins, E. (1978) Research Diagnostic Criteria: rationale and reliability. *Archives of General Psychiatry* 35, 773–782.

Stephens, J.H., Richard, P. & McHugh, P.R. (1997) Long-term follow-up of patients hospitalized for schizophrenia, 1913–40. *Journal of Nervous and Mental Disease* 185, 715–721.

Stephens, J.H., Richard, P. & McHugh, P.R. (1999) Suicide in patients hospitalized for schizophrenia, 1913–40. *Journal of Nervous and Mental Disease* 187, 10–14.

Strian, F., Heger, R. & Klicpera, C. (1982) The time structure of depressive mood in schizophrenic patients. *Acta Psychiatrica Scandinavica* **65**, 66–73.

Subotnik, K.L. & Nuechterlein, K.H. (1988) Prodromal signs and symptoms of schizophrenic relapse. *Journal of Abnormal Psychology* **97**, 405–412.

Summers, F., Harrow, M. & Westermeyer, J. (1983) Neurotic symptoms in the postacute phase of schizophrenia. *Journal of Nervous and Mental Disease* **171**, 216–221.

Szymanski, H.V., Simon, J.C. & Gutterman, N. (1983) Recovery from schizophrenic psychosis. *American Journal of Psychiatry* **140**, 335–338.

Taiminen, T., Syvälahti, E., Saarijärvi, S. et al. (1997) Citalopram as an adjuvant in schizophrenia: further evidence for a sertonergic dimension in schizophrenia. *International Clinical Psychopharmacology* **12**, 31–35.

Tandon, R., Harrigan, E. & Zorn, S.H. (1997) Ziprasidone: a novel antipsychotic with unique pharmacology and therapeutic potential. *Journal of Serotonin Research* **4**, 159–177.

Tapp, A., Tandon, R., Douglass, A. et al. (1994) Depression in severe chronic schizophrenia. *Biological Psychiatry* **35**, 667.

Taylor, M.A. (1992) Are schizophrenia and affective disorder related? A selective literature review. *American Journal of Psychiatry* **149**, 22–32.

Tollefson, G.D. & Andersen, S.W. (1999) Should we consider mood disturbance in schizophrenia as an important determinant of quality of life? *Journal of Clinical Psychiatry* **60** (Suppl. 5), 23–29.

Tollefson, G.D. & Sanger, T.M. (1997) Negative symptoms: a path analytic approach to a double-blind, placebo- and haloperidol-controlled clinical trial with olanzapine. *American Journal of Psychiatry* **154**, 466–474.

Tollefson, G.D., Beasley, C.M. Jr, Tran, P.V. et al. (1997) Olanzapine versus haloperidol in the treatment of schizophrenia and schizoaffective and schizophreniform disorders: results of an international collaborative trial. *American Journal of Psychiatry* **154**, 457–465.

Tollefson, G.D., Sanger, T.M., Beasley, C.M. & Tran, P.V. (1998a) A double-blind, controlled comparison of the novel antipsychotic olanzapine versus haloperidol or placebo on anxious and depressive symptoms accompanying schizophrenia. *Biological Psychiatry* **43**, 803–810.

Tollefson, G.D., Sanger, T.M., Lu, Y. & Thieme, M.E. (1998b) Depressive signs and symptoms in schizophrenia: a prospective blinded trial of olanzapine and haloperidol. *Archives of General Psychiatry* **55**, 250–258.

Tollefson, G.D., Andersen, S.W. & Tran, P.V. (1999) The course of depressive symptoms in predicting relapse in schizophrenia: a double-blind, randomized comparison of olanzapine and risperidone. *Biological Psychiatry* **46**, 365–373.

Trichard, C., Paillère-Martinot, M.-L., Attar-Levy, D. et al. (1998) No sertonin 5-HT$_{2A}$ receptor density abnormality in the cortex of schizophrenic patients studied with PET. *Schizophrenia Research* **31**, 13–17.

Tsuang, M.T. (1978) Suicide in schizophrenics, manics, depressives, and surgical controls. *Archives of General Psychiatry* **35**, 153–155.

Tugg, L.A., Desai, D., Predergast, P. et al. (1997) Relationship between negative symptoms in chronic schizophrenia and neuroleptic dose, plasma levels and side effects. *Schizophrenia Research* **25**, 71–78.

Vandel, B., Vandel, S., Allers, G., Bechtel, P. & Volmat, R. (1979) Interaction between amitriptyline and phenothiazine in man: effect on plasma concentration of amitriptyline and its metabolite nortriptyline and the correlation with clinical response. *Psychopharmcology* **65**, 187–190.

Van Putten, T. (1975) The many faces of akathisia. *Comprehensive Psychiatry* **16**, 43–47.

Van Putten, T. & May, P.R.A. (1978) 'Akinetic depression' in schizophrenia. *Archives of General Psychiatry* **35**, 1101–1107.

Verhoeff, N.P.L.G., Meyer, J.H., Kecojevic, A. et al. (2000) A voxel-by-voxel analysis of [^{18}F]septoperone PET data shows no substantial serotonin 5-HT$_{2A}$ receptor changes in schizophrenia. *Psychiatry Research Neuroimaging* **99**, 123–135.

Vlokh, I., Mikhnyak, S. & Kachura, O. (2000) Zoloft in management of depression in schizophrenia [Abstract]. *Schizophrenia Research* **41**, 209.

Voruganti, L., Cortese, L., Oyewumi, L. et al. (2000) Comparative evaluation of conventional and novel antipsychotic drugs with reference to their subjective tolerability, side-effect profile and impact on quality of life. *Schizophrenia Research* **43**, 135–145.

Waehrens, J. & Gerlach, J. (1980) Antidepressant drugs in anergic schizophrenia: a double-blind cross-over study with maprotiline and placebo. *Acta Psychiatrica Scandinavica* **61**, 438–444.

Walker, A.M., Lanza, L.L., Arellano, F. & Rothman, K.J. (1998) Mortality in current and former users of clozapine. *Epidemiology* **8**, 671–679.

Wassink, T.H., Rose, S., Flaum, M. & Andreasen, N.C. (1997) The prevalence and predictive validity of early depressive symptoms in the course of schizophrenia. *Schizophrenia Research* **24**, 25.

Wassink, T.H., Flaum, M., Nopoulos, P. & Andreasen, N.C. (1999) Prevalence of depressive symptoms early in the course of schizophrenia. *American Journal of Psychiatry* **156**, 315–316.

Weissman, M.M., Pottenger, M., Kleber, H. et al. (1977) Symptom patterns in primary and secondary depression: a comparison of primary depressives with depressed opiate addicts, alcoholics, and schizophrenics. *Archives of General Psychiatry* **34**, 854–862.

Wiersma, D., Nienhuis, F.J., Sloof, C.J. & Giel, R. (1998) Natural course of schizophrenic disorders: a 15-year followup of a Dutch incidence cohort. *Schizophrenia Bulletin* **24**, 75–85.

Winokur, G. (1972) Family history studies. VIII. Secondary depression is alive and well. *Diseases of the Nervous System* **33**, 94–99.

Wise, R.A. (1982) Neuroleptics and operant behavior: the anhedonia hypothesis. *Behavioral and Brain Sciences* **5**, 39–87.

Wistedt, B. & Palmstierna, T. (1983) Depressive symptoms in chronic schizophrenic patients after withdrawal of long-acting neuroleptics. *Journal of Clinical Psychiatry* **44**, 369–371.

Wright, I.C., Ellison, Z.R., Sharma, T. et al. (1999) Mapping of grey matter changes in schizophrenia. *Schizophrenia Research* **35**, 1–14.

Yamagami, S. & Soejima, K. (1989) Effect of maprotiline combined with conventional neuroleptics against negative symptoms of chronic schizophrenia. *Drugs under Experimental and Clinical Research* **15**, 171–176.

Zakzanis, K.K. & Hansen, K.T. (1998) Dopamine D$_2$ densities and the schizophrenic brain. *Schizophrenia Research* **32**, 201–206.

Zisook, S., McAdams, L.A., Kuck, J. et al. (1999) Depressive symptoms in schizophrenia. *American Journal of Psychiatry* **156**, 1736–1743.

Zubin, J. & Spring, B. (1977) Vulnerability: a new view of schizophrenia. *Journal of Abnormal Psychology* **86**, 103–126.

10 Neurocognitive deficits in schizophrenia

T.E. Goldberg, A. David and J.M. Gold

Abnormalities in attentional, associative and volitional cognitive processes have been considered central features of schizophrenia since the original clinical descriptions of Kraepelin (1919/1971) and Bleuler (1950). The application of formal psychological assessment techniques in hundreds of studies in dozens of independent laboratories over the past 70 years has more than amply documented that such abnormalities are common occurrences in patients with the disorder. For example, nearly 60 years ago, Rappaport *et al.* (1945/46) published *Diagnostic Psychological Testing*, an influential work reporting findings from the application of a broad test battery to a wide variety of psychiatric patients. In describing deteriorated chronic schizophrenic patients, they noted that such patients had their greatest impairments in 'judgement, attention, concentration, planning ability and anticipation'. They further commented on the memory difficulties, inadequate concept formation and general intellectual inefficiency of patients with schizophrenia. Although interpreted within a psychodynamic framework and prior to the narrowing of the diagnostic conceptualization of schizophrenia and introduction of modern pharmacotherapy, the empirical observations made in the early 1940s are remarkably consistent with current findings. Indeed, we would suggest that the vast body of data on cognitive functioning in schizophrenia has been remarkably uniform over many years. What has changed is the significance attributed to these results.

In the last 15 years, the routine use of clinical neuropsychological assessment and experimental neuropsychological paradigms has offered a new look to accounts of schizophrenia. Indeed, recent studies have thrown light on several of the more problematic facets of the disorder. In particular, they have made important contributions to understanding the course of cognitive impairment, the specificity of profiles of cognitive impairment to schizophrenia and the prognostic importance of deficits. More recently still, the putative importance of cognitive impairment in understanding cardinal symptoms of schizophrenia and in understanding the genetics of schizophrenia is coming to be appreciated. In this chapter we attempt to address some of the classical issues inherent in neurocognitive approaches to schizophrenia and present newer componential accounts of impairments in attention, working memory and episodic memory. Additionally, there have been several novel applications of neurocognition in schizophrenia, including relating impairments to symptoms and using impairments as intermediate phenotypes in genetic studies, which are reviewed.

Course of cognitive impairment

Subtle attenuations in premorbid developmental milestones and cognitive and academic functions have been demonstrated in schizophrenia that date to the 'prodromal' period or before (David *et al.* 1997; Jones & Cannon 1998; Davidson *et al.* 1999). After clinical onset the course of schizophrenia has sometimes been considered similar to that of progressive dementia in that there is relentless social and presumably cognitive decline. However, there are a great many neuropsychological studies that do not support this view (Heaton & Drexler 1987) and a broad literature can be drawn upon to support a different account which emphasizes features in the course consistent with the notion of 'static encephalopathy'. Within the first few years of their clinical illness, patients typically perform poorly on a wide range of tests which include those assessing memory, executive functions and attentional abilities (Goldberg & Weinberger 1988; Saykin *et al.* 1994; Censits *et al.* 1997; Gold *et al.* 1999). In this period, variability in repeated assessment might also occur, as patients' scores may even improve slightly (Sweeney *et al.* 1991). Longitudinal studies of armed forces personnel, prior to the onset of illness and during its active phase, are consistent with results that suggest relatively abrupt declines in functioning. Thus, on armed forces ability tests, patients performed similarly to their controls in the premorbid period and then displayed significant decrements of near 0.5 standard deviation (SD) after the onset of illness (Lubin *et al.* 1962; Schwartzman & Douglas 1962).

Crucially, deterioration does not appear to occur during the early chronic phase of the illness. It thus appears to be self-arresting. For instance, over intervals of 8 years, the performance of patients did not decline on tests such as the Wechsler Adult Intelligence Scale and Halstead–Reitan measures when assessed longitudinally (Smith 1964; Klonoff *et al.* 1970; Rund 1998). In several large cross-sectional studies using tests known to be sensitive to progressive dementias, using IQ or using variants of the Halstead–Reitan Battery, no differences were found between patients with longer durations of illness and those with shorter durations above and beyond ageing (Goldstein & Zubin 1990; Heaton *et al.* 1994; Hyde *et al.* 1994; Mockler *et al.* 1997). On the other hand, Harvey *et al.* (1998a,b) have strongly argued that some although not all patients suffer a very gradual but demonstrable decline in cognitive abilities throughout adulthood on such screening instruments as the Mini Mental Status Examination, and in late life more striking declines in cognitive and functional status. However, the role of chronic institutionalization is not completely understood.

Several correlation studies have not supported cognitive deteriorations with increasing chronicity. In perhaps the best of these, Gold *et al.* (1999) in a large and well-characterized sample found that associations between duration of illness and cognitive level were weak and non-significant (but see Cuesta *et al.* 1998).

Results which support the notion that schizophrenia is a static encephalopathy are also consistent with the observation of Kraepelin (1919/1971): 'As a rule, if no essential improvement intervenes in at most two or three years after the appearance of the more striking morbid phenomena, a state of weak mindedness will be developed, which usually changes only slowly and insignificantly'. Shakow (1946) also noted that, despite individual variations in course, 'the most frequent type is that which resembles temporally the process of oblivescence, a considerable drop at first with the tapering off through a slowed period to a stable level'.

Core neurocognitive deficits

Despite the difficult methodological issues involved in establishing differential deficits, the clinical interpretation of test data can often point to multiple studies that converge on a set of frequent, severe and selective deficits. In our view, patients with schizophrenia typically demonstrate abnormalities in attention/executive function and memory which stand out against a background of diffuse impairment. Although this view cannot, at present, be proven, the apparent impairments in these cognitive functions are of interest in relation to other neurobiological findings in the illness, such as structural abnormalities of the temporal lobe, dysfunctional activation of the prefrontal cortex and abnormalities in catecholamine function.

Attention

Even the casual observer may often be struck by deficits in the capacity of patients to cull information from their environment. Simply put, patients do not seem to focus attention, to anticipate and to sustain concentration. Moreover, they sometimes appear to be preoccupied with internal stimuli at the expense of salient environmental events, or are easily distracted by external stimuli. While such observations, both historical and clinical, have been broadly supported by numerous studies of sustained and selective attention, the precise nature of the impairments has been more difficult to articulate. One of the early experimental studies of attention, devised by Shakow (1979), found that patients with schizophrenia demonstrate slowed reaction time and, moreover, could not improve their performance even when intervals between warning and stimulus were both predictable and long. Thus, patients appeared to be unable to sustain attention, compromising their readiness to respond across longer time intervals. In another set of attentional paradigms, schizophrenic patients had deficits maintaining vigilance during a continuous performance test involving specific combinations of stimuli (Mirsky 1988). Patients typically failed to respond to target stimuli and also responded inappropriately to lures, thereby making both omission and commission errors. However, the meaning of these studies is unclear. Shakow's results might have been caused by failures in context or working memory, resulting in loss of the warning cue's readying function, while Continuous Performance Test (CPT) errors may be caused in part by deficiencies in encoding information or biasing perceptual modules to targets, such that patients were unable to make decisions based on an adequate representation of the stimulus (Elvevåg *et al.* 2000e).

It is clear that attention is not a unitary construct, but it is unclear whether there is a particular dimension that is maximally impaired in schizophrenia. Posner and Dehaene (1994) developed an elegant model of the components of spatial attention. An initial examination of this model in schizophrenia was potentially promising: Posner *et al.* (1988) reported that schizophrenic patients displayed an asymmetrical slowing in response to stimuli that appeared in the right visual field after so-called invalid cues for a response. However, attempts to replicate this study have not met with success (e.g. Gold *et al.* 1992). Another aspect of attention involves selective attention. In the Stroop test, an exemplar of this class of tests, a prepotent response must be inhibited and a less salient conflicting response made (e.g. stating the colour of the word 'green' when it is printed in red ink). Several studies have found that patients display an increased cost in the incongruent condition or an increased advantage in the congruent condition (Perlstein *et al.* 1998; Elvevåg *et al.* 2000a).

It is also important to consider the extent to which attention is modularized; that is, attentional impairments may or may not disrupt many other cognitive functions. One might assume that poor attention would prevent many types of information from being processed fully. However, correlational studies have generally suggested that attentional dysfunction explains only a small portion of the variance in other cognitive functions (Kenny & Meltzer 1991). Perhaps this should not come as a complete surprise, as patients with well-documented attentional deficit disorders often display many areas of intact cognitive function (Barkley *et al.* 1990). It remains to be seen whether this is because of the properties of the distributed neural system underlying attention (Mesulum 1985) or whether it simply reflects some dissociation between the ecology of the testing situation and the rest of an individual's environment.

Episodic memory

Episodic memory involves binding items and spatiotemporal context to form an episode that can be more or less permanently stored. It is critical in the acquisiton of new information. Its function in schizophrenia was one of the first cognitive abilities to be studied (Hull 1917). The results of numerous studies since then, however, have been difficult to characterize from a cognitive science perspective. Patients with schizophrenia generally remember stories, verbal paired associates and visual designs more poorly than do normal subjects and differences between normal controls and patients may be large (Saykin et al. 1991; Gold et al. 1994). Rate of learning may be abnormal. Thus, Paulsen et al. (1995) found that a large sample of patients exhibited reduced learning slopes when a list of words was repeated over multiple trials. In tests of recognition memory in which retrieval strategies are minimized, patients are generally impaired, but perhaps less so than in free recall (Calev 1984; Gold et al. 1992; Paulsen et al. 1995). Deficits have been attributed not only to consolidation impairments, but to inefficient encoding (Traupmann 1980), poor use of retrieval strategies in effortful recall (Goldberg et al. 1989), rapid forgetting (Sengel & Lovalla 1983; McKenna et al. 1990) and differences between impaired conscious recall and a gross sense of familiarity with the material (Danion et al. 1999).

More recently, Elvevåg et al. (2000b; Elvevåg & Goldberg, unpublished data) have re-examined the possibility that a specific stage of mnemonic processing is disrupted in schizophrenia. They used deep and shallow levels of processing to examine encoding, an 'AB$_R$' paradigm (in which verbal paired associates were first learned and then followed by trials in which pairs were 'shuffled', creating interference and the necessity to 'unlearn') to examine the effects of interference of prior learning, and false memory to examine semantic context effects. They found that these cognitive manipulations exerted the same effect in patients as they did in normal controls, although patients performed more poorly overall. These results suggest that patients do not have qualitative abnormalities in mnemonic processing; rather, consistently poorer performance may be one of degree.

A conservative summary statement is probably in order: schizophrenic patients demonstrate clear deficits in episodic memory measures, i.e. they have difficulty retrieving episodes of experience within distinct spatiotemporal contexts. This is probably a function of multiple factors.

Executive function and working memory

Clinicians have frequently observed that schizophrenic patients have difficulty generating and implementing plans. Patients also appear to have difficulty solving problems whose solutions are not readily apparent, or when they must rely upon novel recom-

binations of existing knowledge. From the neuropsychological standpoint, such deficits are often considered to be 'executive' in nature, in the sense that they involve use of information rather than fundamental processing of the information. Formal tests of analogues of these abilities have usually revealed deficits in patients. For instance, Fey (1951) demonstrated that schizophrenic patients have performance deficits on the Wisconsin Card Sorting Test (WCST) of abstraction, set shifting and response to feedback. More recent studies (Goldberg et al. 1987) have also shown that chronic schizophrenic patients performed poorly on the WCST and had difficulty learning the task even when instructions were provided, suggesting that their capacity to maintain information 'on-line' was reduced.

Studies of verbal tasks also reveal deficits in working memory. Gold et al. (1994) found that schizophrenic patients performed more poorly than patients with temporal lobe epilepsy on tests demanding working memory from the Wechsler Adult Intelligence Scale–Revised. There are multiple reports of poor performance by patients with schizophrenia on variants of the Brown–Peterson task. This task involves remembering a short list of words over a brief delay (e.g. 12 s) during which interpolated distractor activities draw off 'processing resources' and/or prevent covert rehearsal of the to-be-remembered material. Goldberg et al. (1998) showed that patients were inordinately sensitive to interference, large set sizes and notably delay.

In a study involving simultaneous storage and processing of information, Gold et al. (1997) used a working memory task that required ordering short sequences of randomly presented numbers and letters (the so-called letter–number span). Patients fared poorly. Moreover, the degree of impairment was highly correlated with a test of problem solving and rule learning: the WCST. The relationship suggests that both tests, very different in their surface characteristics, may call upon a specialized computational workspace in which material must not only be maintained, but manipulated or transformed.

Several studies of schizophrenia have indicated that patients have impairments on even very basic tests of working memory. Park et al. (1995) showed that on oculomotor delayed response, a probe of prefrontal cortical function adapted from nonhuman primates, patients scored poorly. The finding was confirmed by Fleming et al. (1997) using a test of memory for patterns and locations. Simple short-term working memory for verbal memory indexed by digit span and involving only veridical reproduction of the items and their sequence has been repeatedly found to be impaired in schizophrenia. Indeed, a meta-analysis indicated that the effect size of the difference between normal controls and patients was large and highly significant (Aleman et al. 1999).

Much recent work has focused on a task requiring both intradimensional and extradimensional (ID/ED) set shifting which reflects, at least in part, a componential version of the WCST. In intradimensional shifts, subjects are required to change their response set to an alternative design within a category (e.g. a new exemplar of a line design) while an irrelevant dimension (e.g. shape), which had been introduced earlier, continues to be ignored. At a later stage, an extradimensional shift is demanded as new exemplars are again introduced but subjects are now required to respond to the previously irrelevant dimension (e.g. shapes rather than lines). Subjects make decisions that were based on feedback after each trial. Chronic schizophrenic patients displayed markedly impaired attentional set shifting on the ID/ED task. Pantelis *et al.* (1999) reported that patients with schizophrenia demonstrated a significantly higher rate of attrition at the intradimensional shift stage compared with frontal lobe patients and they were similarly impaired in comparison to frontal lobe patients on the extradimensional shift stage (Pantelis *et al.* 1999). Chronic patients were also impaired on spatial memory span and spatial working memory tasks. The Tower of London test, which involves planning and memory, was impaired in patients with schizophrenia as they made fewer perfect solutions and required more moves and time to complete the task. Thus, patients with schizophrenia showed an overall deficit in executive function, often greater than that observed in patients with frontal lobe lesions (Pantelis *et al.* 1997).

Several studies have indicated that working memory impairment is present in schizophrenia, even in relatively intellectually intact individuals. For instance, Pantelis *et al.* (1999) found that while patients with high IQ performed better than patients with low IQ, performance was still remarkably abnormal. Their performances at the intradimensional shifting stage were below that of normals and markedly below that of normals in extradimensional shifting. Elliott *et al.* (1995) were able to confirm these results, even in patients with preserved intellectual function (IQs greater than 100). Weickert *et al.* (2000) used a different methodology to come to similar conclusions. They found that patients with developmentally compromised intellectual function, normal premorbid intellectual function that declined significantly (the modal subgroup in this study) and with preserved intellectual function (i.e. both current and putative premorbid IQ were normal) displayed deficits compared with a normal control group on WCST's measure of perseveration. Thus, impaired executive function appears to be a core deficit in that it is present irrespective of IQ pattern.

Differential deficits and neuropsychiatry comparative studies

One of the goals of neuropsychological and cognitive research in schizophrenia is to identify abnormalities in particular cognitive processes that are linked to specific brain regions or systems. The neuropsychologically based search for such a 'fundamental' deficit or deficits faces a basic methodological challenge. As noted by Chapman and Chapman (1973), patients with schizophrenia tend to perform more poorly than normal controls on a wide variety of tasks. They demonstrate a 'generalized' deficit whose origin remains undetermined. Such a deficit might conceivably reflect the experience of institutionalization, failures in co-operation or diffuse brain dysfunction. Of greater theoretical

interest, however, is the existence of 'differential' deficits, i.e. deficits more severe than might be anticipated on the basis of the generalized deficit. Such differential deficits could provide evidence of regionally specific neurocognitive impairment with implications for understanding schizophrenic pathology and pathophysiology. Current clinical assessment test batteries are not capable of rigorously supporting inferences of differential deficit. To demonstrate differential deficit adequately, tasks should be matched on the basis of difficulty level and reliability, so that ceiling effects or measurement error do not skew the results. Very few matched tasks have been developed (Calev 1984) and these tasks have generally not been incorporated into standard clinical assessment batteries or experimental procedures. Certainly, findings that patients perform worse on an easier task than a harder task (e.g. semantic fluency is more impaired than letter fluency; Gourovitch *et al.* 1996) strengthen the interpretation of results.

Another aspect of task matching that is frequently overlooked involves the dispersion of test scores. Some tests are constructed such that it is difficult to score more than 2 SD below the normal control mean, while on many other tests it is possible to score several standard deviations below normal (Randolph *et al.* 1993). Therefore, one could conclude incorrectly that an individual's performance on the latter group is worse than on the former group of tests. It should be recognized that when a difference is found between groups, that difference is valid in terms of its existence. On the other hand, claims that one impaired performance is necessarily more deficient than another impaired performance, or that a normal performance is 'truly' normal, are not valid if tasks are not matched. In summary, the interpretation of neuropsychological findings remains largely a matter of clinical judgement, a process which has clear limitations for supporting more specific inferences about areas of maximal dysfunction in a population with widespread cognitive difficulties.

There are no easy solutions to these problems of measurement. One statistical approach involves comparing the residuals from a regression line that is derived from two variables of interest (Chapman & Chapman 1989). In patients with verified neurological disorders, an approach that has been fruitful in identifying differential deficit patterns involves a search for double dissociations (Teuber 1955; Shallice 1988). In this method, two patient groups are compared on two tests. If one group outperforms the other on the first test, but is itself outperformed on the second, then one infers that the groups have a differential profile of performance. This latter approach, underutilized in previous schizophrenia research, has recently been used by Gold *et al.* (1994) in a study of temporal lobe epilepsy and schizophrenia and by Goldberg *et al.* (1990a) in a study of Huntington's disease and schizophrenia. In the former, patients with schizophrenia had worse attentional but better semantic functioning than did patients with left temporal lobe epilepsy. In the latter, patients with schizophrenia had worse attentional but better visual spatial functioning in comparison with patients with Huntington's disease. While the double dissociation approach is not immune to psychometric artefacts (i.e. one test being 'harder' than the other), it appears to have a distinct advantage over studies comparing patients and normal controls.

Nevertheless, strong claims have been made that schizophrenic cognitive impairment reflects generalized impairment. The argument has been made on psychometric grounds through the use of carefully selected tests (Blanchard and Neale 1994) and by way of the use of large normative databases for the Halstead–Reitan Battery (Braff *et al.* 1991). However, careful clinical analysis of results may suggest otherwise. Using tests with well-established brain–behaviour relationships, Kolb and Whishaw (1983) proposed that schizophrenia reflected executive-memory (i.e. frontomedial temporal lobe) dysfunction. In a series of detailed case studies, Shallice *et al.* (1991) observed consistent evidence for executive dysfunction. Weickert *et al.* (2000) showed that the modal patient in a series of 117 consecutively admitted patients exhibited rather circumscribed executive, attentional and memory impairments, although a significant minority of patients exhibited a diffuse pattern of cognitive impairment. Moreover, these results are not subject to criticisms about difficulty level and dispersion, given that they derive from subgroups obtained from a single 'population'. Importantly, deficits in working memory and cognitive control over attentional processes were present even when IQ was preserved.

The identification of a characteristic neurocognitive profile of schizophrenia relative to other disorders provides useful information concerning the fundamental validity of the accumulated neurocognitive findings. Differences in overall global impairment (i.e. level) may have important implications for everyday functioning. Differences in profile of impairment (i.e. shape) may help to sharpen the discussion of anatomical implications of deficits and identify useful measures for intermediate phenotypes in genetic linkage or association studies. Furthermore, these comparative differential deficits derived from comparative studies could provide targets for rehabilitative and pharmacological treatment efforts.

In particular, the comparison of schizophrenic patients and patients with mood disorders offers some insight into the clinical importance of neuropsychological functioning, given the fact that the outcome of schizophrenia is worse in terms of social and vocational functioning than that observed in mood disorders. If the disability of schizophrenic patients reflects neuropsychological impairment, then one would expect formal testing to distinguish the diagnostic groups. The results of a study by Goldberg *et al.* (1993a) support this view. A schizophrenic group performed significantly below affective groups (unipolar and bipolar) on tests of attention and psychomotor speed, verbal and visual memory, and problem solving and abstraction. Values of IQ were also low in the schizophrenic group and appeared to have deteriorated from a normal premorbid level. Moreover, when the analysis was restricted to patients with IQ scores of 90 or more, the patients with schizophrenia still performed more poorly than did the mood disorder group on the WCST and visual memory tests, suggesting that inadequacy of global cognitive competence was not the sole source of the intergroup difference.

While affective psychoses have come under increasing scrutiny in terms of their cognitive relations to schizophrenia, in a recent review of the literature that directly compared patients with bipolar disorder to schizophrenia, Goldberg (1999) concluded that the results provide support for the view that patients with bipolar disorders suffer less severe cognitive impairments than do patients with schizophrenia. While several studies have found the groups to be equivalent in impairment, no study has found bipolar patients to be consistently worse than patients with schizophrenia (with the possible exception of backward masking); indeed, the majority of studies have found that schizophrenic patients have worse cognitive function. With respect to profile, patients with schizophrenia appear to have more severe and more frequent working memory impairments. However, it is important to note that patients with affective psychosis have cognitive impairment.

Concurrent and predictive validity of neuropsychological impairment

Neurocognitive deficits may be a rate-limiting factor in the rehabilitation of patients with schizophrenia. For instance, in a study of patients receiving clozapine, Goldberg *et al.* (1993b) observed that while patients' symptoms improved markedly over the 15-month study period, the patients still required supervised living arrangements and could not work in high-level competitive situations. Because their neuropsychological profile remained impaired and unchanged, neurocognitive deficits might have accounted for some of the continuing disabilities. Strong concurrent relations between the global level of functioning and specific neurocognitive test scores have been found (Goldberg *et al.* 1990b, 1995). In a monozygotic (MZ) twin study in which patients were concordant for schizophrenia (thus controlling for genome, educational and family environment, experience of illness and medication), cognitive measures, which included memory for stories from the Wechsler memory scale, verbal fluency, WCST and IQ, of intratwin pair differences were strongly and significantly associated with differences in social and vocational functioning as measured by the global assessment scale (GAS). In addition, in MZ twins concordant for schizophrenia, a group in whom symptomatology was similar, as was the experience of having a chronic illness, differences in a set of cognitive measures (trails, IQ, WCST and memory quotient) accounted for over 95% of the variance in intrapair differences in GAS scores.

In several important meta-analyses, Green (1996) has convincingly shown that executive and attentional impairments account for about 20% of functional outcome, while both short- and long-term memory account for about 30% and 40%, respectively, of the variance in a variety of functional outcome domains. In this type of analysis, the combined sample sizes were large and the relationships between neurocognition and functional outcome were highly significant. Global indicators of cognitive impairment showed even stronger relationships with outcome.

In contrast, psychotic symptoms (hallucinations and delusions) are not strong predictors and correlates of functional outcome (Green *et al.* 2000). Negative symptoms have higher correlations with functional outcome than positive symptoms, but across studies the relationships are neither stronger nor more consistent than those for neurocognitive deficits (Dickerson *et al.* 1996; Velligan *et al.* 1997; Harvey *et al.* 1998a). The relative contributions of symptoms and neurocognition to functional outcome have only rarely been directly compared with appropriate statistical analyses, including multiple regression. In those studies that have made comparisons, the neurocognitive contributions to outcome were stronger than those from positive symptoms. While negative symptoms covaried to at least a modest extent with neurocognition (Dickerson *et al.* 1996; Velligan *et al.* 1997), their relationship to function appear to be mediated through statistical overlap; i.e. they did not make independent contributions to explain outcome variance.

It is likely that some cognitive domains have direct causal relationships on daily functions, while others may be related to functional outcome through mediators, such as social cognition or the appropriate timely application of knowledge and reasoning to problem solving.

Treatment effects on cognition in schizophrenia: atypical neuroleptic medications

The vast majority of studies published over the last 4 decades examining aspects of neurocognitive performance in patients with schizophrenia have been conducted with samples of patients studied while they were receiving antipsychotic medications. This had led to a persistent concern articulated in the literature that it was not possible to determine, in principle, if the impairments observed were fully attributable to the illness, the impact of antipsychotic medication (and related side-effects) or some combination of the two (Spohn *et al.* 1985; Spohn & Strauss 1989). This concern, coupled with evidence that treatment with conventional antipsychotic agents led to the development of tardive dyskinesia in a significant number of patients, was the context for a series of independent extensive narrative literature reviews written in the 1980s and early 1990s examining the cognitive effects of conventional antipsychotics (Heaton & Crowley 1981; Medalia *et al.* 1988; Spohn & Strauss 1989; Cassens *et al.* 1990; King 1990; Bilder *et al.* 1992). The reviews of this large literature, spanning from the late 1950s through the 1980s, came to remarkably similar conclusions: there was little convincing evidence that treatment with conventional antipsychotics had significant cognitive benefits or costs. Costs observed in motor performance were often attributed to ex-

trapyramidal symptoms, and possible memory 'costs' were often thought to be brought about by the impact of anticholinergic medications used as adjunctive treatments. Benefits were most frequently, but not always, reported on tasks requiring sustained attention or resisting the impact of distracting stimuli. However, new meta-analyses (T.E. Goldberg, unpublished; Keefe & Harvey 2001) suggest modest improvements with typical or atypical neuroleptic medications in higher level cognitive domains. These reviews, combined with studies documenting substantial impairment in neuroleptic naïve first-episode samples (Saykin *et al.* 1994), as well as an attenuated pattern of impairment among untreated non-psychotic first-degree relatives (Cannon *et al.* 1994; Faraone *et al.* 1995; Egan *et al.* 2001), all support the basic notion that the cognitive impairments observed in samples of medicated patients could be reliably attributed to the illness and did not represent medication-related artefacts.

Moreover, while the results from studies examining the cognitive effects of conventional agents appear to be highly reproducible, there are a number of reasons to regard conclusions drawn from this literature with skepticism. As noted by reviewers, the methodological quality of the vast majority of studies in the area was quite poor, limiting confidence in the validity of conclusions that can be drawn. Sample sizes were typically small, doses were frequently higher (or uncontrolled) than contemporary clinical practice, and many studies failed to control for the expected gains brought about by repeated testing (e.g. many studies failed to use either control groups or alternative forms for testing materials). In addition, although the relationship between symptom severity and cognitive performance is typically quite modest, it is clearly unidirectional, with better performance associated with reduced symptom severity in the vast majority of studies (Strauss 1993). Thus, the clinical symptomatic benefits of antipsychotic treatment should again lead to an expectation of enhanced performance, albeit indirect, relative to unmedicated performance levels. Beyond the methodological limitations of the literature, there is an increasing appreciation for the role of dopamine in mediating aspects of cognition, including working memory and the processing of error and reward signals (Müller *et al.* 1998; Schultz 1998). Indeed, it would be surprising if nearly complete blockade of D_2 receptors, as achieved by conventional antipsychotic agents at high doses, did not have cognitive consequences. Recent work in non-human primates demonstrating a substantial deficit in working memory performance following treatment with D_2 blocking agents, an effect that was partially alleviated by treatment with a D_1 agonist, illustrates both the prominent role of dopamine in cortical function and the complexity of receptor interactions in the intact brain (Castner *et al.* 2000).

These lingering qualms about the cognitive effects of conventional antipsychotics have been magnified by the introduction of a number of new generation or 'atypical' antipsychotics. The receptor affinities of these compounds differ from one another substantially (Bymaster *et al.* 1996). However, they share the ability to achieve an antipsychotic effect largely in the absence of extrapyramidal side-effects resulting from striatal D_2 blockade. Although there is ongoing debate about the possible mechanism(s) of action of the newer agents, it is clear that chronic blockade of upwards of 80% of D_2 receptors is not required for antipsychotic efficacy, as had been thought to be the case for conventional antipsychotics (Kapur & Seeman 2000; Kapur et al. 2000a,b). Along with reduced side-effect burden, there are claims that the second-generation agents may offer cognitive advantages relative to conventional agents, and may in fact even be cognitive 'enhancers'. Given this linkage between cognitive impairment and functional outcomes, the demonstration of a clear cognitive benefit resulting from treatment with new generation compounds would represent a dramatic step forward in schizophrenia therapeutics.

The available literature examining the cognitive effects of new generation antipsychotics has many of the methodological problems of the older literature: small (and likely unrepresentative) samples, uncontrolled practice effects in test–retest designs and few examples of random assignment double-blind within subject designs. Given the extensive industry sponsorship of studies examining cognitive effects of new generation compounds, there is an additional concern about possible reporting biases. Despite these limitations, the available literature, as recently reviewed by Keefe et al. (1999) and Meltzer and McGurk (1999), supports a number of broad conclusions. Most importantly, there is fairly consistent evidence that patients treated with new generation compounds demonstrate better cognitive performance than comparator groups (often the baseline performance of the same patients) receiving conventional agents. Such improvements have been noted following treatment with all of the new agents currently on the market including clozapine, olanzapine, risperidone and quetiapine. With one major exception discussed below, these advantages have been documented relative to conventional agents. Without head-to-head trials of new generation compounds, it is premature to draw conclusions about possible differential cognitive efficacy of the new agents, or possible differential effects of individual drugs on specific cognitive functions. Given the limitations of the literature at this point, it is only possible to address broad general issues. Most importantly, it appears that the cognitive benefits of new generation compounds are generally modest, with patients continuing to demonstrate marked impairments in most key domains of cognitive functioning relative to normal control subjects. Unfortunately, only one study has investigated if this subtle cognitive advantage impacts functional outcome. Buchanan et al. (1994) reported that the magnitude of change in memory performance following clozapine treatment was correlated with changes in clinical ratings of quality of life (although memory functioning did not improve significantly). This promising result has yet to be replicated or extended to specific functional outcomes of interest including degree of residential independence or vocational performance.

There is one likely exception to the generalization that new generation agents offer a modest advantage for cognitive performance relative to conventional antipsychotics. Freedman et al. have reported in a series of studies that patients with schizophrenia, and a significant number of their first-degree relatives, demonstrate an electrophysiological abnormality which has been named P50 (Freedman et al. 1997; Adler et al. 1998). This abnormality is elicited when pairs of auditory stimuli are presented; normal subjects demonstrate a reduced eletrophysiological response to the second stimuli, whereas patients fail to modulate/inhibit this response. Unlike conventional antipsychotics, both clozapine and risperidone appear to partially, if not largely, normalize this impairment (Nagamoto et al. 1996; Yee et al. 1998; Light et al. 2000). Thus, it may not be possible to document this genetically transmitted abnormality in patients treated with at least some of the new generation compounds, potentially limiting the further development of this promising and important line of research.

The most provocative study of new generation agents was recently published by Purdon et al. (2000) in a double-blind study comparing the cognitive effects of olanzapine, risperidone and haloperidol. They reported statistically significant advantages of olanzapine relative to both risperidone and haloperidol on a broad array of cognitive measures. Cognitive benefits of olanzapine were observed following 6 weeks of treatment, with further gains noted on later retest occasions. What is particularly noteworthy about this study is that the magnitude of change with olanzapine treatment on multiple tests was quite large: effect sizes >0. 6 were observed on measures of motor performance, verbal learning, perseverative behaviour, non-verbal fluency, visual perception and visual construction. There was much less evidence of a benefit of risperidone relative to haloperidol, in contrast to other published studies (Green et al. 1997; Kern et al. 1998, 1999). There are a number of potential methodological problems with the Purdon et al. study, chief among them the very high attrition rate over the course of the trial complicating the interpretation of results, particularly from the last two testing occasions, resulting in a very small sample. Whatever the limitations, this study raises the possibility that olanzapine may have a substantial cognitive advantage relative to both a conventional agent, haloperidol, and another new generation agent, risperidone. It clearly remains to be determined if the results of this important 'outlier' study can be independently replicated.

However, the issue remains of how to understand the implications of the cognitive advantage of new generation agents. Based on the available literature, it appears that several agents offer at least modest benefits, possibly in somewhat different cognitive domains, perhaps supporting a claim that these agents enhance cognitive function. A number of mechanisms have been speculatively proposed to explain the findings, including the role of 5-HT_{2A}-receptors, acetylcholine and D_1 (Keefe et al. 1999; Meltzer & McGurk 1999). Thus, different specific mechanisms would need to be invoked for the different compounds, given their differing affinities for these receptor systems. Although these mechanisms may prove to be important, it is striking that the most obvious possibility has rarely been discussed: each of the new generation agents achieves antipsychotic effects without inducing D_2-mediated extrapyramidal symptoms. Thus, the common 'cognitive denominator' of these agents may be reduced – or more transient – D_2 blockade relative to conventional agents (Kapur & Seeman 2000). If this speculative formulation were correct, it would suggest that the new generation drugs are advantageous because they do not exact a cognitive cost, whether it be directly on cortical information processing or more indirectly on subcortical motor speed and initiation. This formulation would suggest that the frequently observed advantage of new generation agents relative to conventional antipsychotics on measures of psychomotor speed and response production could be an indirect benefit: it may result from the removal of an adverse effect of high levels of chronic D_2 blockade on frontal–striatal systems. In addition, benefits observed on retesting could represent normal practice effects, with enhanced performance following multiple exposures to a number of testing instruments and procedures. Although a crucial form of learning, the biological implications of a restoration of practice effects vs. the direct enhancement of impaired neural systems may be different. The restoration of practice effects could result from the removal of an iatrogenic impediment; actual enhancement suggests a direct pharmacological benefit.

Pharmacology provides a specific window on the underlying neurobiology of the illness. Indeed, the failure of conventional agents to improve cognitive performance, despite being largely effective in the treatment of positive symptoms, was a critical piece of evidence that the symptomatic and cognitive features of the illness were partially independent. Thus, an accurate understanding of the cognitive effects of new generation agents is critical in guiding future drug development. If the cognitive benefits of new generation agents result from an actual enhancement of cortical function, then these agents might rightfully be considered as 'antischizophrenia' drugs rather than as antipsychotics. Alternatively, if the apparent advantage results from a lack of 'cost', then the mechanisms implicated in the clinical efficacy of the new agents are unlikely to prove to be important in the development of future cognitive enhancement treatment strategies.

Novel approaches

Neuropsychological investigations of psychotic symptoms

Is there a relationship between cognitive deficits and symptoms or syndromes within the schizophrenic group of disorders? Liddle (1987a) examined the relationships between symptoms rated on a symptomatic assessment scale (Krawiecka) in 40 patients with chronic schizophrenia, and demonstrated that symptoms segregated into three syndromes:
1 psychomotor poverty (reduced speech, lack of spontaneous movement and blunting of affect);
2 disorganization (inappropriate affect, poverty of content of speech, and disturbances in the form of thought); and

3 reality distortion (delusions and hallucinations).
Examination of the correlations between syndrome severity and performance on a range of well-standardized clinical neuropsychological tests revealed that each of the syndromes was associated with a specific pattern of neuropsychological impairment (Liddle 1987b). Whereas the psychomotor poverty syndrome was associated with poor performance in tests of conceptual thinking, object naming and long-term memory, the two syndromes linked with the presence of positive symptoms were associated with a different pattern of cognitive dysfunction. The disorganization syndrome was associated with poor performance in tests of concentration, immediate recall and word learning, and the reality distortion syndrome was associated with poor figure ground perception. A similar approach using factor analysis was undertaken by Basso et al. (1998) with 62 schizophrenia patients on whom a wide variety of clinical, demographic and neuropsychological measures were available. Negative symptoms were associated with a range of abnormalities such as impaired global IQ, executive function, motor skill, vigilance, attention and memory indices, while disorganization correlated with a subset of these (IQ, attention and motor tasks). Psychotic symptoms did not correlate with the standard tests.

Other research has focused on specific symptoms to understand their neuropsychological basis. This endeavour requires a shift away from the search for 'deficits' and requires a wider conception of cognitive processes, including excesses as well as deficits, dysfunctions and abnormal interactions (see Halligan & David, 2001) in order to generate mechanistic accounts of symptoms.

Hallucinations

There have been no convincing studies to suggest that auditory verbal hallucinations (AVHs) correlate with deficits on standard neuropsychological tests, unlike, for example, negative symptoms (for review see above and David & Cutting 1994).

Hemisphere dysfunction in auditory hallucinations has been examined utilizing the technique of dichotic listening. This entails competition between the right and left hemispheres in the identification of auditory stimuli presented simultaneously, one to each ear. When the stimuli are words or consonant–vowel syllables, input to the left hemisphere predominates, especially in right-handers. This right ear–left hemisphere advantage appears to be attenuated in patients who are hallucination-prone (Green et al. 1994; Bruder et al. 1995) and correlates with symptom severity (Levitan et al. 1999). This pattern could be interpreted as a left hemisphere abnormality with or without overactivity of the right hemisphere. Recent functional magnetic resonance imaging work has shown that the right hemisphere shows more activity relative to the left in response to external speech (Woodruff et al. 1997), while activity during hallucinations in the single cases studied has a right temporal cortex emphasis (Woodruff et al. 1995; Lennox et al. 1999).

Language and hallucinations

Schizophrenic auditory hallucinations, the characteristic 'voices' talking to or about the subject, have a precise content which is often highly personalized to the voice-hearer (Nayani & David 1996). It has been suggested that consistency of semantic content of AVHs leads the voice-hearer to personify the experience (Hoffman *et al.* 1994). Often, a complex relationship develops between the patient and 'the voices' – usually that of the powerless and the powerful, respectively (Chadwick & Birchwood 1994). This is in contradistinction to the idea that hallucinations are the random productions of a disordered neocortex, but rather that they are intimately linked with language perception and expression systems (David 1994a).

Inner speech

The observation that the universal experience of inner speech resembles some AVHs continues to stimulate neurocognitive research. A single case study of a woman with continuous hallucinations showed that inner speech or, more specifically, short-term maintenance of phonological representations, can coexist with AVHs (David & Lucas 1993). This implies that AVHs are not synonymous with inner speech in any simple sense. A battery of short-term memory tests requiring an intact phonological store was used in a group comparison of schizophrenic patients who had recently reported hallucinations vs. patients who had not (Haddock *et al.* 1995). The authors tested the general hypothesis that any abnormality could affect monitoring of inner speech leading to an increased vulnerability to AVHs. The results showed that all patients performed less well than controls but there was no significant interaction with the presence or absence of hallucinations. Similarly, verbal transformation effect (the sensation that when a word like 'life' is repeated over and over, it turns into 'fly') has been used in this context and most recent findings suggest that hallucinators are no more prone to the effect than controls. However, Haddock *et al.* (1995) demonstrated that this effect is vulnerable to motivational factors (i.e. suggestion). In contrast, a separate case study suggested that thought insertion (a pathological experience akin to hearing voices) does appear to be incompatible with effective short-term or working memory (David 1994b).

Evans *et al.* (2000) carried out an in-depth study of seven patients with no history of AVH and 12 with a strong history of AVH using auditory imagery paradigms which tapped into the functioning of the 'inner ear', the 'inner voice' and the 'inner ear–inner voice' partnership. These included parsing meaningful letter strings, pitch judgements, verbal transformations and a range of tasks requiring phonological judgements. The results showed a wide range of abilities and deficits in both groups but no clear pattern and hence do not support an abnormality in inner speech and phonological processing in patients vulnerable to AVHs. However, problems in attribution of inner speech, for example, or theories of hallucinations based on lower level perceptual or physiological processes are not ruled out (see below).

Reality or source monitoring

The problem of deciding whether one imagined hearing a voice or heard someone else speaking, and, if the latter, deciding who it was, falls under the rubric of source (or reality) monitoring (Johnson *et al.* 1988). Hallucinations and delusions of control can therefore be conceived of as failures of source monitoring – either because of a general failure and hence source confusion or a systematic failure or bias so that imagined voices (planned utterances) tend to be remembered as 'heard'. The first empirical test of this was by Bentall *et al.* (1991) and the results somewhat equivocal, with hallucinators being no more prone to monitoring errors than other groups. Morrison and Haddock (1997) introduced an innovation to this paradigm by examining source monitoring for words with emotional content. They found that such words tended to disrupt source monitoring but only in terms of *immediate* ratings of subjective ownership. Seal *et al.* (1997) manipulated several task parameters including emotional content and found trends toward more self-to-other misattributions in hallucinators (*n* = 6) vs. non-hallucinators (*n* = 11). Other research using similar methodology has shown that patients with schizophrenia may well be prone to making source monitoring errors but the relationship to hallucinations has not emerged (Vinogradov *et al.* 1997). Indeed, a confounding effect of low IQ (Vinogradov *et al.* 1997) and poor verbal memory (Seal *et al.* 1997) has been problematic. In perhaps the most complete study to date, Keefe *et al.* (1999) used a systematic multinomial model to dissect memory level and source and found that patients not only had difficulty remembering both internal and external sources, but showed a bias in reporting that stimuli came from external sources. Unfortunately, only weak relations with various positive symptoms were discerned.

Frith's model (1987, 1992) proposes that source monitoring is achieved by a corollary discharge-like mechanism whereby ownership of a speech act is signalled at the intention stage. The hypothesized failure of this mechanism in AVHs was tested by Cahill *et al.* (1996) using distorted auditory feedback. The aim was to produce a dissonance between external and 'internal' monitoring. Reliance solely on the external route would lead to the attribution of an alien source to the heard speech. By lowering or raising the pitch of the patient's speech, the authors did indeed induce hallucination-like experiences. However, this tendency correlated more strongly with the presence of delusions than hallucinations. Johns and McGuire (1999) repeated the experiment using 10 schizophrenia patients with hallucinations (and delusions) and eight with delusions alone, plus normal volunteers. The results showed that, while uncertainty as to the source of the speech was a feature of both schizophrenia groups, external attribution was more common in the hallucinators, a tendency more evident when derogatory material was heard. Goldberg *et al.* (1997) used delayed auditory feedback on the assumption that the dysfluency this usually causes is a result of the mismatch between planned and perceived speech output. The authors argued that if the speech production is not anticipated (because of a disconnection between intentions and the monitored output) then this adverse effect on speech should be *less* in those with hallucinations compared with those without. The results showed the opposite: speech output was even more affected in the hallucinators and patients with delusions of control. However, the role of attention in this paradigm has been questioned, although it is unclear why this effect would specifically impact hallucinations.

Indirect psychological evidence for a failure in self-monitoring comes from examining speech repairs, especially when these occur rapidly, often within a word, before external acoustic feedback can have come into play. Leudar *et al.* (1994) found that internal error detection occurred much less commonly in schizophrenic patients compared with normal controls. However, there was no difference between patients with and without AVHs.

In summary, inner speech itself appears not to be differentially impaired in hallucinators while there is some inconsistent support for reality monitoring errors. Data on auditory feedback are contradictory.

Delusions

Delusions represent a core feature of psychosis, and are especially evident in schizophrenia. There have been several cognitive models proposed to explain delusion formation. One explanation is that they result from the natural interpretations of abnormal experiences (Maher 1974). However, delusions can occur in the absence of abnormal perceptions and vice versa, and different delusional beliefs can be present in various subjects with abnormal perceptions (Chapman & Chapman 1988). Other theories of delusion formation have therefore emphasized abnormalities in attentional bias, such as increased attention to threatening stimuli in patients with persecutory delusions. Evidence for this includes the significantly longer time that patients with persecutory delusions require to name the print colours of threatening compared with depressive and neutral words in an emotional Stroop test (Kaney & Bentall 1989), and demonstrations of preferential recall of threat-related propositions in a story recall task (Kaney *et al.* 1992). It has also been proposed that patients with persecutory delusions have abnormal attributional processes, making external attributions for negative events and internal attributions for positive events (Kaney & Bentall 1989) and that this acts as a 'self-serving bias' (Kaney & Bentall 1990).

Reasoning

More recent studies have examined the nature of reasoning biases in patients with delusions about non-persecutory themes. Leafhead *et al.* (1996) employed the emotional Stroop paradigm to investigate the attentional bias in a patient with the Cotard delusion, the belief that one is dead. The patient was found to

have increased attention to death-related words. Rossell *et al.* (1998) administered a sentence verification task to patients with delusions. When asked to judge whether statements were real (true), e.g. 'fish swim in rivers', unlikely, e.g. 'passengers have sex on trains' or nonsense (untrue), e.g. 'the bible is a car catalogue', the deluded subjects, whose overall performance matched that of controls, made significantly more incorrect responses to sentences that had an emotional content congruent with their delusional beliefs, especially in the intermediate unlikely category. These findings suggest that reasoning abnormalities in deluded patients become particularly evident with tasks related to the theme of the delusional belief, and also indicate the presence of disturbed higher order semantic processes in these patients. However, it is unclear if delusions cause misinterpretations or misinterpretations cause delusions, or if delusional subjects are relatively preoccupied with certain emotional themes.

Early work suggested that delusions were the consequence of faulty syllogistic reasoning (von Domarus 1944):

I am a man
Napoleon is a man
I am Napoleon.

A recent investigation of logical reasoning ability, including conditional and syllogistic (Evans *et al.* 1993) reasoning tasks, has demonstrated that such reasoning is not impaired in relatively high-functioning deluded patients – at least no more than in non-deluded patients (Kemp *et al.* 1997). Relatively difficult problems were given, such as:

No religious people are criminals
Some priests are criminals
then
Some religious people are not priests (true/false)
or
Some priests are not religious people (true/false).

All subjects tended to be swayed by their common-sense understanding rather than working through the problems logically. In keeping with this, J. Slater, B. Elvevåg and T.E. Goldberg (submitted) found that formal reasoning in patients and normal controls was highly correlated with general intelligence for relationally complex sentences, but not classic working memory measures.

Further studies have emphasized abnormalities in hypothesis testing in deluded patients, with patients with persecutory delusions requiring less information before reaching a conclusion than non-deluded controls – based on judgements of probability of occurrence (Huq *et al.* 1988; Garety *et al.* 1991). Tasks have involved being presented with a bead of one of two colours and judging from which of two jars the bead was most likely to have come, given the known proportion of each coloured bead in the two jars. Deluded patients tended to reach a judgement after a single bead had been presented while controls tended to wait for more beads before deciding the jar of origin. More naturalistic versions of the task have also been devised and the results are similar (Dudley *et al.* 1997). These and similar tasks have shown that patients are more inclined to stick to their hypotheses even in the presence of negative feedback (Young & Bentall 1995). However, recent extensions of this work have failed to confirm the link between performance on such tests and delusions *per se* (Mortimer *et al.* 1996) as opposed to major mental illness.

It is unclear whether these perceptual and reasoning biases lead to predisposition and formation of persecutory delusions or maintain delusions once formed, or are correlates of other cognitive characteristics of delusional patients that are not the causes of the delusions. Indeed, the difficulty in distinguishing between the effects of beliefs on current perception and reasoning and the effects of the latter on belief formation has been highlighted in the investigation of delusional misidentification, in which it has been argued that abnormal beliefs distort current perceptual experiences in a top-down fashion (Fleminger 1994). Delusions may be conceived of as a content-specific reasoning problem. Nevertheless, the extent of reasoning deficits may be slight compared with the fixity and 'irrationality' of abnormal beliefs.

Other approaches to delusions

David and Howard (1994) employed a type of reality monitoring methodology to study cognitively intact patients with delusional memories. The phenomenal characteristics of each person's delusional memory were contrasted with a real memorable event and a fantasy. It was found that delusional memories were more vivid and tangible than even real events (although delusions tended to be 'rehearsed' more mentally) and this vividness could lead to reality confusion. However, a detailed case study approach revealed coincident reasoning aberrations as well, for example, on the cognitive estimates task.

Other psychophysiological methods have been employed to aid the understanding of delusions. Monitoring directed attention in subjects in real time – an 'on-line' measurement of attention – has the advantage over off-line measures in that it allows the presence of 'abnormal' information processing strategies. The measurement of visual scan paths is one method that has potential as a monitor of real-time visual information processing. The visual scan path is, literally, a map which traces the direction and extent of gaze when an individual comprehends a complex scene (Noton & Stark 1971): i.e. a psychophysiological 'marker' of sensory input and directional attention on viewing a stimulus.

A small number of studies have investigated visual scan paths in schizophrenic subjects (Phillips & David 1994). A relationship between symptomatology and viewing strategy has been demonstrated, with the presence of positive symptoms associated with increased scanning and negative symptoms with increased staring (Gaebel *et al.* 1987; Streit *et al.* 1997). While these studies have demonstrated abnormalities in viewing strategies in schizophrenic patients *per se*, others have aimed to investigate specific abnormalities in the visual scan paths (i.e. specific attentional deficits) in deluded schizophrenic patients compared with non-deluded schizophrenics (Phillips & David 1994, 1997, 1998). These studies have demonstrated that deluded schizophrenic patients employ abnormal strategies when viewing salient visual stimuli, e.g. human faces – viewing non-

feature areas to a significantly greater extent than both well-matched non-deluded schizophrenics and normal controls. Such strategies 'normalize' with recovery. One interpretation of these findings is that deluded schizophrenic patients rely on less salient visual information when appraising complex stimuli compared with controls.

Conclusions

The negative symptoms of schizophrenia seem by their very nature to be eminently reducible to cognitive deficits, although there is a danger of circularity (e.g. reduced verbal fluency correlating with poverty of speech). However, linking cognitive abnormalities with positive symptoms has proven to be a challenge. It appears that standard neuropsychological tests lack the specificity and sensitivity to shed light on the cognitive basis of such phenomena as hallucinations and delusions. More successes have been claimed when individual symptoms or symptom complexes have been the focus of investigation coupled with the use of experimental tasks with a sound theoretical basis. Contrasting individual cases with clear-cut phenomenology and relatively few intellectual impairments is a strategy worth employing. Within-subject design with and without the symptoms of interest is another potentially powerful approach. Finally, the remit of neuropsychology needs to expand into social psychology and take account of concepts such as attribution and bias.

Thought disorder

Recent attempts to understand the cognitive underpinnings of thought disorder (i.e. disorganized speech characterized by derailments, tangential responses and poverty of content) in schizophrenia have focused on abnormalities in the semantic memory system. Such formulations generally propose that 'spreading activation' through a network of features or representations based on meaning is abnormal. The construct itself (spreading activation) is usually measured by a cognitive paradigm involving priming, in which one word primes the recognition of a second word because they are related in some way. However, it has been unclear if these abnormalities are caused by failures in controlled processing or automatic processing and even whether the abnormalities reflect too much or too little priming. Moreover, the exact relation of these semantic processing measures to clinical ratings of thought disorder is equivocal. Many of these issues have been covered in detail in recent reviews (Spitzer 1998; Goldberg & Weinberger 2000).

Novel work by Goldberg *et al.* may be helpful in homing in on the signal in this rather noisy area of research. Using changes in medication status in patients (unmedicated vs. medicated) to produce changes in thought disorder, they found that not only did the degree of priming change with medication status independent of changes in reaction time, but also that changes in priming significantly and selectively covaried with clinical ratings of disorganized speech (Goldberg & Weinberger 2000).

Thus, improvements in thought disorder were correlated with increases in priming effects. Several negative findings were also important: neither attention nor working memory improved and neither did verbal comprehension nor naming. These results indicate that thought disorder:

1 is not secondary to general cognitive impairments; but

2 may be caused by a specific abnormality in the semantic system, involving not the integrity of representations but access to connectivity among representations.

In a further refinement of this notion, Elvevåg *et al.* (unpublished data) found that representation (of numbers) in a task requiring numerosity judgements was intact in patients, while priming between 'adjacent' whole numbers was reduced in patients compared with normal controls. However, this work is preliminary and awaits replication.

Cognition as an intermediate phenotype

Genetic linkage studies using diagnosis as a phenotype have generally been disappointing (Egan & Weinberger 1997). One possible reason for this is that individuals do not inherit schizophrenia *per se* but a variety of information processing deficits out of which schizophrenia emerges. In a study of MZ twins discordant for schizophrenia, Goldberg *et al.* (1995) found subtle attenuations of performance in the otherwise well cotwins when compared with normal twins on neurocognitive measures indexing working memory, speed of information processing and episodic memory. More recently, Cannon *et al.* (2000), using population-based samples of discordant MZ and dizygotic (DZ) twins, compellingly demonstrated that compromises in frontal-lobe-type cognitive impairments are heritable in schizophrenia. Indeed, the unaffected twins of MZ and DZ pairs, in whom the other member was schizophrenic, differed in step-wise fashion from normal twins on such tasks as impairment in spatial working memory, divided attention, choice reaction time and intrusion errors.

Investigators in the Clinical Brain Disorders Branch of the National Institue of Mental Health have reported a series of studies of cognitive assessments in a large sample of siblings. Their sample consisted of 147 patients with schizophrenia, 193 of their siblings and 47 controls. The IQ of index cases was 94, for their siblings was 107 and for controls was 108. The percentage of siblings carrying a schizophrenic spectrum diagnosis was relatively low – under 5%. Egan *et al.* (2000) assessed relative risk of the CPT test of attention and encoding, given that prior work from other groups had suggested that this type of test might be sensitive to certain cognitive impairments in relatives of patients. In a version of the test which included flanking distracters, they found that 50% of patients, 24% of siblings and 18% of controls performed 1 SD below the control mean using d' as a dependent measure. Compared with controls, a subgroup of 97 siblings of patients who performed the CPT abnormally also had significantly reduced CPT performance. Examination of a continuous working memory test, the so-called N-back, which demands rapid and precise encoding of stimuli and their temporal order, resistance to interference and maintenance, revealed that relative risk for impairment in siblings was high and that the sibling group as a whole was significantly impaired compared with normal controls, suggesting that such deficits were familial and probably related to genetic risk for schizophrenia (T.E. Goldberg, M.F. Egan and D.R. Weinberger, submitted). Moreover, the impairments were not redundant with diagnosis, because the sibling sample was purified in that individuals with psychosis or spectrum diagnoses were excluded.

Impairments in several other domains of cognition have also been observed in many studies of patients with schizophrenia. These include working memory/executive function, verbal memory, language, oculomotor scanning/psychomotor speed and general intelligence. To assess the suitability of cognitive function for use as phenotypes in genetic studies, relative risk (RR) was estimated in the aforementioned cohort of siblings (Egan *et al.*, 2001). They hypothesized that RR of cognitive dysfunction would be moderate and that different subgroups of families would demonstrate different patterns of impairment. Relative risk was estimated using cut-off scores of 1 and 2 SD below the control mean. Patients performed significantly worse than controls on all tests except Wide Range Achievement Test (WRAT). The entire sibling group demonstrated impaired performance on WCST, verbal fluency and Trails B. Siblings of patients with impaired performance also showed deficits in the verbal list learning and memory for stories. Again using 1 SD as the cut-off for affected status, the RR to siblings was elevated on the Trails B (RR = 3.8). Increased RRs were also seen for list learning, WCST, letter fluency and memory for stories scores (RRs were approximately 2.0, $P < 0.05$). Using 2 SD as the cut-off, RRs were generally higher. Correlations between tests of different cognitive functions were generally weak, suggesting that they measure relatively independent processes; multiple regression analysis also demonstrated that impairment on one test did not predict impairment on another test in the sibling group. In general, siblings had 1–2 impaired scores, schizophrenic cases had 4 and normal controls had 0 or 1 for the following measures: verbal list learning, trailmaking, card sorting and IQ decline. Ultimately, it is hoped that using cognitive phenotypes may reduce clinical and genetic heterogeneity and improve the power of genetic studies of schizophrenia.

Conclusions

This chapter has attempted to demonstrate that cognitive paradigms can be utilized to constrain thinking about schizophrenia (for instance, course), make important observations about what is 'wrong' with patients (in the sense of core impairments) and be used in novel ways to provide novel mechanistic accounts of symptoms or reductionistic accounts of the aetiology of the disorder. The modal pattern of the developmental trajectory of cognitive impairment reflects deterioration from some higher level of functioning and then stabilization, as consistent with a static encephalopathy. Working memory and episodic memory dysfunctions are prominent. Working memory impairments in particular may be found independent of IQ. These impairments are heritable and may provide an intermediate phenotype for association or linkage studies not redundant with diagnosis. Because these deficits may account for some of the social and vocational morbidity associated with schizophrenia, they should probably be considered as targets for various remediation modalities, including novel cognitive-enhancing 'antischizophrenia' medications.

References

Adler, L.E., Olincy, A., Waldo, M. *et al.* (1998) Schizophrenia, sensory gating, and nicotinic receptors. *Schizophrenia Bulletin* **24**, 189–202.

Aleman, A., Hijman, R., de Haan, E.H. & Kahn, R.S. (1999) Memory impairment in schizophrenia: a meta-analysis. *American Journal of Psychiatry* **156**, 1358–1366.

Barkley, R.A., DuPaul, G.J. & McMurray, M.B. (1990) Comprehensive evaluation of attention deficit disorder with and without hyperactivity as defined by research criteria. *Journal of Consulting and Clinical Psychology* **58**, 775–789.

Basso, M.R., Nasrallah, H.A., Olson, S.C. & Bornstein, R.A. (1998) Neuropsychological correlates of negative, disorganized and psychotic symptoms in schizophrenia. *Schizophrenia Research* **31**, 99–111.

Bentall, R., Baker, G. & Havers, S. (1991) Reality monitoring and psychotic hallucinations. *British Journal of Clinical Psychology* **30**, 213–222.

Bilder, R.M., Turkel, E., Lipschutz-Broch, L. & Lieberman, J.A. (1992) Antipsychotic medication effects on neuropsychological functions. *Psychopharmacology Bulletin* **28**, 353–366.

Blanchard, J.J. & Neale, J.M. (1994) The neuropsychological signature of schizophrenia: generalized or differential deficit? *American Journal of Psychiatry* **151**, 40–48.

Bleuler, E. (1950) *Dementia Praecox or the Group of Schizophrenia.* International Universities Press, New York.

Braff, D.L., Heaton, R., Kuck, J. *et al.* (1991) The generalized pattern of neuropsychological deficits in outpatients with chronic schizophrenia with heterogeneous Wisconsin Card Sorting Test results. *Archives of General Psychiatry* **48**, 891–898.

Bruder, G., Rabinowicz, E., Towey, J. *et al.* (1995) Smaller right ear (left hemisphere) advantage for dichotic fused words in patients with schizophrenia. *American Journal of Psychiatry* **152**, 932–935.

Buchanan, R.W., Holstein, C. & Breier, A. (1994) The comparative efficacy and long-term effect of clozapine treatment on neuropsychological test performance. *Biological Psychiatry* **36**, 717–725.

Bymaster, F.P., Calligaro, D.O., Falcone, J.F. *et al.* (1996) Radioreceptor binding profile of the atypical antipsychotic olanzapine. *Neuropsychopharmacology* **14**, 87–96.

Cahill, C., Silbersweig, D. & Frith, C. (1996) Psychotic experiences induced in deluded patients using distorted auditory feedback. *Cognitive Neuropsychiatry* **1**, 201–211.

Calev, A. (1984) Recall and recognition in mildly disturbed schizophrenics: the use of matched tasks. *Psychological Medicine* **14**, 425–429.

Cannon, T.D., Zorrilla, L.E., Shtasel, D. *et al.* (1994) Neuropsychological functioning in siblings discordant for schizophrenia and healthy volunteers. *Archives of General Psychiatry* **51**, 651–661.

Cannon, T.D., Huttunen, M.O., Lonnqvist, J. *et al.* (2000) The inheritance of neuropsychological dysfunction in twins discordant for schizophrenia. *American Journal of Human Genetics* **67**, 369–382.

Cassens, G., Inglis, A.K., Applebaum, P.S. & Gutheil, T.G. (1990) Neuroleptics. effects on neuropsychological function in chronic schizophrenic patients. *Schizophrenia Bulletin* **16**, 477–499.

Castner, S.A., Williams, G.V. & Goldman-Rakic, P.S. (2000) Reversal of antipsychotic-induced working memory deficits by short-term dopamine D_1 receptor stimulation. *Science* **287**, 2020–2022.

Censits, D.M., Ragland, J.D., Gur, R.C. & Gur, R.E. (1997) Neuropsychological evidence supporting a neurodevelopmental model of schizophrenia. *Schizophrenia Research* **24**, 289–298.

Chadwick, P. & Birchwood, M. (1994) The omnipotence of voices: a cognitive approach to auditory hallucinations. *British Journal of Psychiatry* **164**, 190–201.

Chapman, L.J. & Chapman, J.P. (1973) Problems in the measurement of cognitive deficit. *Psychological Bulletin* **79**, 380–385.

Chapman, L.J. & Chapman, J.P. (1988) The genesis of delusions. In: *Delusional Beliefs* (eds T.F. Oltmanns & B.A. Maher), pp. 167–211. Wiley, New York.

Chapman, L.J. & Chapman, J.P. (1989) Strategies for resolving the heterogeneity of schizophrenics and their relatives using cognitive measures. *Journal of Abnormal Psychology* **98**, 571–366.

Cuesta, M.J., Peralta, V. & Zarzuela, A. (1998) Illness duration and neuropsychological impairments in schizophrenia. *Schizophrenia Research* **33**, 141–150.

Danion, J.M., Rizzo, L. & Bruant, A. (1999) Functional mechanisms underlying impaired recognition memory and conscious awareness in patients with schizophrenia. *Archives of General Psychiatry* **56**, 639–644.

David, A.S. (1994a) The neuropsychology of auditory–verbal hallucinations. In: *The Neuropsychology of Schizophrenia* (eds A. David & J. Cutting), pp. 269–312. Lawrence Erlbaum, Hove.

David, A.S. (1994b) Thought echo reflects the activity of the phonological loop. *British Journal of Clinical Psychology* **33**, 81–83.

David, A.S. & Cutting, J.C. (eds) (1994) *The Neuropsychology of Schizophrenia.* Lawrence Erlbaum Associates, Hillsdale, NJ.

David, A.S. & Halligan, P.W. (2000) Cognitive neuropsychiatry: potential for progress. *Journal of Neuropsychiatry and Clinical Neurosciences* **12**, 506–510.

David, A.S. & Howard, R. (1994) An experimental phenomenological approach to delusional memory in schizophrenia and late paraphrenia. *Psychological Medicine* **24**, 515–524.

David, A.S. & Lucas, P. (1993) Auditory–verbal hallucinations and the phonological loop: a cognitive neuropsychological study. *British Journal of Clinical Psychology* **32**, 431–441.

David, A.S., Malmberg, A., Brandt, L., Allebeck, P. & Lewis, G. (1997) IQ and risk for schizophrenia: a population-based cohort study. *Psychological Medicine* **27**, 1311–1323.

Davidson, M., Reichenberg, A., Rabinowitz, J. *et al.* (1999) Behavioral and intellectual markers for schizophrenia in apparently healthy male adolescents. *American Journal of Psychiatry* **156**, 1328–1335.

Dickerson, F., Boronow, J.J., Ringel, N. & Parente, F. (1996) Neurocognitive deficits and social functioning in outpatients with schizophrenia. *Schizophrenia Research* **21**, 75–83.

von Domarus, E. (1944) The specific laws of logic in schizophrenia. In: *Language and Thought in Schizophrenia*, pp. 104–114. University of California Press, Berkeley, CA.

Dudley, R.E.J., John, C.H., Young, A.W. & Over, D.E. (1997) Normal and abnormal reasoning in people with delusions. *British Journal of Clinical Psychology* **36**, 243–258.

Egan, M.F. & Weinberger, D.R. (1997) Neurobiology of schizophrenia. *Current Opinions in Neurobiology* 7, 701–707.

Egan, M.F., Goldberg, T.E., Gscheidle, T. *et al.* (2000) Relative risk of attention deficits in siblings of patients with schizophrenia. *American Journal of Psychiatry* 157, 1309–1316.

Egan, M.F., Goldberg, T.E., Gscheidle, T. *et al.* (2001) Relative risk for cognitive impairments in siblings of patients with schizophrenia. *Biological Psychiatry* 50, 98–107.

Elliott, R., McKenna, P.J., Robbins, T.W. & Sahakian, B.J. (1995) Neuropsychological evidence for frontostrial dysfunction in schizophrenia. *Psychological Medicine* 25, 619–630.

Elvevåg, B., Duncan, J. & McKenna, P.J. (2000a) The use of cognitive context in schizophrenia: an investigation. *Psychological Medicine* 30, 885–897.

Elvevåg, B., Egan, M.F. & Goldberg, T.E. (2000b) Paired-associate learning and memory interference in schizophrenia. *Neuropsychologia* 38, 1565–1575.

Elvevåg, B., Weinberger, D.R., Egan, M.F. & Goldberg, T.E. (2000c) Memory for temporal oderd in schizophrenia. *Schizophrenia Research* 46, 187–193.

Elvevåg, B., Weinberger, D.R. & Goldberg, T.E. (2000d) Short-term memory for serial order in schizophrenia: a detailed examination of error types. *Neuropsychology* 15, 128–135.

Elvevåg, B., Weinberger, D.R., Suter, J.C. & Goldberg, T.E. (2000e) Continuous performance test and schizophrenia: a test of stimulus-response compatibility, working memory, response readiness, or none of the above? *American Journal of Psychiatry* 157, 772–780.

Evans, C., McGuire, P. & David, A.S. (2000) Is auditory imagery defective in patients with auditory hallucinations? *Psychological Medicine* 30, 137–148.

Evans, J.StB.T., Newstead, S.E. & Byrne, R.M.J. (1993) *Human Reasoning.* Erlbaum, Hove.

Faraone, S.V., Seidman, L.J., Kremen, W.S. *et al.* (1995) Neuropsychological functioning among the non-psychotic relatives of schizophrenic patients: a diagnostic efficacy analysis. *Journal of Abnormal Psychology* 104, 286–304.

Fey, E.T. (1951) The performance of young schizophrenics and young normals on the Wisconsin Card Sorting Test. *Journal of Consulting Psychology* 15, 311–319.

Fleming, K., Goldberg, T.E., Binks, S. *et al.* (1997) Visuospatial working memory in patients with schizophrenia. *Biological Psychiatry* 41, 43–49.

Fleminger, S. (1994) Top-down processing and delusional misidentification. In: *The Neuropsychology of Schizophrenia* (eds A.S. David & J.C. Cutting), pp. 161–167. Lawrence Erlbaum, Hove.

Freedman, R., Coon, H., Myles-Worsley, M. *et al.* (1997) Linkage of a neurophysiological deficit in schizophrenia to a chromosome 15 locus. *Proceedings of the National Academy of Sciences, USA* 94, 587–592.

Frith, C.D. (1987) The positive and negative symptoms of schizophrenia reflect impairments in the perception and initiation of action. *Psychological Medicine* 17, 631–648.

Frith, C. (1992) *Cognitive Neuropsychology of Schizophrenia.* Erlbaum, Hove.

Gaebel, W., Ulrich, G. & Frick, K. (1987) Visuomotor performance of schizophrenic patients and normal controls in a picture viewing task. *Biological Psychiatry* 22, 1227–1237.

Garety, P.A., Hemsley, D.R. & Wessely, S. (1991) Reasoning in deluded schizophrenic and paranoid patients: biases in performance on a probabilistic inference task. *Journal of Nervous and Mental Disease* 179, 194–201.

Gold, J.M., Randolph, C., Coppola, R. *et al.* (1992) Visual orienting in schizophrenia. *Schizophrenia Research* 7, 203–209.

Gold, J.M., Hermann, B.P., Wyler, A. *et al.* (1994) Schizophrenia and temporal lobe epilepsy: a neuropsychological study. *Archives of General Psychiatry* 51, 265–272.

Gold, J.M., Carpenter, C., Randolph, C., Goldberg, T.E. & Weinberger, D.R. (1997) Auditory working memory and Wisconsin Card Sorting Test performance in schizophrenia. *Archives of General Psychiatry* 54, 159–165.

Gold, S., Arndt, S., Nopoulos, P., O'Leary, D.S. & Andreasen, N.C. (1999) Longitudinal study of cognitive function in first-episode and recent-onset schizophrenia. *American Journal of Psychiatry* 156, 1342–1348.

Goldberg, T.E. (1999) Some fairly obvious distinctions between schizophrenia and bipolar disorder. *Schizophrenia Research* 39 (2), 161–162.

Goldberg, T.E. & Weinberger, D.R. (1988) Probing prefrontal function in schizophrenia with neuropsychological paradigms. *Schizophrenia Bulletin* 14, 179–183.

Goldberg, T.E. & Weinberger, D.R. (2000) Thought disorder in schizohrenia: a reappraisal of older formulations and an overview of some recent studies. *Cognitive Neuropsychiatry* 5, 1–19.

Goldberg, T.E., Weinberger, D.R., Berman, K.F., Pliskin, N. & Podd, M. (1987) Possible evidence for dementia of the prefrontal type in schizophrenia? *Archives of General Psychiatry* 44, 1008–1014.

Goldberg, T.E., Weinberger, D.R., Pliskin, N.H., Berman, K.F. & Podd, M. (1989) Recall memory deficits in schizophrenia: a possible manifestation of frontal lobe dysfunction. *Schizophrenia Research* 2, 251–225.

Goldberg, T.E., Berman, K.F., Mohr, E. & Weinberger, D.R. (1990a) Regional cerebral blood flow and cognitive function in Huntington's disease and schizophrenia. *Archives of Neurology* 47, 418–422.

Goldberg, T.E., Ragland, D.R., Gold, J.M. *et al.* (1990b) Neuropsychological assessment of monozygotic twins discordant for schizophrenia. *Archives of General Psychiatry* 47, 1066–1072.

Goldberg, T.E., Gold, J.M., Greenberg, R. *et al.* (1993a) Contrasts between patients with affective disorder and patients with schizophrenia on a neuropsychological screening battery. *American Journal of Psychiatry* 150, 1355–1362.

Goldberg, T.E., Greenberg, R. & Griffin, S. (1993b) The impact of clozapine on cognition and psychiatric symptoms in patients with schizophrenia. *British Journal of Psychiatry* 162, 43–48.

Goldberg, T.E., Torrey, E.F., Gold, J.M. *et al.* (1995) Genetic risk of neuropsychological impairment in schizophrenia: a study of monozygotic twins discordant and concordant for the disorder. *Schizophrenia Research* 17, 77–84.

Goldberg, T.E., Gold, J.M., Coppola, R. & Weinberger, D.R. (1997) Unnatural practices, unspeakable actions: a study of delayed auditory feedback in schizophrenia. *American Journal of Psychiatry* 154, 858–860.

Goldberg, T.E., Patterson, K., Taqqu, Y., Wilder, K. & Weinberger, D.R. (1998) Capacity limitations in schizophrenia: tests of competing hypotheses. *Psychological Medicine* 28, 665–673.

Goldstein, G. & Zubin, J. (1990) Neuropsychological differences between young and old schizophrenics with and without associated neurological dysfunction. *Schizophrenia Research* 3, 117–120.

Gourovitch, M.L., Weinberger, D.R. & Goldberg, T.E. (1996) Verbal fluency deficits in patients with schizophrenia: semantic fluency is differentially impaired as compared with phonologic fluency. *Neuropsychology* 6, 573–577.

Green, M.F. (1996) What are the functional consequences of neurocognitive deficits in schizophrenia? *American Journal of Psychiatry* **153**, 321–330.

Green, M.F., Hugdahl, K. & Mitchell, S. (1994) Dichotic listening during auditory hallucinations in patients with schizophrenia. *American Journal of Psychiatry* **151**, 357–362.

Green, M.F., Marshall, B.D.J., Wirshing, W.C. *et al.* (1997) Does risperidone improve verbal working memory in treatment-resistant schizophrenia? *American Journal of Psychiatry* **154**, 799–804.

Green, M.F., Kern, R.S., Braff, D.L. & Mintz, J. (2000) Neurocognitive deficits and functional outcome in schizophrenia: are we measuring the 'right stuff'? *Schizophrenia Bulletin* **26**, 119–136.

Haddock, G., Slade, P.D. & Bentall, R.P. (1995) Auditory hallucinations and the verbal transformation effect: the role of suggestions. *Personality and Individual Differences* **19**, 301–306.

Halligan, P.W. & David, A. S. (2001) Cognitive neuropsychiatry: towards a scientific psychoathology. *Nature Reviews. Neuroscience* **2**, 209–215.

Harvey, P.D., Howanitz, E., Parrella, M. *et al.* (1998a) Symptoms, cognitive functioning, and adaptive skills in geriatric patients with life-long schizophrenia: a comparison across treatment sites. *American Journal of Psychiatry* **155**, 1080–1086.

Harvey, P.D., Parrella, M., White, L. *et al.* (1998b) Convergence of cognitive and adaptive decline in late-life schizophrenia. *Schizophrenia Research.* **35**, 77–84.

Heaton, R.K. & Crowley, T.J. (1981) Effect of psychiatric disorders and their somatic treatments on neuropsychological test results. In: *Handbook of Clinical Neuropsychology* (eds S. Filskov & T.J. Boll), pp. 481–525. John Wiley, New York.

Heaton, R.K. & Drexler, M. (1987) Clinical neuropsychological findings in schizophrenia and aging. In: *Schizophrenia and Aging: Schizophrenia, Paranoia and Schizophreniform* (eds N.E. Miller & G.D. Cohen), pp. 145–161. Guilford Press, New York.

Heaton, R., Paulsen, J.S., McAdams, L.A. *et al.* (1994) Neuropsychological deficits in schizophrenics: relationship to age, chronicity and dementia. *Archives of General Psychiatry* **51**, 469–476.

Hoffman, R.E., Oates, E., Hafner, J., Hustig, H.H. & McGlashan, T.H. (1994) Semantic organization of hallucinated 'voices' in schizophrenia. *American Journal of Psychiatry* **151**, 1229–1230.

Hull, C.L. (1917) The formation and retention of associations among the insane. *American Journal of Psychology* **28**, 419–435.

Huq, S.F., Garety, P.A. & Hemsley, D.R. (1988) Probabilistic judgments in deluded and non-deluded subjects. *Quarterly Journal of Experimental Psychology* **40A** (4), 801–812.

Hyde, T.M., Nawroz, S., Goldberg, T.E. *et al.* (1994) Is there cognitive decline in schizophrenia: a cross-sectional study. *British Journal of Psychiatry* **164**, 494–500.

Johns, L.C. & McGuire, P.K. (1999) Verbal self-monitoring and auditory hallucinations in schizophrenia. *Lancet* **353**, 469–470.

Johnson, M.K., Foley, M.A. & Leach, K. (1988) The consequence for memory of imagining in another person's voice. *Memory and Cognition* **16**, 337–342.

Jones, P. & Cannon, M. (1998) The new epidemiology of schizophrenia. *Psychiatric Clinics in North America* **21**, 1–25.

Kaney, S. & Bentall, R.P. (1989) Persecutory delusions and attributional style. *British Journal of Medical Psychology* **62**, 191–198.

Kaney, S. & Bentall, R.P. (1990) Persecutory delusions and the self-serving bias: evidence from a contingency judgment task. *Journal of Nervous and Mental Disease* **180**, 773–780.

Kaney, S., Wolfenden, M., Dewey, M.E. & Bentall, R.P. (1992) Persecutory delusions and the recall of threatening and non-threatening propositions. *British Journal of Clinical Psychology* **31**, 85–87.

Kapur, S. & Seeman, P. (2000) Antipsychotic agents differ in how fast they come off the dopamine D_2 receptors: implications for atypical antipsychotic action. *Journal of Psychiatry and Neuroscience* **25**, 161–166.

Kapur, S., Zipursky, R., Jones, C. *et al.* (2000a) Relationship between dopamine D_2 occupancy, clinical response, and side effects: a double-blind PET study of first-episode schizophrenia. *American Journal of Psychiatry* **157**, 514–520.

Kapur, S., Zipursky, R., Jones, C. *et al.* (2000b) A positron emission tomography study of quetiapine in schizophrenia: a preliminary finding of an antipsychotic effect with only transiently high dopamine D_2 receptor occupancy. *Archives of General Psychiatry* **57**, 553–559.

Keefe, R.S.E. & Harvey, P.D. (2001) Studies of cognitive change in patients with schizophrenia following novel and antipsychotic treatment. *American Journal of Psychiatry* **158**, 176–284.

Keefe, R.S.E., Silva, S.G., Perkins, D.O. & Lieberman, J.A. (1999) The effects of atypical antipsychotic drugs on neurocognitive impairment in schizophrenia: a review and meta-analysis. *Schizophrenia Bulletin* **25**, 201–222.

Kemp, R., Chua, S., McKenna, P. & David, A.S. (1997) Reasoning and delusions. *British Journal of Psychiatry* **170**, 398–405.

Kenny, J.T. & Meltzer, H.Y. (1991) Attention and higher cortical functions in schizophrenia. *Journal of Neuropsychiatry* **3**, 269–275.

Kern, R.S., Green, M.F., Marshall, B.D. *et al.* (1998) Risperidone vs. haloperidol on reaction time, manual dexterity, and motor learning in treatment-resistant schizophrenia patients. *Biological Psychiatry* **44**, 726–732.

Kern, R.S., Green, M.F., Marshall, B.D. *et al.* (1999) Risperidone vs. haloperidol on secondary memory: can newer antipsychotics medications aid learning? *Schizophrenia Bulletin* **25**, 223–232.

King, D.J. (1990) The effect of neuroleptics on cognitive and psychomotor function. *British Journal of Psychiatry* **157**, 799–811.

Klonoff, H., Hutton, G.H. & Fibiger, C.H. (1970) Neuropsychological patterns in chronic schizophrenia. *Journal of Nervous and Mental Disease* **150**, 291–300.

Kolb, B. & Whishaw, I.Q. (1983) Performance of schizophrenic patients on tests sensitive to left or right frontal temporal, and parietal function in neurologic patients. *Journal of Nervous and Mental Disease* **171**, 435–443.

Kraepelin, E. (1919/1971) *Dementia Praecox and Paraphrenia* (ed. G.M. Robertson), Translated by R.M. Barclay & R.E. Krieger. Huntington, New York.

Leafhead, K.M., Young, A.W. & Szulecka, T.K. (1996) Delusions demand attention. *Cognitive Neuropsychiatry* **1**, 5–16.

Lennox, B.R., Bert, S., Park, B.G., Jones, P.B. & Morris, P.G. (1999) Spatial and temporal mapping of neural activity associated with auditory hallucinations. *Lancet* **353**, 644.

Leudar, I., Thomas, P. & Johnston, M. (1994) Self-monitoring in speech production: effects of verbal hallucinations and negative symptoms. *Psychological Medicine* **24**, 749–761.

Levitan, C., Ward, P.B. & Catts, S.V. (1999) Superior temporal gyral volumes and laterality correlates of auditory hallucinations in schizophrenia. *Biological Psychiatry* **46**, 955–962.

Liddle, P.F. (1987a) The symptoms of chronic schizophrenia: a re-examination of the positive–negative dichotomy. *British Journal of Psychiatry* **151**, 145–151.

Liddle, P.F. (1987b) Schizophrenic syndromes, cognitive performance and neurological dysfunction. *Psychological Medicine* **17**, 49–57.

Light, G.A., Geyer, M.A., Clementz, B.A. *et al.* (2000) Normal P50 suppression in schizophrenia patients treated with atypical antipsychotic medications. *American Journal of Psychiatry* **157**, 767–771.

Lubin, A., Gieseking, G.F. & Williams, H.L. (1962) Direct measurement of cognitive deficit in schizophrenia. *Journal of Consulting, Psychology* **26**, 139–143.

Maher, B.A. (1974) Delusional thinking and perceptual disorder. *Journal of Individual Psychology* **30**, 85–95.

McKenna, P.J., Tarnlvn, D., Lund, C.E. *et al.* (1990) Amnesic syndrome in schizophrenia. *Psychological Medicine* **20**, 967–972.

Medalia, A., Gold, J. & Merriam, A. (1988) The effects of neuroleptics on neuropsychological test results in schizophrenia. *Archives of Clinical Neurology* **3**, 249–271.

Meltzer, H.Y. & McGurk, S.R. (1999) The effects of clozapine, risperidone, and olanzapine on cognitive function in schizophrenia. *Schizophrenia Bulletin* **25** (2), 233–256.

Mesulum, M.M. (1985) *Principles of Behavioral Neurology*. F.A. Davis Company, Philadelphia, PA.

Mirsky, A.F. (1988) Research on schizophrenia in the NIMH Laboratory of Psychology and Psychopathology, 1954–87. *Schizophrenia Bulletin* **14**, 151–156.

Mockler, D., Riordan, J. & Sharma, T. (1997) Memory and intellectual deficits do not decline with age in schizophrenia. *Schizophrenia Research* **26**, 1–7.

Morrison, A.P. & Haddock, G. (1997) Cognitive factors in source monitoring and auditory hallucinations. *Psychological Medicine* **27**, 669–679.

Mortimer, A.M. *et al.* (1996) Delusions in schizophrenia: a phenomenological and psychological exploration. *Cognitive Neuropsychiatry* **1**, 289–304.

Müller, U., von Cramon, D.Y. & Pollmann, S. (1998) D_1- versus D_2-receptor modulation of visuospatial working memory in humans. *Journal of Neuroscience* **18**, 2720–2728.

Nagamoto, H.T., Adler, L.E., Hea, R.A. *et al.* (1996) Gating of auditory P50 in schizophrenics: unique effects of clozapine. *Biological Psychiatry* **40**, 181–188.

Nayani, T.H. & David, A.S. (1996) The auditory hallucination: a phenomenological survey. *Psychological Medicine* **26**, 177–189.

Norton, D. & Stark, L. (1971) Eye movements and visual perception. *Scientific American* **224**, 35–43.

Pantelis, C., Barnes, T.R., Nelson, H.E. *et al.* (1997) Frontal–striatal cognitive deficits in patients with chronic schizophrenia. *Brain* **120**, 1823–1843.

Pantelis, C., Barber, F.Z., Barnes, T.R. *et al.* (1999) Comparison of set-shifting ability in patients with chronic schizophrenia and frontal lobe damage. *Schizophrenia Research* **37**, 251–270.

Park, S., Holzman, P.S. & Goldman-Rakic, P.S. (1995) Spatial working memory deficits in the relatives of schizophrenic patients. *Archives of General Psychiatry* **52**, 821–828.

Paulsen, J.S., Heaton, R.K., Sadek, J.R. *et al.* (1995) The nature of learning and memory impairments in schizophrenia. *Journal of International Neuropsychology Society* **1**, 88–99.

Perlstein, W.M., Carter, C.S., Barch, D.M. & Baird, J.W. (1998) The Stroop task and attention deficits in schizophrenia. a critical evaluation of card and single-trial Stroop methodologies. *Neuropsychology* **12**, 414–425.

Phillips, M.L. & David, A.S. (1994) Understanding the symptoms of schizophrenia using visual scan paths. *British Journal of Psychiatry* **165**, 673–675.

Phillips, M.L. & David, A.S. (1997) Visual scan paths are abnormal in deluded schizophrenics. *Neuropsychologia* **35**, 99–105.

Phillips, M.L. & David, A.S. (1998) Abnormal visual scan paths: a psychophysiological marker of delusions in schizophrenia. *Schizophrenia Research* **29**, 235–245.

Posner, M.I. & Dehaene, S. (1994) Attentional networks. *Trends in Neuroscience* **17**, 75–79.

Posner, M.I., Early, T.S., Reiman, E., Pardo, P.J. & Dhawan, I.M. (1988) Asymmetries in hemispheric control of attention in schizophrenia. *Archives of General Psychiatry* **45**, 814–821.

Purdon, S.E., Jones, B.D.W., Stip, E. *et al.* (2000) Neuropsychological change in early phase schizophrenia during 12 months of treatment with olanzapine, risperidone, or haloperidol. *Archives of General Psychiatry* **57**, 249–258.

Randolph, C., Goldberg, T.E. & Weinberger, D.R. (1993) The neuropsychology of schizophrenia. In: *Clinical Neuropsychology*, 3rd edn (eds K.M. Heilman & E. Valenstein), pp. 499–522. Oxford, New York.

Rappaport, D., Gill, M. & Schafer, R. (1945/46) *Diagnostic Psychological Testing*. Year Book, Chicago.

Rossell, S.L., Shapleske, J. & David, A.S. (1998) Sentence verification and delusions: a content-specific deficit. *Psychological Medicine* **28**, 1189–1198.

Rund, B.R. (1998) A review of longitudinal studies of cognitive functions in schizophrenia patients. *Schizophrenia Bulletin* **24**, 425–435.

Saykin, J.A., Gur, R.C., Gur, R.E. *et al.* (1991) Neuropsychological function in schizophrenia: selective impairment in memory and learning. *Archives of General Psychiatry* **48**, 618–624.

Saykin, A.J., Shtasel, D.L., Gur, R.E. *et al.* (1994) Neuropsychological deficits in neuroleptic naïve patients with first-episode schizophrenia. *Archives of General Psychiatry* **51**, 124–131.

Schultz, W. (1998) Predictive reward signal of dopamine neurons. *Journal of Neurophysiology* **80**, 1–27.

Schwartzman, A.E. & Douglas, V.I. (1962) Intellectual loss in schizophrenia. II. *Canadian Journal of Psychology* **16**, 161–168.

Seal, M.L., Crowe, S.F. & Cheung, P. (1997) Deficits in source monitoring in subjects with auditory hallucinations may be due to differences in verbal intelligence and verbal memory. *Cognitive Neuropsychiatry* **2**, 273–290.

Sengel, R.A. & Lovalla, W.R. (1983) Effects of cueing on immediate and recent memory in schizophrenics. *Journal of Nervous and Mental Disease* **171**, 426–430.

Shakow, D. (1946) The nature of deterioration in schizophrenic conditions. *Nervous and Mental Disease Monographs*, 70.

Shakow, D. (1979) *Adaptation in Schizophrenia: the Theory of Segmental Set*. John Wiley, New York.

Shallice, T. (1988) *From Neuropsychology to Mental Structure*. Cambridge University Press, Cambridge.

Shallice, T., Burgess, P.W. & Frith, C.D. (1991) Can the neuropsychological case-study approach be applied to schizophrenia? *Psychological Medicine* **21**, 661–673.

Smith, A. (1964) Mental deterioration in chronic schizophrenia. *Journal of Nervous and Mental Disease* **39**, 479–487.

Spitzer, M. (1997) A cognitive neuroscience view of schizophrenic thought disorder. *Schizophrenia Bulletin* **23**, 29–50.

Spohn, H.E. & Strauss, M.E. (1989) Relation of neuroleptic and anticholinergic medication to cognitive function in schizophrenia. *Journal of Abnormal Psychology* **98**, 367–380.

Spohn, H.E., Coyne, L., Lacoursiere, R. *et al.* (1985) Relation of neuroleptic dose and tardive dyskinesia to attention, information-processing, and psychophysiology in medicated schizophrenics. *Archives of General Psychiatry* **42**, 849–859.

Strauss, M.E. (1993) Relations of symptoms to cognitive deficits in schizophrenia. *Schizophrenia Bulletin* **19**, 215–231.

Streit, M., Woelwer, W. & Gaebel, W. (1997) Facial-affect recognition and visual scanning behaviour in the course of schizophrenia. *Schizophrenia Research* **24**, 311–317.

Sweeney, J.A., Haas, G.L., Keilp, J.G. & Long, M. (1991) Evaluation of the stability of neuropsychological functioning after acute episode of schizophrenia: 1-year follow-up, study. *Psychiatry Research* **38**, 63–76.

Teuber, H.L. (1955) Physiological psychology. *Annual Review of Psychology* **9**, 267–298.

Traupmann, K.L. (1980) Encoding processes and memory for categorically related word by schizophrenic patients. *Journal of Abnormal Psychology* **89**, 704–716.

Velligan, D.I., Mahurin, R.K., Diamond, P.L. *et al.* (1997) The functional significance of symptomatology and cognitive function in schizophrenia. *Schizophrenia Research* **25**, 21–31.

Vinogradov, S., Willis-Shore, J., Poole, J.H. *et al.* (1997) Clinical and neurocognitive aspects of source monitoring errors in schizophrenia. *American Journal of Psychiatry* **154**, 1530–1537.

Weickert, T.W., Goldberg, T.E., Gold, J.M. *et al.* (2000) Cognitive impairments in patients with schizophrenia displaying preserved and compromised intellect. *Archives of General Psychiatry* **57**, 907–913.

Woodruff, P., Brammer, M., Mellers, J. *et al.* (1995) Auditory hallucinations and perception of external speech. *Lancet* **346**, 1035.

Woodruff, P.W.R., Wright, I.C., Bullmore, E.T. *et al.* (1997) Auditory hallucinations and the temporal cortical response to speech in schizophrenia: a functional magnetic resonance imaging study. *American Journal of Psychiatry* **154**, 1676–1682.

Yee, C.M., Nuechterlein, K.H., Morris, S.E. & White, P.M. (1998) P50 suppression in recent-onset schizophrenia: clinical correlates and risperidone effects. *Journal of Abnormal Psychology* **107**, 691–698.

Young, H.F. & Bentall, R.P. (1995) Hypothesis testing in patients with persecutory delusions: comparison with depressed and normal subjects. *British Journal of Clinical Psychology* **34**, 353–369.